The SAGES Manual for Navigating a Successful Military Surgical Career

Andrew T. Schlussel
Danielle B. Holt • Robert B. Lim
Tamara J. Worlton
E. Matthew Ritter
Editors

The SAGES Manual for Navigating a Successful Military Surgical Career

Springer

Editors
Andrew T. Schlussel
HCA Florida Jacksonville
Surgical Specialists
Jacksonville, FL, USA

Robert B. Lim
Department of Surgery
Wake Forest University at
Charlotte
Charlotte, NC, USA

E. Matthew Ritter
Surgery
Indiana University
Indianapolis, IN, USA

Danielle B. Holt
Surgery
Uniformed Services University
of the Health Sciences
Bethesda, MD, USA

Tamara J. Worlton
Surgery
Uniformed Services University
of the Health Sciences
Bethesda, MD, USA

ISBN 978-3-031-88489-4 ISBN 978-3-031-88490-0 (eBook)
https://doi.org/10.1007/978-3-031-88490-0

This Springer imprint is published by the registered company Springer Nature Switzerland AG
The registered company address is: Gewerbestrasse 11, 6330 Cham, Switzerland

Foreword

A Patient's Perspective

I am the beneficiary of best-in-the-world military medicine and combat casualty care.

In April 2012, I deployed to Afghanistan as a Brigade Commander—this was my 11th operational or combat deployment since beginning my Army career in May 1988, my 7th post-9/11 deployment, and my 4th deployment to Afghanistan. I had been in numerous engagements with enemy forces, but had always been lucky enough to avoid being wounded. On the 8th of August 2012, my luck ran out.

On that day, two insurgents wearing explosive vests conducted a suicide attack against the dismounted patrol that I was part of, killing four Americans and seriously wounding several others. Ball bearings from one of the explosive vests shredded all three arteries in my left leg below the knee. As the Department of State officer assisted me with applying my tourniquet to control the bleeding from my leg, I thus began a long journey of treatment and recovery. A journey that included 3 months at Walter Reed Military Medical Center, 2 months at Brooke Army Medical Center's Center for the Intrepid and 30 surgeries, and that continues today over 11 years later.

At every step of my journey, I have been the recipient of the highest level of medical skill, the kindest compassion, and the surest professionalism and judgement. A flight medic that saved my life by diverting my medevac flight before I bled out. A forward surgical team that stabilized my bleeding. A vascular surgeon that saved my leg by grafting a vein and restoring blood flow to my lower extremity. A team of surgeons and nurses that eradicated infection. Physical therapists that got me on my feet and moving again. A prosthetist and trainer that enabled me to walk and run again with an innovative new device. The cumulative quality of care I received made a qualitative difference in outcome, with Walter Reed's chief of orthopaedics telling me on the eve of my discharge that he 'would never have predicted the condition of your leg now given your circumstances on arrival three months ago'.

My medical care made a difference in my physical condition, just as my faith, family, and friends made a difference in navigating the many great unknowns present at every turn of my journey. My wife—present from the moment I regained consciousness in Landstuhl Regional Medical Center in Germany and my foremost caregiver and advocate, my children—my constant companions, and a deep network of Army colleagues, gave me a constant hope that each day would be better than the one before.

Then in July 2013 at Fort Campbell, 11 months after the attack, wearing a novel external orthosis, I was able to walk the ¼ mile trooping the formation of a Brigade Combat Team of Soldiers during my outgoing change of command ceremony. Proof positive that the suicide insurgents did not and would not hold sway over my destiny. I was humbled to be able to continue active duty service for another 9 years to include passing the APFT, passing the new ACFT, running the Army 10-Miler, and completing two more combat deployments. Outside of the Army, I was blessed to be able to continue an active lifestyle with my family.

My journey of recovery could have taken many different directions. But the skill and care of military medical professionals—medics, nurses, doctors, surgeons, technicians, therapists, and trainers—over an 11-year span ensured I had the greatest opportunities for success. What these caregivers did absolutely matters to me and my family every day. What you will do for those trusted to your care will absolutely matter too. You may never fully comprehend how your actions will impact lives, but I guarantee you will make a difference. Remember that as you utilize this manual and the helpful advice and lessons it contains.

Thank you!

Pensacola, FL, USA Daniel Walrath

Prologue: Military Committee History

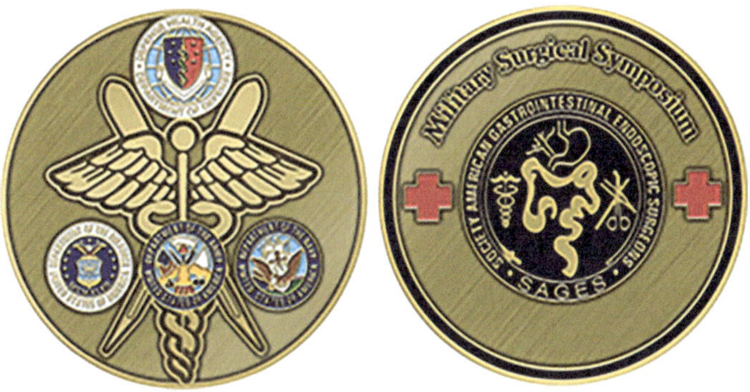

The Society of American Gastrointestinal and Endoscopic Surgeons (SAGES) has a long history with our surgical colleagues in the military. Rick Satava, Steven Bowers, Rob Lim, Matt Ritter, Gordy Wisbach, Henry Lin, Andrew T. Schlussel, and Mary O'Donnell (to name a few) have been instrumental in strengthening the offerings of SAGES to our members in the military.

In 2009, a Military Task Force was established to create a dedicated forum for our military members to help address issues pertinent to military surgeons. Evolving into a standing committee, it has become an essential resource for all SAGES Military Members. The Military symposium then started in 2010, and is now a staple at the SAGES annual meeting, facilitating a forum for military surgeons to discuss combat care, as well as laparoscopic, endoscopic, and general surgery. The committee has successfully secured complimentary Annual Meeting registration for active duty military personnel and substantially reduced Membership dues for military surgeons.

As SAGES continues to foster their professional relationship with the military, many of our staff and membership have developed deeply personal connections with the military community. Below are just two brief examples.

> On a personal note, I've had a heart for those heeding the call to military service, but especially when surgeons make that commitment. They make personal and professional sacrifices to serve, which are largely unknown or not fully understood by their non-military surgical colleagues. My brother has made his career in the Army National Guard, and was recently promoted to the rank of Brigadier General in military intelligence. Seeing the service and sacrifice first hand gave me greater appreciation of my SAGES colleagues who did the same. SAGES is honored to have such a strong presence of military surgeons in our membership and annual meeting, and to serve as a societal home to them. One of the walls in our West Los Angeles office proudly holds a flag sent by Rob Lim following his deployment to Afghanistan, flown in honor of SAGES.
> **—Sallie Matthews, SAGES Executive Director**

> Like many others, I chose the military as an escape route, enlisting in the Marine Corps immediately after high school. It offered a departure from the aimless comfort of my young, sheltered life, opening up a world of adventure and new expectations. My military service was brief but it laid the groundwork for everything significant in my life. My family and my work with SAGES are direct extensions of my time in the Corps. Staffing the SAGES Military Committee allows me to honor the military and repay it for all that it has given me.
> **—Ed Rosado, SAGES Director of IT/Education, Military Committee Staff**

As you read this manual, SAGES hopes to have provided a "how-to" guide for military surgery, the opportunities it provides, and navigating the challenges that come through deployment and re-acclamation upon return. Without hesitation we will state that SAGES can and will be your home through all phases of your military service, and beyond. As eloquently stated by Rob Lim, "SAGES provides world class education for the US Military and asks nothing in return."

Disclaimer for the Society of American Gastrointestinal and Endoscopic Surgeons (SAGES) Manual

The contents of this manual are intended exclusively for educational and informational purposes only, and nothing contained within constitutes medical advice. Neither this manual nor its contents have been subject to formal peer-review. The information provided herein does not represent, nor should it be interpreted as, the official position, view, or endorsement of the Society of American Gastrointestinal and Endoscopic Surgeons (SAGES) or its governing body. This manual is not intended for use in diagnosing or treating any health problem, condition, or disease. Individuals seeking personal medical advice should consult an appropriate licensed professional.

Neither SAGES, nor its officers, directors, employees, members, nor any of the contributors to this manual, make any representation or warranty, express or implied, regarding the accuracy, completeness, fitness for any intended purpose, or suitability of the information contained herein for any specific use or function. Neither access to, nor use of, this manual creates or implies any physician-patient relationship, and reliance on any information provided, contained, or implied herein is solely at the user's own risk.

Department of Defense Disclosure

The views and opinions expressed herein are those of the authors and do not represent the official policy or position of the US Army, US Air Force, US Navy, the Uniformed Services University of the Health Sciences, or the Department of Defense.

Contents

Contributors

Eric P. Ahnfeldt Department of Surgery, Uniformed Services University of Health Sciences, Bethesda, MD, USA

Paul B. Allen Sr. Department of Physician Assistant Studies, University of Texas Health Sciences Center, San Antonio, TX, USA

Oak Ridge Institute of Science and Education, Oak Ridge Associated University, Oak Ridge, TN, USA

Scott B. Armen Division of Trauma, Acute Care, and Critical Care Surgery, Department of Surgery, Penn State University College of Medicine, Hershey, PA, USA

Joseph Aryankalayil Department of General Surgery, Walter Reed National Military Medical Center, Bethesda, MD, USA

Rex E. Atwood Department of Surgery, Uniformed Services University of Health Sciences, Bethesda, MD, USA

Kenneth S. Azarow Department of Surgery, Oregon Health and Science University, Portland, OR, USA

Jason Babcock David Grant Medical Center, Fairfield, CA, USA

Jeffrey A. Bailey Joint Trauma System, US Department of Defense, JBSA Fort Sam Houston, San Antonio, TX, USA
Section of Acute and Critical Care Surgery, Washington University in Saint Louis, Saint Louis, MO, USA
Uniformed Services University of the Health Sciences, Bethesda, MD, USA
Washington University, St. Louis, MO, USA

Bradley C. Bandera University of Nevada School of Medicine, Ioannis A. Lougaris Veterans' Administration Medical Center, Reno, NV, USA

Kelly Beeken, MD, FACOG Martin Army Community Hospital, Fort Benning, GA, USA

Marissa Beiling Department of Surgery, Oregon Health and Science University, Portland, OR, USA

Linda C. Benavides Committee on Surgical Combat Casualty Care, DoD Center of Excellence for Trauma, Joint Base San Antonio-Fort Sam Houston, TX, USA
Department of Surgery, Madigan Army Medical Center, Joint Base Lewis-McChord, WA, USA

John Blickle Uniformed Services University, Bethesda, MD, USA
National Capital Consortium, Washington, DC, USA

M. J. Bradley Department of Surgery, Uniformed Services University, Bethesda, MD, USA

Matthew Bradley Walter Reed National Military Medical Center, Uniformed Services University of the Health Sciences, Bethesda, MD, USA

Joel Brockmeyer Department of Surgery, D.D. Eisenhower Army Medical Center, Fort Eisenhower, GA, USA

Shaun R. Brown Joint Trauma System, Fort Sam Houston, San Antonio, TX, USA
Uniformed Services University of the Health Sciences, Bethesda, MD, USA
Army War College, Washington, DC, USA

Zachary W. Brown Department of Surgery, Naval Medical Center, Portsmouth, VA, USA

Pamela L. Burgess University of Minnesota School of Medicine, Colon and Rectal Surgery Associates, Minneapolis, MN, USA

Katherine Cameron RAF Lakenheath, Brandon, England, UK

Jeremy W. Cannon Division of Traumatology, Surgical Critical Care and Emergency Surgery, Department of Surgery, Perelman School of Medicine at the University of Pennsylvania, Philadelphia, PA, USA
Department of Surgery, F. Edward Hébert School of Medicine at the Uniformed Services University, Bethesda, MD, USA

Joseph Caravalho Jr., MD The Henry M. Jackson Foundation for the Advancement of Military Medicine, Bethesda, MD, USA

Christy Y. Chai Operative Care Line, Michael E. DeBakey Veteran Affairs Medical Center, Houston, TX, USA
Division of General Surgery and Surgical Oncology, Michael E. DeBakey Department of Surgery, Baylor College of Medicine, Houston, TX, USA

Pamela Choi Department of Surgery, Uniformed Services University of Health Sciences, Bethesda, MD, USA
Naval Medical Center San Diego, San Diego, CA, USA

Tiffany C. Cox Department of Surgery, Uniformed Services University of Health Sciences, Bethesda, MD, USA

Miguel Cubano Department of Surgery, Uniformed Services University of Health Sciences, Bethesda, MD, USA

Micaela Cuneo Brooke Army Medical Center, Fort Sam Houston, TX, USA

Joshua Dilday Division of Trauma and Acute Care Surgery, Medical College of Wisconsin, Milwaukee, WI, USA

Samuel Douglas Department of HPB/Surgical Oncology—Alabama Oncology, Birmingham, AL, USA

Jenifer Edmondson Darnell Army Medical Center, Ft. Cavazos, TX, USA

Theodore D. Edson Department of Surgery, Naval Medical Center, San Diego, CA, USA

E. A. Elster Department of Surgery, Uniformed Services University, Bethesda, MD, USA
School of Medicine, Uniformed Services University, Bethesda, MD, USA

Andrew C. Eppstein Section of General Surgery, Surgery Service, Division of General Surgery, Department of Surgery, Richard L. Roudebush Veterans Affairs Medical Center, Indianapolis, IN, USA

Mark Ervin Oak Ridge Institute of Science and Education, Oak Ridge Associated University, Oak Ridge, TN, USA

Michele M. Gage Uniformed Services University, Bethesda, MD, USA
Division of Surgical Oncology, Walter Reed National Military Medical Center, Bethesda, MD, USA

Margaret E. Gallagher Blanchfield Army Community Hospital, Fort Campbell, KY, USA

W. Bryan Gamble Department of Surgery, Uniformed Services University of Health Sciences, Bethesda, MD, USA
Trauma/Surgical Critical Care, Brooke Army Medical Center, San Antonio, TX, USA

Brian J. Gavitt Wright-Patterson Medical Center, Wright-Patterson AFB, OH, USA
Joint Trauma System, Fort Sam Houston, San Antonio, TX, USA
Uniformed Services University of the Health Sciences, Bethesda, MD, USA
88th Surgical Operations Squadron, Wright Patterson Air Force Base, Cincinnati, OH, USA

David A. Gerber Department of Surgery, University of Cincinnati, Cincinnati, OH, USA

Kimberly Gerling Johns Hopkins Hospital, Baltimore, MD, USA

Suzanne Gillern Tripler Army Medical Center, Honolulu, HI, USA

John Christopher Graybill Joint Trauma System, Fort Sam Houston, San Antonio, TX, USA
Walter Reed National Military Medical Center, Bethesda, MD, USA
Uniformed Services University of the Health Sciences, Bethesda, MD, USA

Kirby R. Gross, MD Cooper Medical School of Rowan University, Camden, NJ, USA

Jennifer M. Gurney Joint Trauma System, US Department of Defense, JBSA Fort Sam Houston, TX, USA

Kayleigh M. Herrick-Reynolds Department of Surgery, Walter Reed National Military Medical Center, Bethesda, MD, USA

Danielle B. Holt Office of Admissions, Uniformed Services University, Bethesda, MD, USA
Department of Surgery, Uniformed Services University, Bethesda, MD, USA

Ashley E. Humphries Uniformed Services University, Bethesda, MD, USA
Department of Orthopedic Surgery, Walter Reed National Military Medical Center, Bethesda, MD, USA

Farah A. Husain University of Arizona College of Medicine-Phoenix, Obesity and Metabolic Disorders Service Line, Banner University Medical Group, Phoenix, AZ, USA

Romeo C. Ignacio Jr. Department of Trauma, Rady Children's Hospital San Diego, San Diego, CA, USA
Division of Pediatric Surgery, Rady Children's Hospital San Diego, San Diego, CA, USA

Kyle J. Iverson Keesler Medical Center, Biloxi, MS, USA

William Jordan Orthopaedic Surgery and Sports Medicine, Woodlands Center for Special Surgery, The Woodlands, TX, USA

Chonna L Kendrick, MD, FACS Department of General Surgery, Carl R. Darnall Army Medical Center, Fort Cavazos, TX, USA

1st Cavalry Division Sustainment Brigade, Fort Cavazos, TX, USA

Fred Kobylarz Eisenhower Army Medical Center, Fort Eisenhower, GA, USA

Robert W. Krell Brooke Army Medical Center, Fort Sam Houston, TX, USA

Walter B. Kucera Department of Surgery, Naval Medical Center San Diego, San Diego, CA, USA

Department of Surgery, Uniformed Services University of Health Sciences, Bethesda, MD, USA

Chungeun Lee Keesler Medical Center, Biloxi, MS, USA

Brian C. Lein USUHS Department of Surgery, F Edward Hebert School of Medicine, Bethesda, MD, USA

Robert B. Lim Department of Surgery, Wake Forest University, Atrium Health Carolinas, Charlotte, NC, USA

Christopher Mahoney Eglin AFB, Valparaiso, FL, USA

Matthew J. Martin Division of Trauma and Acute Care Surgery, Keck School of Medicine, USC Medical Center, Los Angeles, CA, USA

Division of Upper GI and General Surgery, Keck School of Medicine, USC Medical Center, Los Angeles, CA, USA

Kresimira Milas University of Arizona College of Medicine—Phoenix, Phoenix, AZ, USA

Margaret M. Morgan Division of Trauma and Acute Care Surgery, University of Colorado Health Memorial, Colorado Springs, CO, USA

Division of Trauma and Acute Care Surgery, UCHealth Memorial Hospital Central, Colorado Springs, CO, USA

Matthew D. Nealeigh, DO, MHPE, FACS CDR, MC, USN Uniformed Services University, Walter Reed National Military Medical Center, Bethesda, MD, USA

Mary O'Donnell Department of Surgery, Uniformed Services University of Health Sciences, Bethesda, MD, USA

Breanne Parets Keesler Medical Center, Biloxi, MS, USA

Eric Petersen University of Arizona College of Medicine—Phoenix, Phoenix, AZ, USA

Adam M. Pickett Anderson Orthopedic Clinic, Arlington, VA, USA

Jason S. Radowsky Department of Surgery, Walter Reed National Military Medical Center, Bethesda, MD, USA
Department of Surgery, Uniformed Services University of the Health Sciences, Bethesda, MD, USA

M. H. Remondelli School of Medicine, Uniformed Services University, Bethesda, MD, USA

Adam M. Robinson Jr. VA Pacific Islands Health Care System, Honolulu, HI, USA

Erik Roedel Madigan Army Medical Center, Tacoma, WA, USA

Robert M. Rush Trauma and Acute Care Surgery Service, PeaceHealth St. Joseph's Medical Center, Bellingham, WA, USA
Division of Healthcare Simulation Science, Department of Surgery, UW Medicine, Seattle, WA, USA

Andrew T. Schlussel HCA Florida Jacksonville Surgical Specialists, Jacksonville, FL, USA

M. Keith Sellers Walter Reed National Military Medical Center, Bethesda, MD, USA

M. M. Shields Department of Surgery, Uniformed Services University, Bethesda, MD, USA

Kaleigh Stabenau University of Arizona College of Medicine—Phoenix, Phoenix, AZ, USA

Matthew D. Tadlock Department of Surgery, Naval Medical Center San Diego, Uniformed Services University of the Health Sciences, San Diego, CA, USA
Committee on Surgical Combat Casualty Care, DoD Center of Excellence for Trauma, Joint Base San Antonio-Fort Sam Houston, San Antonio, TX, USA
Department of Surgery, Naval Medical Center, San Diego, CA, USA
Department of Surgery, Uniformed Services University of the Health Sciences, Bethesda, MD, USA

Jemorie Teixeira VA Pacific Islands Health Care System, Honolulu, HI, USA

Robert W. Tracey Uniformed Services University, Bethesda, MD, USA
Department of Orthopedic Surgery, Walter Reed National Military Medical Center, Bethesda, MD, USA

Diego Vicente, MD Uniformed Services University of the Health Sciences, Bethesda, MD, USA

Aaron Wickard Department of Surgery, Naval Medical Center San Diego, San Diego, CA, USA

Gordon Wisbach Department of General Surgery, Navy Medicine Readiness and Training Command—San Diego, San Diego, CA, USA
Department of Surgery, Uniformed Services University, Bethesda, MD, USA

Tamara J. Worlton, MD Uniformed Services University of the Health Sciences, Bethesda, MD, USA
Center for Global Health Engagement (CGHE), Uniformed Services University of the Health Sciences, Bethesda, MD, USA

Acronyms

AAMC	American Association of Medical Colleges
ACC	Air Combat Command
ACFT	Army Combat Fitness Test
ACGME	Accreditation Council for Graduate Medical Education
ACHE	American College of Healthcare Executives
ACLS	Advanced Cardiac Life Support
ACME	Advanced Combat Medical Experience
ACO	Accountable Care Organization
ACS	American College of Surgeons
ACS	Army Community Services
ACSCOT	American College of Surgeons Committee on Trauma
AD	Active Duty
ADCON	Administrative Control
ADSO	Active-Duty Service Obligation
AE	Aeromedical Evacuation
AFFORGEN	Air Force Force Generation
AFIT	Air Force Institute of Technology
AFRICOM	Africa Combatant Command
AFRRI	Armed Forces Radiobiology Research Institute
AFSOC	Air Force Special Operations Command
AIM	Assignment Interactive Module
AMC	USAF Air Mobility Command

AMCAS	American Medical College Application Service
AMCT3	Army Military-Civilian Trauma Team Training
AMEDD	Army Medical Department
AO	Area of Responsibility
AOR	Area of Responsibility
AOSA	Association of Out Surgeons and Allies
APA	Auxiliary Personnel, Attack
APD	Associate Program Director
APOLLO	Applied Proteogenomics Organizational Learning Outcomes
APP	Advanced Practice Provider
AQDs	Additional Qualification Designators
ARG	Amphibious Ready Groups
AROC	Advanced Readiness Officer Course
ARSC	Austere Resuscitative Surgical Care
AST	Austere (or Air) Surgical Team
AT	Annual Training
ATLS	Advanced Trauma Life Support
ATOM	Advanced Trauma Operative Management
ATTC	Army Trauma Training Center
ATTD	Army Trauma Training Detachment
AWOL	Absent Without Leave
BAH	Basic Allowance for Housing
BAS	Basic Allowance for Sustenance
BAS	Battalion Aid Stations
BG	Brigadier General
BOG	Boots on the Ground
BOLC	Basic Officer Leadership Course
BOLC-A	Basic Officer Leadership Course-A
BROC	Basic Readiness Officer Course
BRS	Blended Retirement System
BUMED	US Navy Bureau of Medicine and Surgery
CAC	Common Access Card
CATF	Commander, Amphibious Task Force
CCATT	Critical Care Aeromedical Transport Team
CCC	Captains' Career Course
CCCRP	Combat Casualty Care Research Program

CCMD	Combatant Command
CDMRP	Congressionally Directed Medical Research Programs
CDP	Center for Deployment Psychology
CENTCOM	US Central Command
CGHE	Center for Global Health Engagement
CGSC-ILE	Command General Staff College Intermediate Level Education
CHAMP	Consortium for Health and Military Performance
CHeCS	Crew Health Care System
CHPE	Center for Health Professions Education
CHSR	Center for Health Services Research
CM	Crew Module
CMO	Chief Medical Officer
CMPH	Center for Military Precision Medicine
CMS	Centers for Medicare & Medicaid Services
CMS	Combat Medical Skills
CoC	Commission on Cancer
COIN	Counter insurgency operations
COLA	Cost-of-Living Adjustment
CONUS	Continental United States
CoSCCC	Committee on Surgical Combat Casualty Care
CoT	Committee on Trauma
CPG	Clinical Practice Guideline
CPRS	Computerized Patient Record System
CPT	Current Procedural Terminology
CRADA	Cooperative Research and Development Agreements
CRC	CONUS Replacement Center
CRSR	Center for Rehabilitation Sciences Research
CRTS	Casualty Receiving and Treatment Ship
CSA	Combat Support Agency
CSH	Combat Support Hospital
CSS	Commander Support Staff
CSTARS	Center for Sustainment of Trauma And Readiness Skills

C-STARs	Center for the Sustainment of Trauma and Readiness Skills
CSTS	Center for the Study of Traumatic Stress
CVN	Aircraft Carrier
DADT	Don't Ask, Don't Tell
DCC	Direct Commissioning Course
DCCS	Deputy Commander Clinical Services
DCI	Departments of Clinical Investigation
DCR	Damage Control Resuscitation
DCS	Damage Control Surgery
DEERS	Defense Enrollment Eligibility Reporting System
DHA	Defense Health Agency
DHHQ	Defense Health Headquarters
DIMO	Defense Institute for Medical Operations
DM	Definitive Medical Care Facility
DMCF	Definitive Medical Care Facility
DMMAC	Deputy Military Medical Action Council
DNBI	Deaths from Non-Battle Injury
DoD	Department of Defense
DoDTR	Department of Defense Trauma Registry
DSO	Diversity, Equity, and Inclusion
DSS	Director of Surgical Services
DVA	Department of Veteran Affairs
DVCIPM	Defense and Veterans Center for Integrative Pain Management
EAMC	Eisenhower Army Medical Center
EAST	Eastern Association for the Surgery of Trauma
ECLSS	Environmental Control and Life Support Systems
EDRP	Education Debt Reduction Program
EFMP	Exceptional Family Member Program
EMDP2	Enlisted to Medical Degree Preparatory Program
EMEDS	Expeditionary Medical Support System
EMF	Expeditionary Medical Facility
eMSM	Enhanced Multi-Service Markets
EOB	Explanation of Benefits

ERSA	External Resource Sharing Agreements
ERSS	Expeditionary Resuscitative Surgical System
ETFs	Exchange-Traded Funds
ETO	European Theater of Operations
ETS	Expiration – Term of Service
FCCS	Fundamental Critical Care Support
FDA	Food and Drug Administration
FEDVIP	Federal Employees Dental and Vision Insurance Program
FEGLI	Federal Employees' Group Life Insurance
FEHB	Federal Employee Health Benefits
FERS	Federal Employees' Retirement System
FITREP	Fitness Report
FORCECOM	FORCES Command
FRSD	Forward Resuscitative Surgical Detachment
FRSS	Forward Resuscitative Surgical System
FSS	Fee-for-Service
FST	Fleet Surgical Team
FST	Forward Surgical Team
FTIS	Full Time In-Service
GEO	Graduate Education Office
GHE	Global Health Engagement
GHERI	Global Health Engagement Research Initiative
GHSP	Global Health Specialist Program
GIO	Globally Integrated Operations
GME	Graduate Medical Education
GMO	General Medical Officer
GST	Ground Surgical Team
GWOT	Global War on Terror
HADR	Humanitarian Assistance and Disaster Relief
HCA	Humanitarian and Civic Assistance
HCDP	Human Capital Development Plan
HCO	Healthcare Operations
HJF	Henry M. Jackson Foundation for the Advancement of Military Medicine
HMO	Health Maintenance Organizations
HO	Host Nation

HPERB	Health Professions Education Requirements Board
HPSP	Health Professions Scholarship Program
HR	Human Resources
HSS	Health Service Support
IACUC	Institutional Animal Care and Use Committee
IDCRP	Infectious Disease Clinical Research Program
IG	Inspector General
ILC	Intermediate Leadership Course
ILE	Intermediate Level Education
IMET	International Military Education and Training
IRA	Individual Retirement Account
IRB	Institutional Review Board
IRR	Individual Ready Reserve
ISR	Institute for Surgical Research
ISS	International Space Station
J1	Personnel
J8	Budget and Finance
JEMO	Joint Expeditionary Medical Officer
JGMESB	Joint Graduate Medical Education Selection Board
JKSA	Joint Knowledge, Skills, and Activity
JMESI	Joint Medical Executive Skills Institute
JP 4-02	Joint Publication 4-02, Health Service Support
JPME	Joint Professional Military Education
JROCM	Joint Requirements Oversight Council Memorandum
JTET	Joint Trauma Education and Training
JTS	Joint Trauma System
JTTR	Joint Theater Trauma Registry
JTTS	Joint Theater Trauma System
KSA	Knowledge, Skills, and Abilities
LCME	Liaison Committee on Medical Education
LNO	Command Liaison Officers
LRMC	Landstuhl Regional Medical Center
LSCO	Large-Scale Combat Operations
LST	Landing Ship, Tanks

M2MM	Molecules to Military Medicine
MAMC	Madigan Army Medical Center
MASCAL	Mass Casualty
MASH	Mobile Army Surgical Hospital
MCC	Murtha Cancer Center
MCCRP	John P. Murtha Cancer Center Research Program
MCPs	Military-Civilian Partnerships
MEDCEN	Medical Centers
MEDCOM	US Army Medical Command
MEDDAC	Medical Department Activities
MEDEVAC	Medical Evacuation
MEDRETES	Medical Readiness Training Exercises
MEPS	Military Entrance Processing Station
MERT	Medical Emergency Response Team
MFST	Mobile Field Surgical Team
MHS	Military Health System
MHSER	MHS Executive Review Board
MHSSPACS	Military Health System Partnership with the American College of Surgeons
MID	Moral Injury and Distress
MMPL	Military Medical Practice and Leadership
MODS	Medical Operational Data System
MOUs	Memorandums of Understanding
MSC	Medical Services Corps
MTBI2	Military Traumatic Brain Injury Initiative
MTF	Military Treatment Facility
MTOE	Modified Tables of Organization and Equipment
MUCH	Military Unique Curriculum in Honduras
MWR	Morale, Welfare, and Recreation
NATT	Navy Adaptive Trauma Team
NCDMPH	National Center for Disaster Medicine and Public Health
NCO	Non-Commissioned Officers
NDAA	National Defense Authorization Act
NGOs	Non-Governmental Organizations
NMA	National Medical Association

NMCSD	Naval Medical Center San Diego
NMRC	Naval Medical Research Center
NMRTC	Navy Medicine Readiness and Training Command
NPS	Naval Postgraduate School
NSQIP	National Surgical Quality Improvement Program
NTDB	National Trauma Data Bank
NTTC	Navy Trauma Training Center
OASD[HA]	Office of the Assistant Secretary of Defense for Health Affairs
OCONUS	Outside the Continental United States
ODE	Off-Duty Employment
OEF	Operation Enduring Freedom
OIC	Officer-In-Charge
OIF	Operation Iraqi Freedom
OND	Operation New Dawn
OPCON	Operational Control
OPM	US Office of Personnel Management
OPPE	Ongoing Professional Practice Evaluation
OPTEMPO	Operations Tempo
OR	Operating Room
OTS-A	Officer Training School-Abbreviated
OTSG	Office of the Surgeon General
PCBI	Pacific, China, Burma, India
PCS	Permanent Change of Station
PD	Program Director
PEPFAR	President's Emergency Plan for AIDS Relief
PHA	Periodic Health Assessment
PI	Principal Investigators
PME	Professional Military Education
PMI	President's Malaria Initiative
PN	Partner-Nation
POA	Power of Attorney
POI	Point of Injury
PPG	Personnel Policy Guidance
PRA	Probabilistic Risk Assessments
PRD	Projected Rotation Date

PRD	Projected Rotation Date
PROMETHEUS	PROject for Military Exposures and Toxin History Evaluation in U.S. Service Members
PTO	Paid Time Off
R2LM	Role 2 Light Maneuver
RDT&E	Research, Development, Testing, and Evaluation
RF	Radio Frequency
RIP	Relief-In-Place
RNLTD	Report No Later Than Date
ROFR	Right of First Refusal
RTC IP	Report to Congress
RVU	Relative Value Unit
SAGES	Society of American Gastrointestinal and Endoscopic Surgeons
SAMMC	San Antonio Military Medical Center
SC2i	Surgical Critical Care Initiative
SCC	Senior Service Colleges
SCC	Subclinical Cognitive Decline
SDP	Savings Deposit Program
SEI	Special Experience Identifier
SELRES	Selected Reservist
SHAPE	Simulation Healthcare Advanced Practice Environment
SIMCEN	Val G. Hemming Simulation Center
SMAAC	Senior Military Medical Action Council
SMEE	Subject Matter Expert Exchanges
SOCCET	Special Operations Critical Care Evacuation Teams
SOE	Summer Operational Experiences
SOF	Special Operations Forces
SOFA	Status of Forces Agreement
SOM	School of Medicine
SOMOS	Society of Military Orthopaedic Surgeons
SOS	Squadron Officer School
SOST	Special Operations Surgical Teams
SPEARR	Small Portable Expeditionary Aeromedical Rapid Response

SRM	Sustainment, Restoration, and Modernization
SSH	Simulation in Healthcare
STaRC	Strategic Trauma Readiness Center
STP	Shock Trauma Platoon
SWMDO	Surface Warfare Medical Department Officer
T3	Tactical Combat Casualty Care
TAA	Training Affiliation Agreements
TAD	Temporary Additional Duty
TAP	Transition Assistance Program
TCCC	Tactical Combat Casualty Care
TCCET	Tactical Critical Care Evacuation Team
TCCET-E	Tactical Critical Care Evacuation Team Enhanced
TD	Temporary Duty
TDA	Tables of Distribution
TDY	Temporary Duty
TMA	Talent Management System
TMD	Trauma Medical Director
TMS	Talent Management System
TNC	Trauma Nurse Coordinators
TPM	Trauma Program Manager
TPU	Troop Program Unit
TSP	Thrift Savings Plan
TTPs	Tactics, Techniques, and Procedures
TY	Transitional Year
UME	Undergraduate Medical Education
USAFA	United States Air Force Academy
USAFSAM	United States Air Force School of Aerospace Medicine
USAISR	United States Army Institute for Surgical Research
USC	United States Code
USG	United States Government
USMA	United States Military Academy
USMC	United Stated Marine Corp
USNA	United States Naval Academy
USU	Uniformed Services University

USUHS	Uniformed Services University of Health Sciences
VA	Veteran Affairs
VAMCs	VA Medical Centers
VASQIP	VA Surgical Quality Improvement Program
VHA	Veterans Health Administration
vMPF	Virtual Military Personnel Flight
VSP	Visiting Surgeon Program
VTU	Voluntary Training Unit
WAMC	Womack Army Medical Center
WBAMC	William Beaumont Army Medical Center
WBB	Walking Blood Bank
WFP	World Food Program
WRNMMC	Walter Reed National Military Medical Center
wRVU	work relative value units
YMAV	Year/Month Available to Move

Introduction

1

Robert B. Lim

The decision to join the military was the best one of my professional career. Unfortunately, I did not know it then back in 1987 when I became an ROTC cadet at Davidson College or when I accepted an HPSP scholarship as a medical student at New York Medical College in 1992. Back then, it was a way to pay for my education. I did not understand it in 2002 when I finished my general surgery residency at William Beaumont Army Medical Center. I learned some of it during my first 3 combat deployments and after I finished my minimally invasive surgery fellowship at Beth Israel Deaconess Medical Center/Harvard Medical School, however, I really did not appreciate the magnitude of my decision until after I had been on active duty for about a decade. And even during the second decade, there was so much more to understand. The sheer volume of leaders and times that the military affects people in politics, the number of retired or prior service members who use the Veterans Administration system for healthcare, the number of dependents who rely on military medical care, the number of civilian people who are needed to run the VA and the military medical system, and the number of future and young

R. B. Lim (✉)
Department of Surgery, Wake Forest University, Atrium Health Carolinas, Charlotte, NC, USA
e-mail: robert.lim@atriumhealth.org

A. T. Schlussel et al. (eds.), *The SAGES Manual for Navigating a Successful Military Surgical Career*,
https://doi.org/10.1007/978-3-031-88490-0_1

physicians that are directly influenced by their leader's decisions is truly overwhelming. It hurts my brain to think of all the possibilities and permutations. It is the largest medical system in the world and is present on all 7 continents. At times, one can feel like a drop in the ocean.

Surgically a military surgeon could operate on a state-of-the-art robot system doing an advanced surgical procedure or they could be operating in a tent, without any environmental control, and without electricity. One can work in a community hospital where they are the only surgeon or in a medical center supported by two services like San Antonio Military Medical Center, which is staffed by the Army and Air Force. Deployments can require one to provide medical care in deserts, the ocean, the mountains, a jungle, in a sandstorm, at 30,000 ft. above sea level, and behind enemy lines. Now, this probably does not appeal to many providers, but it does highlight the fact that a military career covers the full gamut of clinical experiences. Similarly, a military career can provide and sometimes catapult one's career to all aspects of a professional career including an administrative leadership one, an academic one, a research-based one, and a clinical one. In many cases, the military can provide the framework for all of them together. The crux of the information in this book is that all possibilities are open with a military career. There are no doubt unique obstacles to military service but there are also unique opportunities.

Currently, there are about 380 million people in the United States, and around 2.8 million serve on active duty, in the reserves, and the national guard. This includes the Coast Guard and the newly formed Space Force. That means that *less than 1 percent* of the entire US population serves in national defense. Conversely, the United States spends roughly over $800 billion dollars on defense annually, which includes its medical mission, is the world's highest expenditure, and is more than double what China spends on its military, despite having almost 4 times as many people. Defense is very important to the United States and its policies, and thus, good medical care is needed if the United States is to complete its missions. Every beneficiary has access to care regardless of socioeconomic status, making it the largest socialized medicine system in the world. Unlike socialized medicine, though, it is expected to be current, readily available, and not rationed. Further, the medical mission cannot be subsidized, because its providers need to be ready, sometimes with only a moment's notice, to deploy anywhere around the world. In addition to the clinical skills, they need an uncanny resilience to face danger, to accept a lot of things out of their control, to be away from loved ones for undetermined periods of time, and even to be patient and restrained when things are spiraling around them. Many times, clinical skills are the easiest part of the job. One of my mentors Dan Jones, MD, who was a professor of surgery at Harvard and is now the chief of surgery at Rutgers Medical School, once told me, "You military guys do the jobs that we (other surgeons) don't want to do or cannot do."

Recently I had the privilege of attending the retirement of a military surgical legend, COL Stephen Hetz, MD. In addition to his 30 years on active duty, he continued to train and mentor military surgeons for almost an additional 15 years. At his celebration, 2 decades of his former residents, and several former partners came to honor him. In my estimation, there were over 100 surgeons present, representing thousands of years of clinical duty. Only the now deceased COL Norman Rich, MD, who started the Uniformed Services University of the Health Sciences (the military's medical school), has had more influence on military medicine. Dr. Hetz's influence aided the care of likely hundreds of thousands of patients, through dozens of armed conflicts. It also spurred the advancements of his trainees and colleagues who went on to become United States Army Medical Command commanders, hospital commanders, professors of surgery, chiefs of surgery, famed researchers, and not least, just plain ol' solid, reliable, professional clinicians. Dr. Hetz's teachings and his passed-along acumen will positively help surgeons and patients for at least another 45 years. I'm sad that some of his wisdom will not directly come from him via a chapter in this book, but it is safe to say that many authors here will have some Hetz influence in their words.

But as much as the night was about Stephen Hetz, to me, it was also about the military's surgical mission and its importance to the

United States. In that room were decades of knowledge and mastery-level surgical skills. There was also unwavering commitment to the United States, and perseverance to a mission much higher than themselves and the patients in front of them. It was also about making combat care better for the next surgeon and the next injured soldier or service member. It was also about assuring these soldiers that their loved ones will get the highest quality care while they are deployed and that they themselves will get great care when they are not deployed or when they are retired. It was also about being there for one another and letting them know that when it was their time to deploy, we would take care of their patients, their families, and their friends. Because soon we might deploy and need the same things from them. There was a togetherness and camaraderie that would last a lifetime because we were the ones who could and would do the things other surgeons would not.

There are an estimated 53,000 surgeons in the United States today with an average annual salary of around $338,854 (https://datausa.io/profile/soc/surgeons; www.zippia.com/surgeon-jobs/demographics). By contrast there are about 1000 military surgeons with an average annual salary around $250,190 or about 26% less than the average civilian salary. There are some tax breaks and financial benefits that lower this difference, and no one should feel that military surgeons are poor as this salary would still have them in the top 10% of all wages. It is worthwhile to specifically look at general surgeons as those surgeons in the military are the ones who typically deploy to combat or to austere care situations. The numbers are more staggering for general surgeons, as there are about 17,324 general surgeons in the United States while there are roughly 350 such surgeons among the United States Army, Air Force, and Navy combined. The average salary for a civilian general surgeon is estimated at $434,400, meaning there is now a 42% difference in salary. So, while many surgeons join the military to pay for medical school, most do not remain in the military for money. They remain that less than 1% of people who do it for the military.

Now, there is a lot to dislike about the military and those things will be discussed in this book too. They include frequent deployments, low case volume, dealing with poor leadership, and the feeling of just being a number. For these and for many other reasons, surgeons do not make a long career of being a military surgeon nor make it to their retirement in the military. This book explores that also because knowing when to get out can be a difficult decision for anyone. Anyone who serves in the armed forces should be lauded as much as the ones who spent 30 years in uniform. Even if they only did one deployment where they did only one case in a country that wasn't at war, they still served this nation's best interest and were ready to help those who needed it. Even if they only backfilled for another surgeon while that surgeon deployed, they enabled that surgeon to be away from their patients and for that surgeon to help those who were deployed. Even if they never deployed and only trained other surgeons to finish residency and become board-certified, they helped make sure that the injured would get good care. Even if they never deployed and never trained a resident, they cared for servicemembers and their families, which enabled them to fight and defend the United States. There are still less than 1 percent of US citizens who served and less than 2% of surgeons who served.

While I did not appreciate this as much when I was a younger officer, there are plenty of people who do; and they would like to help the military surgeon. SAGES, the Society of American Gastrointestinal and Endoscopic Surgeons, has been an avid supporter of the military for almost 15 years. In addition to helping publish this textbook, they offer free registration to its annual meeting for all active-duty surgeons. At the annual meeting, SAGES also provides the military a venue to house its military-specific surgical education, so it can provide its education to young and future military surgeons. Why would a surgical society that is historically based on laparoscopic and endoscopic surgery want to help military surgeons whose needs are based on the combat environment and open surgical techniques? Because they too understand that not everyone answers the call to serve and those that do protect their families and the United States. And how did SAGES realize this? The founding president of SAGES, Gerald Marks, MD, served as a corpsman in World War II. The brother of its Executive Director, Sallie Matthews, is a Lieutenant General in the Army National Guard and flew helicopter missions in Iraq and Afghanistan. SAGES boasts 3 presidents who served on active duty: Frederick Greene, MD, Rick Satava, MD, and Steven Schwaitzberg, MD. My aforementioned mentor, Dr. Jones's father and son both served on active duty. It's likely one of the reasons he chose me as a fellow. Several other surgical societies offer benefits and discounts to the military including the Excelsior Surgical Society of the American College of Surgeons, the American Association of Surgery for Trauma and Acute Care, and even the American Society of Metabolic and Bariatric Surgeons, whose former president, Robin Blackburn, MD, served on active duty. There is thus a long history of military involvement in surgery and a recognized need to assist the military surgeon that goes beyond financial compensation.

This textbook hopes to help military surgeons and those who are considering a military career to navigate the unique aspects of the military's clinical work including deployment. It also outlines a path to an academic career and a career toward becoming a general or an admiral. It also highlights the distinctions among the different services and how reserve duty differs from active duty. It also unabashedly talks about operational surgery and being part of a unit that may not be in awe of the fact that you are a surgeon. One of the challenges of operational medicine is going from being in charge of everything in one's clinic and operating room to taking orders from someone whom you outrank and having them tell you where and when you can and cannot go. It is humbling and will challenge your concept of teamwork.

This textbook will address some of the unique aspects of military life like both spouses serving in the military and starting a family in the military. It also discusses how to maximize one's finances and how to prepare for retirement from active duty. There is no more powerful and prominent meritocracy in the world than in military service, but I would imagine that persons who are not white, not male, and not heterosexual still feel some apprehension about joining and belonging to an institution that has a history of discriminating against them. It is the hope of the editors that this book will provide information to help military surgeons choose the best path for themselves. It is information that I believe all of the authors wish they had when they embarked on their careers.

So why was commissioning in the military the best decision for me? First of all, let me reiterate that it was the best decision for *me,* which is probably not the best for everyone. I've always been a romantic and I've always felt that surgery was romantic—there was no greater expression of love than sacrificing oneself for another. Surgeons sacrifice their time, sometimes their physical and emotional well-being, and sometimes their families to become better at their craft and to ensure that their patients have a good outcome. Surgery in the military is even more romantic. Military surgeons sacrifice money, have extended and unknown periods of time away from their families, and put themselves in harm's way for the good of a nation. But along the way, they make great friendships that span a lifetime because of the adversity like combat they have experienced together. They become natural leaders because they will be put in charge of others whose safety and professional development will depend on them. They become strong administrators because their jobs will demand that they do more tasks with fewer resources. All the while, they will have to be excellent clinicians because the national defense depends on it. It was the best move for me because it taught me all these things. I certainly would not be where I am today without the military.

Finally, it enabled me to be the surgeon I always wanted to be. I wanted to be able to help the sickest when others could not. I retired from active duty in 2019, but for personal reasons, I found myself in Ukraine a week after Russia invaded it in 2022. A friend of mine ran a surgery-based, nongovernmental organization called the Global Surgical and Medical Support Group that had been asked by the Ukraine Minister of Defense to provide combat care training for its citizens and military fighting the war. As Ukraine was not a NATO country, the United States military could not enter the Ukrainian border without escalating the war with Russia, and therefore, active-duty military surgeons could not assist Ukraine in this crisis. Civilian surgeons may have the clinical expertise, but few would have the experience and comfort to function in the uncertainty of the combat environment. In fact, probably only 2% (or less) of US surgeons would feel comfortable traveling to a war-torn and potentially nuclear warzone. An ex-military surgeon, though, is uniquely qualified for this mission. Without my military training and experience, I would not have thought for one second that I would go there. Soon after I arrived there, several of my ex-military friends wanted to know if they could go and how they could help. This led to more ex-military and some civilian surgeons to travel to Ukraine. Together we provided combat casualty training to thousands of Ukraine citizens and to its army. We provided training on caring for victims of massive casualty events and biochemical warfare. We assisted the surgeons of Ukraine with operations, and we even got the Ukraine government to change their laws regarding blood transfusion. This was possible because of the military surgeon.

Who knows when and what the next war will bring. The United States enjoyed air superiority during the wars in Iraq, Afghanistan, and Syria, which will not be the case in a war against Russia. Evacuation times are likely to be longer due to Russia's ability to strike from several miles away with heavier ordinance. Should there be a war with China, there are likely to be maritime challenges, which also were not seen during the wars in the Middle East. Whatever the situation, though, the military surgeon will be prepared, trained, and ready to play their part in national defense. Any surgeon who serves on active duty should take great pride in that even if they do not fully understand the impact. It is my hope that this textbook will help surgeons understand that and successfully navigate their time in service to this country.

Part I

The Early Years

History of Military Surgery

2

Andrew T. Schlussel, Fred Kobylarz, Kyle J. Iverson, Breanne Parets, Chungeun Lee, Aaron Wickard, and Matthew D. Tadlock

Introduction

Military medicine, and specifically military surgery, differs from its civilian counterpart due to the multistage provision of care necessitated by battlefield confines and mission objectives [1]. Military medicine is often practiced in austere environments without access to all the resources and luxuries of modern medicine;

A. T. Schlussel
HCA Florida Jacksonville Surgical Specialists, Jacksonville, FL, USA
e-mail: andrew.schlussel@hcahealthcare.com

F. Kobylarz
Eisenhower Army Medical Center, Fort Eisenhower, GA, USA

K. J. Iverson · B. Parets · C. Lee
Keesler Medical Center, Biloxi, MS, USA
e-mail: kyle.j.iverson.mil@health.mil; breanne@weski.co

A. Wickard
Department of Surgery, Naval Medical Center San Diego, San Diego, CA, USA

M. D. Tadlock (✉)
Department of Surgery, Naval Medical Center San Diego, Uniformed Services University of the Health Sciences, San Diego, CA, USA

A. T. Schlussel et al. (eds.), *The SAGES Manual for Navigating a Successful Military Surgical Career*,
https://doi.org/10.1007/978-3-031-88490-0_2

thus, not everything is translatable to civilian settings. However, because military medicine requires ongoing and expedient innovation and improvement as wars, global conflicts, and tactical conditions continually evolve, the military tends to be a leader in cutting edge research and development [1, 2]. As such, lessons learned by military medicine providers remain integral to the advancement of medicine as a whole. Throughout history, each branch of the military has made notable contributions to the field of medicine. This chapter reviews some of this history and is divided into three sections. Each section provides a broad overview of the history medical and surgical care in the U.S. Army, Air Force, and Navy and gives an introduction to the current surgical capabilities in each service.

What Is a Surgeon?

Before discussing the history of medical and surgical care in the U.S. military it is important to give a brief history the word "surgeon." In the military, the title "surgeon" typically indicates a military medical leadership role, not necessarily one who practices the art and science of surgical care. The word "surgeon" is derived from the Greek *kheirourgos,* meaning "working or done by hand." In the modern world, all practitioners who provide surgical care are physicians first, but throughout history, wound care and surgical procedures have been performed by a diverse group of practitioners including, surgeons, soldiers, priests, barbers, and apothecaries, not necessarily physicians. To dress and treat wounds, set fractured bones or to "balance" humors by bloodletting these practitioners had to use their hands. Therefore, the modern practice of surgery and all of its subspecialties ultimately evolved from the management of wounds and traumatic injuries.

History of the United States Army Medical Corps

Fred Kobylarz and Andrew T. Schlussel

Introduction

As one embarks on the journey to become a military officer and a surgeon, one must understand the history of the United States Army Medical Corps to understand best the successes and failures that brought us to where we are today and guide our future. The U. S. Army Medical Corp's history is rooted in many aspects of modern-day medicine and surgery. Its creation is the oldest, with its inception by the Continental Army to fight the Revolutionary War. The U.S. Army is the largest of all services, comprised of the Regular Army, Army National Guard, and Army Reserves, its present influence still touches all corners of the world. Today, the U.S. Army Medical Corp upholds the same values and goals, "To Conserve Fighting Strength" and ensures our nation's service members can win wars and return home [3].

Early Milestones and the Civil War

The United States Army Medical Corps has a history of accomplishments that demonstrate bravery, innovation, and dedication to the service of its country. The history of the Army Medical Corps began on July 25, 1775, when the Continental Congress established the Medical Department. Notable milestones include the 1778 publication of the first American pharmacopoeia by Army surgeons, and the 1818 appointment of Joseph Lovell as the first Surgeon General, which marked the beginning of a succession of Surgeons General and the formal Corps organization in the Army Medical Department (AMEDD). In 1833, Surgeon William Beaumont's pioneering work on the digestive process laid the foundation for modern gastroenterology.

Although not a direct medical development, the Civil War served as a pivotal moment for significant advancements in wartime policy. In 1863, the Lieber Code, also referred to as General Order No. 100, was issued by President Lincoln. This order was one of the earliest formalized sets of rules governing warfare, outlining protections for prisoners of war, prohibiting unnecessary suffering, safeguarding noncombatant civilians, and ensuring medical care for enemy combatants. These principles were later incorporated into international humanitarian law and influenced subsequent agreements, including the Geneva Conventions [4].

In 1862, during the Civil War, Dr. Jonathan Letterman, often called the "Father of Battlefield Medicine," developed the principles of organized battlefield care, including the use of triage and dedicated medical evacuation systems, which continued to influence military medical protocols. Other key twentieth-century achievements include Major Walter Reed's 1900 discovery that the Aedes mosquito transmits yellow fever and the 1909 introduction of typhoid vaccination by Major Frederick Russell, significantly reducing morbidity and mortality among soldiers [5, 6].

Modernization and the World Wars

Both World Wars proved to be pivotal moments for the Army Medical Corps. With the rapid mobilization and deployment of American forces around the globe came significant advancements in military medical practices. This period also introduced the new age of antibiotics and advanced resuscitation techniques. In 1940, Captain Douglas Kendrick, at the Army Medical School (which later became the Walter Reed Army Institute of Research), studied whole blood preservation and the use of albumin to treat shock. He pioneered systems for the storage and deployment of plasma on the battlefield. Newer methods would emerge for treating traumatic wounds and shock, and the notable advantages of whole blood would revolutionize surgery [5, 6].

During the majority of World War I, laparotomy was not a universal intervention for abdominal wounds, and when performed, this was often delayed for over 6 h. Toward the end of the First

World War, as antibiotics were developed, fluid resuscitation was available, and laparotomies became more popularized, the mortality rate was reduced from 87% to 40% [7]. During World War II, Royal Army Medical Corps surgeon Dr. William Ogilvie advocated that a colostomy should be created for all colonic injuries [8]. These recommendations were so valued by the U.S. Army Medical Corp of that time that in 1943, the U.S. Surgeon General made it mandatory for all surgeons to make a colostomy, and violation would be subject to a court martial [9].

As with all wars, during World War II, surgeons had an opportunity to improve their overall surgical management of trauma patients, not only operatively but also with the discovery and use of antibiotics, knowledge of appropriate fluid resuscitation, and the importance of whole blood in treating hemorrhagic shock. By the end of the war, these advancements led to a significant reduction in mortality rates.

In 1943, Congress authorized the commissioning of women as military doctors. Major Margaret D. Craighill became the first woman to receive a Regular Army commission in the Medical Corps. Dr. Craighill served as the Chief Surgeon with the newly established Women's Army Corps (WAC) and traveled across the globe reporting on the performance of WAC personnel. Her feedback helped dispel the myth that women were unsuited to military roles [5, 6, 10].

In 1945, Captain Edwin Pulaski established a medical research unit at Halloran General Hospital, Staten Island, NY, to study antibiotic use in surgery. The U.S. Army Surgical Research Unit would later relocate to Fort Sam Houston, Texas, in 1947, where it evolved into the Burn Center at Brooke Army Medical Center, now known as the Institute of Surgical Research [5, 6].

Colonel Michael DeBakey volunteered for the armed forces and served on the Army Surgeon General's staff from 1945 to 1946. He published numerous papers on treating chest wounds and vascular injuries, leading to the development of mobile army surgical hospitals (MASH units). DeBakey also helped establish the system for treating returning military personnel, which evolved into the Veterans Affairs Medical Center System [11].

As one of the most prominent and innovative thoracic surgeons of his time, Colonel Edward D. Churchill played a pivotal role in advancing Army medicine during World War II as the Chief Surgical

Consultant in the Mediterranean Theater of Operations. He pioneered the practice of early debridement and delayed primary closure for contaminated wounds, significantly reducing infection rates and improving patient recovery. Churchill advocated for the use of whole blood transfusions on the battlefield, establishing regional blood banks to ensure this critical resource was readily available. He also restructured the medical evacuation process by developing a streamlined chain of evacuation, with specific responsibilities assigned to each hospital, ensuring timely and effective surgical care for injured soldiers. Churchill's contributions to wartime medical care have been preserved through his memoirs and diaries, establishing standards in military medical practices that continue to influence treatment in current conflicts [12].

Korean and Vietnam Conflicts

The Korean and Vietnam Wars further tested the resilience and capabilities of the Army Medical Corps. During these conflicts, the emphasis on rapid evacuation and advanced surgical techniques in the field saved numerous lives. In 1951, the first helicopter ambulance flew in Korea. By the end of the conflict in 1953, over 17,000 casualties had been airlifted by helicopter. In 1958, the Army Medical Department helped publish the North Atlantic Treaty Organization (NATO) manual "Emergency War Surgery." At the time of this writing, the 6th Edition of the Emergency War Surgery was in production. The 5th Edition is available at https://medcoe.army.mil/borden-tb-ews [13].

In Vietnam, the MUST (Medical Unit, Self-Contained, Transportable) significantly improved efficiency and speed by providing a mobile "instant" hospital easily transported by truck or aircraft. It was common for medical personnel to work under fire, and many Vietnam medics, like their predecessors from previous wars, earned the Medal of Honor for heroism. During this time, Army Colonel Norman Rich emerged as a pioneering vascular surgeon. His work in refining vascular surgical techniques, particularly for arteriovenous injuries to the extremity, emphasized the importance of venous and arterial system repairs. His clinical work and his establishment of the Vietnam Vascular Registry at Walter Reed General Hospital helped usher in new advances in managing vascular injuries and limb salvage [5, 6, 14].

Following the Vietnam War, the Army Medical Corps continued to evolve, integrating new technologies, expanding infrastructure, and focusing on reorganization. In 1988, the first Composite Health Care System (CHCS) was tested at Fort Knox, KY. CHCS was a comprehensive computer system for military hospitals across the three Services, a step toward the goal of a paperless hospital. The Gulf War in the early 1990s highlighted the importance of medical preparedness and the use of telemedicine. During the conflict, a small task force from the Uniformed Services University of the Health Sciences developed a telemedicine program, but its impact was limited due to a lack of interest from commanders and insufficient experience among medics. During subsequent conflicts in Somalia in 1993, military physicians used telemedicine to treat eye wounds and fractures. These provers were able to send x-rays and photographs to colleagues at Walter Reed Army Medical Center to assist with a diagnosis [15]. These capabilities have continued to grow and evolve with advancements in technology.

Global War on Terror and Beyond

The dawn of the twenty-first century brought new challenges with the Global War on Terror. The conflicts in Iraq and Afghanistan saw a resurgence in the importance of trauma surgery and emergency medical care. Dr. Richard Jadick, a Navy surgeon who served with the Marines during the Battle of Fallujah, demonstrated the critical role of forward surgical teams. Jadick's efforts in setting up makeshift trauma centers close to the front lines significantly increased survival rates for wounded soldiers. For his actions, he was awarded the Bronze Star with Combat "V" [16]. Dr. John B. Holcomb, a trauma surgeon and Army Colonel, played a pivotal role during this era. Holcomb's work on improving hemorrhage control and resuscitation via tourniquet use hemostatic dressings had a profound impact on battlefield medicine, leading to better outcomes for wounded soldiers. More importantly, he recognized the strategic, operational and tactical need for the development of a deployed trauma system. Under his leadership, the Joint Theatre Trauma System and the Joint Theater Trauma Registry were established in the U.S. Central Command area of operations to help standardize combat casualty care and identify and promulgate life-saving best practices. Ultimately his work and the work of many pioneering Tri-Service trauma surgeons, resulted in the creation of the Joint Trauma System, the Department of Defense (DoD) Center of Excellence for trauma and the DoD Trauma Registry. His contributions were recognized with numerous awards, and he continues to influence trauma care and support The Joint Trauma System as a civilian surgeon and researcher [17].

Current Route from Injury to Definitive Care (Fig. 2.1)

Current military doctrine is a culmination of modern resources and improved techniques from past lessons learned. The echelons, or roles, of care in Army Medicine represent a structured system designed to provide escalating levels of support to wounded soldiers from the point of injury to definitive treatment. This system is organized as follows.

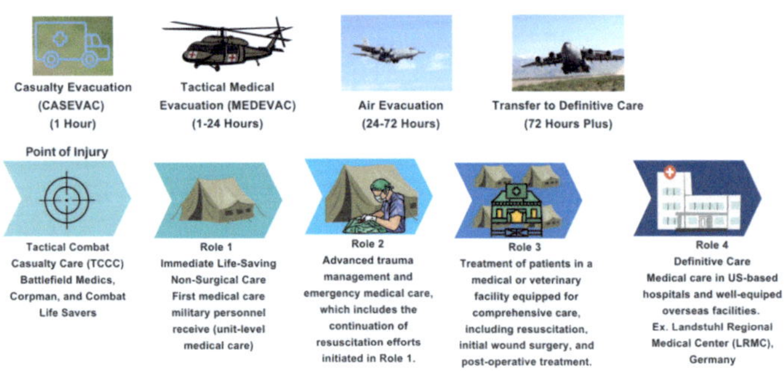

Fig. 2.1 Roles of care from point of injury to definitive care

Point of Injury and Role 1: Immediate Life-Saving Measures

At the point of injury, care begins with Tactical Combat Casualty Care (TCCC), administered by battlefield medics, corpsmen, or combat life savers. This level focuses on immediate, life-saving interventions, such as hemorrhage control, airway management, and stabilization for evacuation. The goal is to keep the casualty alive until they can be moved to a location with more appropriate resources [18, 19].

Role 2: Forward Resuscitative Surgical Care

Casualties are typically evacuated to Role 2 facilities within 1–24 h, such as a Forward Resuscitative Surgical Detachment (FRSD), previously known as a Forward Surgical Team (FST). Here, more advanced life-saving measures, including emergency surgery, are performed. The focus is on damage control surgery and resuscitation to stabilize the patient for further evacuation [18, 19].

Role 3: Field Hospital

Over the next 24–72 h, the casualty is airlifted to a Role 3 facility, such as a Field Hospital (FH), formerly known as a Combat Support Hospital (CSH) or Mobile Army Surgical Hospital (MASH). These facilities provide comprehensive surgical and medical interventions, including intensive care units (ICUs), to further stabilize and treat the patient before being transferred to a more permanent medical facility [18, 19].

Role 4: Definitive Care

Once stabilized, the patient is transferred to a Role 4 facility, such as Landstuhl Regional Medical Center (LRMC) in Germany. These hospitals are well equipped and offer a robust level of definitive surgical and medical care, preparing the patient for further treatment and some rehabilitation [18, 19].

Full Range of Care

Finally, the patient may be transferred to a facility such as Walter Reed National Military Medical Center in Bethesda, MD. While technically considered a Role 4 capability. Military medical centers in the United States provide the full spectrum of medical care, including long-term rehabilitation, comprehensive subspecialty medical and surgical care, and specialized resources required for recovery [18, 19].

Conclusion: A Legacy to Uphold

The history of the United States Army Medical Corps in the modern era is rich with examples of individual bravery and success in the face of incredible adversity. The contributions of military surgeons and medical officers have advanced the field of medicine and ensured the survival and recovery of countless soldiers. Today's young officers and doctors have big shoes to fill. As they embark on their careers, they carry forward the proud tradition of the Army Medical Corps, facing new challenges and opportunities to innovate. The legacy of past medical officers serves as both an inspiration and a reminder of their duty to others.

History of the United States Air Force Medical Service

Breanne ParetsChungeun Lee, and Kyle J. Iverson

The Air Force Separates from the Army Air Corp

The United States Air Force (USAF) separated from the Army to become an independent branch in September 1947 after the

National Security Act of 1947 became law. However, medical care for the USAF remained the responsibility of the Army for nearly two additional years [20].[3] Beginning in 1948, Major General Malcolm C. Grow—who later became the first Surgeon General of the USAF—advocated for an independent medical structure that supported the particular mission of the USAF. Aviation technology had been advancing rapidly since World War I, and pilots needed care tailored to their increasing physical demands. In addition, World War II emphasized the utility of aeromedical evacuation in reducing war-zone fatality rates, and the USAF presented a unique potential for expanding aeromedical evacuation capabilities [20]. Maj Gen Grow's position aligned with the perspective of the 1947 Hawley Board, an interdepartmental medical committee established by the Secretary of Defense to examine hospital requirements of the armed forces, who reported that "the medical service of an armed force is a necessary and integral part of the force. To separate it from the force is wholly or largely to destroy its usefulness" [21]. Momentum for an independent Air Force medical service continued to build with support from the Air Force Chief of Staff, the Air Force Association, and the American Medical Association until Maj Gen Grow successfully convinced the Army and President Truman's administration of the need. The Air Force Medical Service (AFMS) was officially established on 1 July 1949, with the primary goal of ensuring the health and readiness of Airmen [22]. Since then, the AFMS has continued to evolve with the changing needs of the military and promoted innovative research that contributes to medicine.

Air Force Medical Service Developments

Korean War (1950–1953)

The Korean War was the first opportunity for the AFMS to demonstrate its wartime value. Perhaps the most distinguished accomplishment was the USAF's ability to provide long-range aeromedical evacuation during the war, not only for American troops but for all United Nations forces in Korea [23]. At the beginning of the war, the young AFMS was unprepared and undertrained, but necessity and high demand forced rapid growth and development [23]. By the end of the war, the AFMS had established itself as an effective global aeromedical evacuation system offering in-transit medical care provided by USAF medical personnel aboard various aircraft, including H-5 helicopters and C-47 s [2, 24]. The USAF also built aeromedical staging facilities in combat areas and created portable, customizable medical assemblies that could be flown in and set up to function as field hospitals [24]. Thus, injured military members, civilians, and prisoners of war received not only necessary pre-hospital care at the front lines but also rapid transport to Mobile Army Surgical Hospitals and military or United Nations allied hospitals around the world for definitive management. Evacuating casualties from combat areas by air reduced the casualty death rate by 50% compared to World War II [24].

Other medical improvements made during the Korean War can be seen today in both the military and civilian settings. For instance, the use of plastic bags for blood storage, shipping, and administration in place of glass bottles proved to be equal, if not superior, in blood quality and cost. Blood collected in plastic bags did not have to be discarded due to hemolysis, and the bags did not have to be refrigerated before collecting blood. The cost of each equipment unit also decreased from $1.48 to $0.45 [25]. In addition, the United States organized a nationwide collection and delivery program to move life-saving blood halfway around the world for combat support. In the largest blood shipment operation in the history of United States military medicine, the Whole Blood Processing Laboratory at Travis Air Force Base in California handled 397,711 pints of whole blood, shipping 340,427 of them to Korea for distribution to United Nations medical units [26].

Vietnam War (1962–1974)

Aeromedical evacuation continued to advance during the Vietnam War, and rapid evacuations by helicopter and subsequently jets moved casualties to hospitals around the world for definitive care much more quickly than was ever before possible [27]. The USAF introduced the C-9A Nightingale during the Vietnam War. Named after the British Nurse Florence Nightingale (1820-1910), the founder of modern nursing who pioneered military nursing care during the Crimean War, it was the first plane specifically intended for aeromedical evacuation. The aircraft was designed to safely carry stretchers, gurneys, ambulatory patients, and other special medical equipment to facilitate in-flight medical care [28]. The C-9A's initial role in Vietnam demonstrated the value of having a designated aircraft for patient transfers and prompt medical care in flight.

Gulf War (1990–1991)

The overall medical deployment during the initial stage of the Gulf War was much faster and larger than during the Vietnam War, largely due to air-transportable clinics and hospitals [29]. Medical teams were rapidly deployed and arrived in the theater just 2 days after the first combat units [23]. In August and September of 1990, the USAF set up medical facilities in the Arabian Peninsula that had both surgical and chemical decontamination capabilities and were equipped for up to 30 days without the need for resupply [23]. By the combat stage of the war, 31 deployed air-transportable clinics provided initial triage and medical evaluation, and 15 air-transportable hospitals supplied the bulk of in-theater hospital beds and medical personnel for the USAF [29]. These air-transportable medical facilities proved to be critical, as there were no contingency hospitals positioned in the Arabian Peninsula prior to the Gulf War [23]. In 1983, the Air Force Surgeon General approved a program to increase the capacity of air-transportable hospitals from 24 beds, which was the standard at the time, to 50 beds. Throughout the 1990s, these air-transportable clinics and hospitals continued to be re-engineered and tailored for use in various humanitarian and peacekeeping missions around the world [23].

The speed and comprehensive deployment of the AFMS during Operations Desert Shield and Desert Storm demonstrated the exceptional state of preparation at the time. This success is attributable to the USAF's prioritization of and dedication to medical readiness since the late 1970s [23]. For example, in response to rising worldwide terrorism directed at the United States, the AFMS initiated the Medical Red Flag Program. Beginning in 1979 at Keesler Air Force Base, this program included a series of annual readiness exercises designed for medical providers to gain hands-on exposure to battlefield casualty management [23, 30].

Despite the AFMS's overall success in rapid medical deployment and care for the American forces during the Gulf War, it became clear during this time that aeromedical evacuation capabilities were constrained by the acuity of patients needing transport. For instance, the AFMS was unable to transport patients on a ventilator or those with any other critical care needs [31]. To overcome these limitations, efforts were directed toward the formalization of Critical Care Air Transport Teams (CCATTs), which were officially adopted into the USAF aeromedical evacuation system in 1996, shortly after the Gulf War (see below for more detail) [32].

Global War on Terror (2001–2021)

As American troops deployed to Afghanistan, the AFMS once again demonstrated its rapid deployment capabilities, this time with the new Expeditionary Medical Support (EMEDS) system. Compared to a 25-bed Air Transportable Hospital from the Gulf War era, a 25-bed EMEDS was one-third the size and weight. It could be transported in its entirety—complete with personnel, equipment, and shelters—on one C-130. Additional specialty capabilities could be added to the basic EMEDS according to local needs. The AFMS remained the predominant medical support for the first 60 days of Operation Enduring Freedom [23].

Throughout the Global War on Terror, the AFMS underwent significant modernization to adapt to changing mission requirements and tactical environments. This involved retiring old practices and legacy systems and incorporating new equipment and methods. For instance, the C-9A Nightingale was phased out from active service in 2003, and C-130 s, C-141 s, and KC-135 s took over its role in aeromedical evacuation. A newly designed patient support pallet, able to support six patient litters or a combination of three seats and three litters, accommodated the provision of high-quality patient care aboard cargo aircraft [23]. Operations in Afghanistan and Iraq produced a new emphasis on having surgical and aeromedical evacuation capabilities far forward to further facilitate expeditious access to advanced trauma care and evacuation to higher levels of care. Single-surgeon teams were positioned in austere locations to provide damage control resuscitation and damage control surgery as close to the point of injury as possible, and CCATTs demonstrated the ability to evacuate even the most critically ill and injured patients with minimal delay [23, 33, 34]. Landstuhl Regional Medical Center in Germany emerged as a major hub for treating ill and injured troops in a quickly accessible location outside of the combat zone en route to the United States. An innovative tracking system, TRAC2ES, was also introduced to track patients throughout the aeromedical evacuation process. These efforts collectively contributed to historically unprecedented casualty survival rates [23].

Just as AFMS medics were present at the onset of the Global War on Terror, they were also present at its conclusion. As American forces prepared to withdraw from Afghanistan in 2021, the AFMS shifted its focus to humanitarian efforts associated with Operations Allies Refuge and Allies Welcome. AFMS personnel offered medical aid to evacuees in Afghanistan before travel to the United States, en route at various travel hubs, and at EMEDS deployed within the United States to serve as reception centers [23].

Present-Day Air Force Medical Capabilities

Roles of Care

An essential tenet of military medicine is the need to efficiently "triage, treat, evacuate, and return soldiers to duty" [1]. This is accomplished through multiple stages of care with progressive capabilities, beginning on the battlefield and ending in a hospital in the United States. Formally, there are four roles of care (Roles 1–4). There were previously five levels, or echelons, of care, but the DoD adopted NATO terminology midway through the Global War on Terror. Role 1 entails first aid delivered immediately at the point of injury, including self-aid, buddy aid, and care given by a combat lifesaver (nonmedical military personnel with advanced first aid training). Role 1 also may include some medical personnel who are able to provide basic triage and sick calls, but it does not include any surgical or patient-holding capabilities. Role 2 offers advanced trauma resuscitation and limited inpatient bed space as a continuation of care provided in Role 1. This includes the ability to transfuse blood products, obtain limited imaging and labs, and perform advanced resuscitation procedures and damage control surgery prior to evacuation [35]. Role 3 facilities are field hospitals comparable to civilian trauma centers but located within the combat zone [36]. They are manned and supplied to provide medical, surgical, and trauma care for any patient acuity and offer not only resuscitation and damage control surgery but also specialty surgery and advanced post-operative care [35]. Role 4 differs from Role 3 in that it offers definitive medical and surgical care outside of the combat zone, either at robust overseas hospitals, such as Landstuhl Regional Medical Center in Germany or at hospitals within DoD medical centers in the United States [1, 35]. This multistage provision of care optimizes casualty survivability and mission readiness while maintaining tactical and operational feasibility. The USAF's substantial aeromedical evacuation and critical care transport capabilities are essential to supporting this model.

Ground Surgical Teams

Ground Surgical Teams (GSTs) have become the mainstay of USAF surgical care in the modern deployment setting. A GST comprises six members: a general surgeon, an anesthesiologist or Certified Nurse Anesthetist (CRNA), an emergency medicine (EM) physician, a critical care or EM nurse, a surgical technician, and a Medical Service Corpsman (MSC). GSTs are single-surgeon teams capable of providing early intervention following battlefield injuries. In general, putting up a hospital near the front lines is not feasible, but a GST is designed to operate as a functional hospital unit that can be placed far forward.

USAF forward surgical capabilities have evolved through time to create the modern-day GST. Fielded in 1984, the Flying Ambulance Surgical Team (FAST), composed of 20 members, was a prototype for caring for USAF combat casualties. Based on lessons learned from various military operations over the next decade, smaller Mobile Field Surgical Teams (MFSTs) were introduced in 1995 and became the standard by 1998. Consisting of five individuals, the MFSTs were responsible for providing emergency and surgical care, while separate Expeditionary Critical Care Teams (ECCTs) took over perioperative and critical care management [37].

During the early years of the Global War on Terror, the small size and portability of the MFSTs enabled them to support the military's mission very effectively [37]. Around the same time, Special Operations Surgical Teams (SOSTs) were created to support Special Operations Forces (SOF) (see below for more detail). Even as traditional combat operations in Afghanistan and Iraq decreased, demand for austere surgical care remained high. To meet that demand, the next-generation Ground Surgical Team (GST) was established as a counterpart to SOSTs for the regular forces [34]. The first GST was deployed in 2017, replacing MFSTs and ECCTs [34, 37]. Members of GSTs attend 3 weeks of specialized training before deployment [34]. When mobilized, they are expected to expeditiously provide "damage control surgery, damage control resuscitation, and emergency care of injured or critically ill patients in dynamic, austere environments outside of established support and patient movement capabilities" [37]. GSTs are equipped with field packs containing the supplies needed to perform up to 10 surgeries and to provide 12 h of postoperative critical care for three patients. Their goal is first to provide the care and interventions necessary to save life, limb, and eyesight, and ultimately to stabilize the critically injured for evacuation [37].

Special Operations Surgical Teams

Special Operations Surgical Teams (SOSTs) are another asset utilized by the USAF to bring medical care still closer to the front lines. SOSTs are extremely lightweight, mobile teams with advanced medical and tactical training designed to be speedily deployable to provide expert trauma and surgical care in any place and at any time. They are specifically intended to support Special Operations Forces (SOF) on various missions all over the world [38].

The idea behind SOSTs originated in 2001 and SOSTs were mobilized by 2003 [39]. SOSTs, like GSTs, are six-member teams that include a general surgeon, an anesthesiologist or

CRNA, an emergency physician, a critical care or EM nurse, and a surgical technician. The difference between the two is that the final member of a SOST is a respiratory therapist, rather than an MSC [40]. New SOST appointees undergo an extensive preselection process and, if chosen, they complete 10–12 months of advanced operational medical training and SOF-caliber tactical training [38].

SOSTs operate with the limited resources they can carry with them in backpacks, making them entirely independent of any established healthcare system or facility. This gives them great mobility and leaves a much smaller footprint than any other surgical asset [39]. SOSTs can be fully operational in as little as 15 min after arrival on site. They set up in hostile environments on the battlefield or very near to it [38]. This capability radically minimizes the time from the point of injury in combat to skilled resuscitation and surgical intervention, giving special operators, host nation fighters, and other victims of crisis their best chance at survival [39].

Critical Care Air Transport Team

Critical Care Air Transport Teams (CCATTs) are a capability unique to the USAF and are essential to combat casualty evacuation [41]. CCATTs are specialized teams consisting of three members: a critical care or EM physician, a critical care nurse, and a respiratory therapist. These teams accompany aeromedical evacuation aircrew to transform aircraft into flying intensive care units [32].

The CCATT concept was developed by a former Air Force Surgeon General, Lieutenant General (Dr.) Paul K. Carlton, in the 1980s and further developed during Operation Desert Shield and Operation Desert Storm when it became apparent that even though large receiving hospitals were set up to care for combat casualties away from the front lines, they were underutilized because there was no way to safely transport critically ill or injured patients from the field to those hospitals. Thus, the Army had to increase the capabilities of field hospitals closer to the front, as they did during the Vietnam War [31]. Such hospitals leave a large footprint and are very expensive to construct, man, and defend [41]. Lt Gen Carlton and Colonel Chris Farmer proposed CCATT in response as a more modern mechanism of transport to meet the needs of all the branches in the modern battlefield [31]. CCATT gained momentum during various conflicts in the 1990s and was officially approved in 1996 [32].

Aeromedical evacuation crews with CCATT capabilities can land aircraft at small forward airfields to pick up injured patients close to the point of injury. These patients continue to receive the life-saving medical care they need en route as they are transported to higher echelons of care thus revolutionizing casualty care. A single CCATT can care for up to three critical patients or six stabilized patients [32]. They are qualified on multiple platforms, meaning they can complete their mission on almost any aircraft [42]. They receive specialized training to equip them to provide care in small spaces with loud noises, low light, turbulence, and changes in temperature and air pressure that occur during flight [32].

During the Vietnam War, it could take over a month for wounded service members to reach hospitals in the United States, and during the Gulf War, it took 10–14 days for casualties to be evacuated to Europe. Now, thanks to CCATT and improved aeromedical evacuation capabilities, transport time from the battlefield to tertiary hospitals can be achieved in as little as 48–72 h [23, 32]. As modern missions continue to emphasize leaving a small footprint, CCATT will become more and more essential [41].

Conclusion

Providing medical care is a high priority for the USAF, as evidenced by the fact that roughly 9% of its active duty members and nearly 60,000 total force individuals are in the AFMS [43–45]. At present, medical care for the United States Space Force remains under the AFMS [46]. Future development may include the formation of a separate medical service specific to the Space Force to fit its unique needs. While, the size of the United States Armed Forces and their mission may change with time, the need for medical care and readiness will remain.

A Brief History of the United States Navy Medical Corps and Overview of Current Capabilities

Aaron Wickard and Matthew D. Tadlock

Origins of Surgery at Sea

Travel by sea has been integral to the evolution of civilization. Since ancient times sailors have navigated the ocean, and the world's navies have enabled global migration, exploration, commerce, and war. In Classical Greece, Athenian sea power was an integral part of history's first known democracy. The Roman Republic did not realize empire until its Navy achieved maritime mastery of the Mediterranean [47]. British sea power enabled England to become the world's largest empire from the late sixteenth century through WWI at the beginning of the twentieth century. Indeed, after the Revolutionary War, U.S. Navy structure, tactics, traditions, and naval medicine evolved from that of the Royal Navy.

Shipboard medical care has been a staple of combat naval operations since the time of the ancient Greeks. In Homer's classic *The Iliad* circa 800 B.C, a surgeon named Machaon is described, whose skill and renown as a military surgeon elevated him to the level of a deity in the ancient world [48]. The Middle Ages and the Age of Sail marked the rise of barber surgeons who not only treated common medical conditions but specialized in treating surgical conditions and injuries from naval combat and routine naval operations with their hands [49]. The city-state of Venice utilized the first known embarked shipboard surgeons to augment their medical capabilities while deployed in foreign ports and at sea. Perhaps the first known ship's surgeon was

Venetian barber-surgeon Master Gualtieri. Venetian archives from 1300 indicate that he treated many wounded on Venetian galleys and had a long career paid by the city-state [50, 51]. Venetian vessels trading throughout Europe likely disseminated the practice of embarked barber surgeons.

The British Royal Navy was the first to coin the terms "ship's surgeon" and "surgeon's mate" with the creation of a structured naval medical service in 1512. Laying the groundwork for future British sea power, King Henry VIII began refitting warships with two tiers of heavy guns in 1540, revolutionizing naval warfare and forever changing injury patterns managed by naval surgeons. 1540 was also a significant year in the history of surgery, as Henry VIII formally incorporated the Guild of Surgeons with the Company of Barbers to form the Royal College of Barber-Surgeons. This institution would last over 200 years and evolve into the current Royal College of Surgeons. Eventually, Royal Navy Surgeons were formally certified, and their surgical instruments and medicine chests were inspected before deployments [52, 53]. By the early seventeenth century, Dutch, Spanish, Portuguese, and French navies all had ship surgeons in regular service.

Beginnings of U.S. Naval Medicine

The first American naval surgeons were civilians who answered wanted ads in New England area newspapers seeking "properly qualified" surgeons to serve on the privateer vessels comprising General George Washington's "ad hoc" Continental Navy of the Revolutionary War [54]. The U.S. Navy was formally established in 1798 after Congress passed the Naval Act of 1794 which authorized the construction of six frigates to assist with coastal defense of the new country and power projection abroad. One of these originally authorized frigates was the USS *Constitution*. Commissioned in 1797, it is still in active service and can be visited in its home port at the Charleston Naval Yard, near Boston. Experienced military medical personnel were scarce, and the first surgeons temporarily appointed to American warships came from the U.S. Army. By 1798, Army surgeons and surgeon's mates serving on U.S. warships were formally appointed to the Navy. George Balfour started his military career in the U.S. Army in 1792, and by 1798 he was appointed Surgeon of the USS *Constellation.* In 1799, Balfour and Surgeon's Mate Isaac Henry became the first formal U.S. Navy physicians to serve in naval combat during the *Constellation's* engagement with the French ship *L'Insurgente* in the Caribbean Sea [55].

Naval hospitals were established in 1811 with the first operational naval hospital, Naval Hospital Portsmouth, opening in 1830. The first naval hospitals were located near the busiest shipyards on the East Coast in Washington D.C., New York City, Portsmouth, Boston, and Philadelphia. In these early years, a small Board of Naval Commissioners provided oversight and administration of the U.S. Navy. As it grew in size and technology changed, a more formal and specialized bureaucracy was needed. In 1842 Congress established five functional Navy bureaus, one of which was the Bureau of Medicine and Surgery (BUMED) [55]. Of the original five, only BUMED and the Bureau of Naval Personnel (BUPERS) formally exist in the U.S. Navy today.

With the beginning of the Civil War in 1861, Navy Medicine expanded its expeditionary ability by establishing the first hospital ship; a captured Confederate gunboat steamer named the USS *Red Rover* which was retrofitted with an operating room and ward beds. Unlike unarmed modern hospitals, the *Red Rover* was armed with a 32-pounder gun to protect itself while supporting operations along the Mississippi River [56].

Modernization in the Twentieth Century

Modernization of the U.S. Navy medical force began during the global conflicts of the twentieth century. The battleship had emerged as the supreme naval asset with the ability to inflict massive damage and high casualties. Navies began incorporating more robust shipboard medical care including dedicated spaces for a sick bay, isolation ward, pharmacy, radiography, and an operating room. Specific dispersed casualty care locations well stocked with medical supplies known as Battle Dressing Stations were incorporated into Navy policy [57]. Not included in these advances was a dedicated embarked anesthesiologist. The use of spinal anesthesia, sodium thiopental, ether, chloroform, or even a simple tourniquet and refrigeration, unchanged since the Civil War, were managed by the surgeons themselves to perform a variety of operations. A corpsman at the head of the bed monitored the patient's pallor and pulse to assess the hemodynamics of the patient. By WWII resuscitation of critically injured patients at sea began with freeze-dried plasma, typically available within 5 min, then augmented with fresh whole blood from walking blood banks which was available in as little as 20 min [58, 59].

The first hospital ship specifically designed and built to provide medical care at sea was the USS *Relief* (AH-1) which was commissioned in 1920 [60]. These ships were initially used as "floating ambulances" during WWI, serving as medically capable patient transports ferrying patients from the battlefield to hospitals back in the United States. During the European and African Campaigns in WWII, the Navy continued the "scoop and sail" model utilizing medically augmented Tank Landing Ships (LST) to shuttle wounded to hospital ships stationed offshore over relatively short distances. Over time, particularly in the Pacific Theatre of Operations (PTO), some LSTs were converted to medically and surgically capable combatant vessels. During the PTO island hoping campaigns these medically augmented LSTs provided initial damage control resuscitation and damage control surgery, until these capabilities were established on land. In contrast, during the early conflicts within the PTO, hospital ships were initially utilized to transport patients out of the theater after initial stabilization. The increased casualty capacity of hospital ships, coupled with the increased efficacy of U.S. naval air power, and the need to support long-range, high-causality amphibious operations during the Pacific Campaign of WWII, medical doctrine shifted toward hospital ships providing damage control surgery and resuscitation within the combat zone [61]. During the Battle of Iwo Jima, hospital ships were brought to on station within 1 day of the invasion to decrease the time to definitive care for critically wounded casualties [62]. The Korean War saw the first use of rotary wing aircraft for casualty evacuation with the USS

Consolation (AH-15) stationed off the coast of Korea [63]. During the Vietnam War, emphasis again was placed on rapid patient aeromedical evacuation and point of injury care by Field Corpsmen attached to Marine Corps units.

The first female physicians in the Navy were commissioned in the Medical Corps (MC) of the U.S. Navy Reserves during WWII between 1943 and 1945. In 1948, psychiatrist Dr. Frances Willoughby became the first female MC officer to be commissioned to active duty in the Navy. The first woman MC officer to go to sea was anesthesiologist Dr. Bernice Rosenthal Walters, serving on the hospital ship USS *Consolation* in 1950. However, women were not allowed to serve on U.S. combatant vessels until 1993 when Congress repealed Title 10 USC 6015. Four years later, Dr. Beth Jaklic became the first woman Ship Surgeon serving aboard the aircraft carrier USS *George Washington* (CVN-73) in 1997 [64].

At the end of the twentieth century, U.S. Navy surgeons on combatant vessels began to integrate a new surgical capability into their toolkit when Dr. Miguel Cubano performed the first laparoscopic surgery, an inguinal hernia repair, in 1995 on the aircraft carrier USS *Abraham Lincoln* (CVN-72) with telemedicine assistance [65]. Given that U.S warships do not have computed tomography capability afloat like French and British aircraft carriers, diagnostic laparoscopy is an important diagnostic tool for contemporary U.S. Navy surgeons to help diagnose or rule out hollow-viscous injury after blunt abdominal trauma or when there is diagnostic uncertainty during the management of emergency general and gynecological surgical conditions.

U.S. Marine Corps Health Service Support

The U.S. Marine Corps (USMC) does not have its own embedded medical corps. As such, naval caregivers have been taking care of sick and injured marines on land and sea since the Continental Navy and Continental Marines were formed during the Revolutionary War. The Marine Corps did not formally become part of the Department of the Navy until 1834. During WWI, U.S. Navy medical personnel provided care to U.S. Marines on the front line with courage and skill with Navy Corpsmen being awarded two Medals of Honor, 55 Navy Crosses, and 31 Distinguished Service Medals [66]. Corpsmen serving in USMC units are affectionately referred to as "Doc." During WWII Corpsmen who served with the Fleet Marine Force attended USMC boot camp with the Marines they would be taking care of in Pacific and European theaters of operation.

U.S. Military engagements at the turn of the twenty-first century focused on expeditionary, land-based, counter-insurgency efforts with the Navy supporting the USMC through Expeditionary Maneuver Warfare. Medical care during Operation Enduring Freedom (OEF) and Operation Iraqi Freedom I/II (OIF) necessitated an inland presence of forward, austere surgical care augmented by sea-based logistics. The manifestation of these doctrinal changes was seen during the initial surge of troops into Afghanistan following September 11, 2001, when a battalion aid station with damage control surgical capabilities was established at Camp Rhino in the Registan Desert of Afghanistan. This forward surgical capability, located 400 miles away from its ship-based supply chain in the Arabian Sea, evaluated and stabilized casualties near the point of injury before transporting them to care either aboard Casualty Receiving Treatment Ships (CRTS) or at the Role 3 U.S. Air Force Theater Hospital in Seeb, Oman [67]. To further decrease the time to surgical intervention for injured Marines, more mobile surgical care was supported by the Forward Resuscitative Surgical Systems (FRSS). The goal of these units was to treat patients requiring life-saving surgical intervention before evacuation without fixed medical treatment facilities. These units could treat up to 18 surgical patients without resupply and were paired with a Shock Trauma Platoon (STP), a forward emergency room capable of providing damage-control resuscitation and life-saving procedures to stabilize critically ill and injured patients prior to surgery or transport [68–71].

Navy Medicine and Surgery in the Twenty-first Century

Doctrinally the U.S. Navy's deployable Role 3 medical capabilities include hospital ships and large field hospitals known as Expeditionary Medical Facilities (EMF). While the Role 3 EMFs have not been utilized in the recent past, U.S. Navy medicine broadened its scope of care in support of multinational military efforts in Afghanistan by assuming control of the Role 2-Extended field hospital at Kandahar Airfield. Between October 2009 and September 2020, the Navy-lead hospital provided advanced surgical and medical care, treating 2,100 patients per year between 2009 and 2012. In May 2010, the hospital became a Role 3 Multinational Medical Unit (MMU) providing the only neurosurgery, ophthalmology, oral and maxillofacial surgery, and interventional radiology capabilities in southern Afghanistan [72]. During OIF and OEF, U.S. Navy Role 2 surgical teams also deployed throughout Iraq and Afghanistan supporting U.S. Army units during numerous Individual Augmentee deployments. At the time of this writing the U.S. Navy continues to provide a shore-based Role 2 capability supporting U.S. Army operations in Iraq.

In the twenty-first century, the Navy's two hospital ships, the USNS *Comfort* and USNS *Mercy*, provide regular medical and surgical care to host nations during elective humanitarian assistance and emergent disaster response missions with partner nations around the world. These missions enable rapid disaster relief responses with partner nations after devastating earthquakes, hurricanes, and other natural disasters. U.S. Navy hospital ships provide the full spectrum of Role 3 medical care. The first robot-assisted laparoscopic surgery at sea, a cholecystectomy, was performed aboard the USNS *Mercy* off the coast of Sri Lanka in 2018 [73].

Overview of Current U.S. Navy Surgical Capabilities

The modern at-sea expeditionary surgical capabilities that exist today were developed on battleships, aircraft carriers, and LSTs during WWI and WWII. These capabilities were refined through the Korean, Vietnam, and Cold Wars. Naval Health Service Support to Sailors and Marines has been critical to the U.S. Navy enabling freedom of navigation and commerce at sea around the world. Current U.S. Navy medical capabilities are based on the NATO Roles of care used throughout the U.S. Department of Defense. Each Role is part of a patient care continuum with progressively escalating medical capabilities starting at the point of injury through definitive treatment utilizing a variety of land and maritime-based platforms (Table 2.1) [74, 75]. Within each Role of care (particularly Role, 1, 2, and 3), each medical capability exists within a spectrum of care depending on the unit or capability being supported. For example, point-of-injury care by a single corpsman deployed with their USMC combat unit is considered Role 1 care. However, USMC battalion aid stations led by a general physician and multiple corpsmen, which have significantly more organic medical capability, are still considered Role 1 care. Similarly, a cruiser or destroyer (CRUDES) provides Role 1 capabilities led by an Independent Duty Corpsman (IDC). However, smaller amphibious ships such as a Landing Transport Dock ship (LPD) have more medical capability and are led by a general practice physician. Both are considered Role 1 capabilities unless they are augmented by an embarked surgical team.

Likewise, U.S. Navy Role 2 medical care exists within a spectrum. Depending on mission requirements and the operational platforms being supported, patient capacity and capabilities can vary between the different units providing Role 2 Naval Health Service Support. Single surgeon Role 2 capabilities include the Expeditionary Resuscitative Surgical Systems (ERSS), aircraft carrier surgical teams (CVN), and Fleet Surgical Teams (FST). The ERSS is a seven-person team with a light footprint; team members carry their own equipment and supplies and can rapidly augment Role 1 platforms on both land and sea to provide austere resuscitative surgical care (ARSC) including damage control resuscitation and damage control surgery. However, these teams are dependent on what they bring with them (e.g., blood and consumables) and the organic shipboard resources for crucial elements of care including sterilization and additional blood products [76]. Capital ships, including large-deck amphibious ships and aircraft carriers, have designated surgical spaces and advanced resuscitative capabilities native to the ship. CVN surgical teams are part of a larger ships

Table 2.1 Overview of current U.S. maritime medical capabilities

Roles of care	Platform		Patient capacity	Capabilities	Organic medical department personnel
Role 1	DDG, CG, LSD[a], submarine		1 patient	TCCC	Corpsman, IDC, physician[a]
Role 2	Aircraft carrier (CVN)		1 OR, 3 ICU beds, 51 ward beds	DCR, DCS, WBB, blood products (5 units whole blood)	1 General surgeon, 1 CCRN, 1 Anesthesia provider, 1 OMFS, 1 PA, 2 IDCs, 39 HM
	Casualty receiving treatment ship (CRTS)[b]	LHD	2 ORs (flex 6 ORs), 16 ICU beds, 45 ward beds	DCR, DCS, prolonged patient care w/FST, blood products (400 PRBC, 40 FFP)	2 Medical officer, 24 HM
		LHA	2 ORs, 3 ICU beds, 23 ward beds	DCR, DCS, prolonged patient care w/FST, blood products (400 PRBC, 40 FFP)	2 Medical officers, 19 HM
		LPD	1 OR (flex 2 ORs), 3 ICU beds, 24 ward beds	DCR, DCS w/FST, blood products (45 PRBC, 10 FFP)	1 Medical officer, 11 HM
	Expeditionary resuscitative surgical system (ERSS)		Capacity based on the modular variant, range 1–4 surgeries	DCR, DCS, brings own AMAL, l patient holding up to 72 h depending on AMAL, ship being augmented, severity of injury, and number of patients. ~40 total units of blood products	1 General surgeon, 1 EM physician, 1 CCRN, 1 PA/IDC, 1 HM, 1 CRNA, 1 Surgical tech
	Fleet surgical team (FST)		Capacity based on type of CRTS augmenting	DCR, DCS, ERC, and AMAL maintain by ship personnel	1 General surgeon, 1 CCRN, 1 CRNA, 2 Surgical techs, 1 ORRN, 1 IM physician, 1 psychiatrist, 1 BHT, 1 OIC MD, 1 MRCO, 1 SEL(CPO), 1 RT, 1 Lab Tech, 1 Rad Tech, 2 HM
	Expeditionary medical unit (EMU)		2 ORs, 4 ICU beds, 6 ward beds	DCR, DCS, component blood products (60 units)	30–120 personnel depending on size of Role 2/mission capability requirements
	USMC surgical platoon		Up to 50 casualties and 10–18 surgeries in 48 h without re-supply	DCR, DCS, ERC. Blood products are variable depending on mission. FRSS+STP w/80 units of plasma and blood cells (~40 each)	Comprised of FRSS/STP: 2 Surgeons (general/ortho), 1 Anesthesiologist, 2 EM physicians, 3 PA/ICD, 1 CCRN, 2 EM RNs, 13 HMs, 2 Surgical techs

Role 3	Hospital ship (T-AH)	12 ORs, 100 ICU beds, 1,000 ward beds[c]	DCR, DCS, prolonged patient care, advanced imaging, specialist care, component blood products (5,000 units)	1,214 personnel when fully staffed
	Expeditionary medical facility (EMF)	4 ORs, 20 ICU beds, 130 or 30 ward beds	DCR, DCS, prolonged patient care, advanced imaging, specialist care, blood products (300 PRBC, 192 FFP)	150-bed EMF includes 454 personnel when fully staffed
	Forward hospital	Full shore-based medical facility		
Role 4	Military treatment facility	Full shore-based medical facility (NMCSD, NMCP, WRNMMC, LRMC)		

[a] Only LSD embarks with physicians
[b] Only Role 2 DCS with FST or other surgical team embarked
[c] Dependent on nurse staffing. Approximately ½ of ward beds are "top bunk" minimal-care, walking-wounded beds

company, have access to laparoscopic and endoscopic equipment, and have the ability to sterilize surgical equipment. Current CVN medical capabilities remain mostly unchanged from those in service after WWII with the exception of more modern endoscopy and laparoscopic capabilities. Fleet Surgical Teams (FST), can only embark on amphibious ships, specifically LHAs, LHDs, and LPDs (Table 2.1); however, they only become part of the ship's medical department leading up to a deployment. In contrast to the ERSS, all FST surgical equipment and consumables are already on board the amphibious warship and are managed by the ship's medical department. The large deck amphibious warships (LHA, LHD) that FSTs augment are known as Casualty Receiving and Treatment Ships (CRTS) and can be augmented with up to 84 more caregivers to increase operative and patient-holding capability. These teams include additional general, orthopedic, and oral-maxillofacial surgeons as well as the support staff to run more operating rooms simultaneously [77]. The LHD and LHA represent the evolution of the medically augmented LSTs utilized to transport troops, vehicles, and supplies for amphibious operations in both the European and Pacific theatres of operation during WWII.

Blood product availability varies widely in Role 2 capable ships (Table 2.2). CRTS have varying amounts of frozen blood products though these products are not immediately available due to thawing and are susceptible to loss during preparation. For

Table 2.2 Blood product availability on U.S. Navy ships

Ship class	Blood products
Aircraft carrier (CVN)	– Walking blood bank program – 5 units whole blood
Landing helicopter dock (LHD)	– 400 PRBC – 40 FFP
Landing helicopter assault (LHA)	– 400 PRBC – 40 FFP
Landing platform dock (LPD)	– 45 PRBC – 10 FFP
Expeditionary fast transport (EFP) flight II	Capability not yet defined

emergencies and mass casualty events, each CRTS has a walking blood bank capability. CVNs recently began storing whole blood onboard the ship; however, this capability is minimal, and the walking blood bank program is still the primary source of fresh whole blood for resuscitation during mass casualty events [75].

The USMC utilizes a modular and scalable model to provide, land-based Role 2 forward resuscitative care near the point of injury by incorporating an STP and FRSS into a Surgical Platoon capable of performing damage control resuscitation and surgery, prolonged patient care, and en route care (ERC). Like the ERSS, the USMC FRSS/STP brings their own equipment with them wherever they go. However, the footprint, weight and cube, capability, and patient capacity are significantly larger than the ERSS [68]. The U.S. Navy also has a Role 2 Expeditionary Medical Unit (EMU) that is task organized to provide a more robust Role 2 capability than ERSS, FST, and CVN surgical teams. The EMU resembles the USMC FRSS/STP when supporting ground combat operations but can also embark on the new variant of catamaran-hulled Expeditionary Fast Transport (EPF) ships [78]. The Flight II EPF, first delivered in January 2024, provides high-speed, shallow-draft patient transport and stabilization capabilities afloat. Further modifications to this ship to improve surgical capabilities and capacity will be included in the Bethesda-class configuration known as the Expeditionary Medical Ship (EMS) scheduled to be delivered in 2026 [79].

Further stabilization, advanced imaging, and specialty care occur at Role 3 facilities which can be either land-based (EMF) or sea-based (hospital ships). EMFs are deployable, in-theater hospitals with the ability to be fully constructed and operational within 10 days once all equipment and personnel are in the theater [80]. The U.S. Navy currently has two hospital ships, USNS *Mercy* and USNS *Comfort*, which boast capabilities similar to land-based treatment facilities and can be forward deployed in support of combat or humanitarian missions. Stabilized patients are transported to either a Military Treatment Facilities (MTF) stateside or Landstuhl Regional Medical Center (LRMC), the only Role 4 treatment facility outside of the United States. While each of the naval capabilities described in this chapter has specific required operational capabilities designed for projected operational environments, ultimately each is modular and scalable such that, when mobilized, they can adapt to provide world-class health care to Sailors, Soldiers, Marines, and Airmen deployed in any expeditionary environment during crisis and contingency operations on land and sea.

Guided-missile Destroyer (DDG), Guided-missile Cruiser (CG), Landing Ship Dock (LSD), Landing Helicopter Dock (LHD), Landing Helicopter Assault (LHA), Landing Craft Control (LCC), Landing Platform Dock (LPD), Tactical Combat Casualty Care (TCCC), Independent Duty Corpsman (IDC), Damage Control Resuscitation (DCR), Damage Control Surgery (DCS), operating room (OR), intensive care unit (ICU), walking blood bank (WBB), Critical care nurse (CCRN), nurse anesthetist (CRNA), oral and maxillofacial surgery (OMFS), physician assistant (PA), corpsman (HM), authorized medical allowance list (AMAL), en-route care (ERC), internal medicine (IM), emergency medicine (EM), behavioral health technician (BHT), officer in charge (OIC), physician (MD/DO), senior enlisted leader (SEL), chief petty officer (CPO), medical regulating control officer (MRCO), perioperative nurse (ORRN), respiratory therapist (RT), forward resuscitative surgical system (FRSS), shock trauma platoon (STP), packed red blood cells (PRBC), fresh frozen plasma (FFP), Naval Medical Center San Diego (NMCSD), Naval Medical Center Portsmouth (NMCP), Walter Reed National Military Medical Center (WRNMMC), Landstuhl Regional Medical Center (LRMC), United States Marine Corps (USMC).

Disclaimer The opinions and assertions expressed herein are those of the author(s) and do not reflect the official policy or position of the United States Army, Air Force, Navy, Uniformed Services University of the Health Sciences, or the Department of Defense.
This research was supported (in whole or in part) by HCA Healthcare and/or an HCA Healthcare affiliated entity. The views expressed in this publication represent those of the author(s) and do not necessarily represent the official views of HCA Healthcare or any of its affiliated entities.

References

1. Burris DG, Dougherty PJ, Elliot DC, et al. Emergency war surgery. 3rd revision. Department of Defense; 2004.
2. Bricknell MCM. Observations from the Korean War for modern military medicine. Uisahak. 2023;32(3):787–828. https://doi.org/10.13081/kjmh.2023.32.78.
3. U.S. Army Medical Center of Excellence. About us. https://medcoe.army.mil/about-us. Accessed 10 Dec 2024.
4. Lieber F. Instructions for the Government of Armies of the United States in the Field. General Orders No. 100. Washington, DC: War Department. April 24, 1863
5. Army Medical Department. Development guide for the medical corps. https://web.archive.org/web/20060815094112/http://www.cs.amedd.army.mil/medicalcorps/developmentguide.pdf2. Accessed 15 Aug 2006.
6. Army Medical Department. About AMEDD history. https://achh.army.mil/regiment/about-ameddhistory. Accessed 2 Aug 2024.
7. Bowlby A, Wallace C. The development of British surgery at the front. Br Med J. 1917;1(2944):705–21. https://doi.org/10.1136/bmj.1.2944.705. PMID: 20768605; PMCID: PMC2348578
8. Ogilvie WH. Abdominal wounds in the Western Desert. Bull U S Army Med Dep. 1946;6(4):435–45. PMID: 20275008
9. Sharpe JP, Magnotti LJ, Fabian TC, Croce MA. Evolution of the operative management of colon trauma. Trauma Surg Acute Care Open. 2017;2(1):e000092. https://doi.org/10.1136/tsaco-2017-000092. PMID: 29766094; PMCID: PMC5877907
10. National Library of Medicine. Dr. Joseph Lovell. https://cfmedicine.nlm.nih.gov/physicians/biography_72.html. Accessed 2 Aug 2024.
11. Baylor College of Medicine. Legacy of excellence. https://www.bcm.edu/about-us/our-campus/debakey-museum/legacy-of-excellence. Accessed 2 Aug 2024.
12. Churchill ED. In: Cannon JW, Elster EA, editors. Surgeon to soldiers: diary and records of the surgical consultant, allied force headquarters, World War II. 2024th ed. Wolters Kluwer Health; 2024.
13. Emergency War Surgery. 5th ed. Office of the Surgeon General, U.S. Army; 2018.
14. American College of Surgeons. Colonel Norman M. Rich, MD, FACS, receives inaugural distinguished military lifetime achievement award. https://www.facs.org/for-medical-professionals/news-publications/news-and-articles/bulletin/2019/11/colonel-norman-m-rich-md-facs-receives-inaugural-distinguished-military-lifetime-achievement-award/. Accessed 2 Aug 2024.

15. Lanoue G. Telemedicine: a lifeline for troops. In: Frontline: the heart of the matter. PBS; 1996. https://www.pbs.org/wgbh/pages/frontline/shows/heart/readings/telemedicine.html. Accessed 21 Nov 2024.
16. Zoroya G. A navy doctor Goes on call in hell. NPR March 7, 2007. https://www.npr.org/2007/03/07/7754799/a-navy-doctor-goes-on-call-in-hell. Accessed 2 Aug 2024.
17. Holcomb JB. The warrior's combat surgeon: col (ret) John B. Holcomb. J Trauma. 2009;66(4 Suppl) https://journals.lww.com/jtrauma/citation/2009/04001/the_warrior_s_combat_surgeon__col__ret___john_b_.2.aspx. Accessed 2 Aug 2024
18. Emergency War Surgery. The survivalist's medical desk reference. 5th ed. U.S. Department of the Army; 2019.
19. U.S. Army. Tactical combat casualty care handbook. https://api.army.mil/e2/c/downloads/2023/01/19/31e03488/17-13-tactical-casualty-combat-care-handbook-v5-may-17-distro-a.pdf. Accessed 25 Aug 2024.
20. Creation of the Air Force Medical Service. Air force medical service. https://www.airforcemedicine.af.mil/AFMSHeritage/#:~:text=The%20effective%20date%20of%20the,a%20part%20of%20the%20AFMS. Accessed 12 Aug 2024.
21. Romero M. Celebrating 75 years of the air force medical service. Air force medical service. Published July 1, 2024. https://www.airforce medicine.af.mil/News/Display/Article/3818522/celebrating-75-years-of-the-air-force-medical-service/. Accessed 11 Aug 2024.
22. Nanney JS. The U.S. army air forces in world war ii: army air forces medical services in world war II. Air force history and museums program. Published 1998. https://media.defense.gov/2010/Sep/23/2001330103/-1/-1/0/AFD-100923-014.pdf. Accessed 13 Aug 2024.
23. Nanney JS, Frechette JR. The air force medical service 1949–2024: a commemorative history. Published 2024. https://www.airforcemedicine.af.mil/Portals/1/Documents/AFMS-75th-Anniversary/The-Air-Force-Medical-Service-1949-2024-A-Commemorative-History.pdf. Accessed 6 Sept 2024.
24. Holstein P. Air force medicine in the Korean War. Air force medical service. Published December 18, 2017. https://www.airforce medicine.af.mil/News/Display/Article/1399024/air-force-medicine-in-the-korean-war/. Accessed 11 Aug 2024.
25. Baker MS. Military medical advances resulting from the conflict in Korea, part 1: systems advances that enhanced patient survival. Mil Med. 2012;177(4):423–9. https://doi.org/10.7205/MILMED-D-11-00311.
26. The blood, plasma, and related programs in the Korean War. AMEDD Center of History and Heritage. https://achh.army.mil/history/book-korea-blood-chapter20. Accessed 12 Aug 2024.
27. Holstein P. Air force medicine during the Vietnam War. Air Force Medical Service. Published January 25, 2018. https://www.airforcemedicine.af.

mil/News/Display/Article/1421624/air-force-medicine-during-the-vietnam-war/. Accessed 12 Aug 2024.
28. C9A/C Nightingale. Air mobility command museum. https://amcmuseum.org/at-the-museum/aircraft/c-9ac-nightingale/. Accessed 13 Aug 2024.
29. AFMS Operations During the Gulf War: Operations Desert Shield, Desert Storm. Air Force Medical Service. Published January 21, 2021. https://www.airforcemedicine.af.mil/News/Article/645788/afms-operations-during-the-gulf-war-operations-desert-shield-desert-storm/. Accessed 11 Aug 2024.
30. Taylor J. This month in AFMS history: medical red flag begins. Air Force Medical Service. Published November 18, 2016. https://www.airforcemedicine.af.mil/News/Article/1008715/this-month-in-afms-history-medical-red-flag-begins/. Accessed 6 Sept 2024.
31. Hymel KM. The air force medical service in the persian gulf war and the need for critical care. Joint Base San Antonio. Published January 20, 2021. https://www.jbsa.mil/News/News/Article/2476780/the-air-force-medical-service-in-the-persian-gulf-war-and-the-need-for-critical/. Accessed 11 Aug 2024.
32. AFMS Capability: Critical Care Air Transport Team. Air Force Medical Service. https://www.airforcemedicine.af.mil/Platforms/AFMS-Capability-Critical-Care-Air-Transport-Team/. Accessed 12 Aug 2024.
33. Morgan J. Understanding ground surgical teams. Air Force Medical Service. Published April 19, 2022. https://www.airforcemedicine.af.mil/News/Display/Article/3003277/understanding-ground-surgical-teams/. Accessed 11 Aug 2024.
34. Edmonds R, Hansen D. Aligning air force ground surgical team (GST) training with deployment exercises. Mil Med. 2022;188(5–6):997–1002. https://doi.org/10.1093/milmed/usac043.
35. Cubano MA, Butler F, Cap AP, et al., editors. Emergency war surgery. 5th revision. Fort Sam Housten, TX: Office of the Surgeon General; 2018.
36. Bagg MR, Covey DC, Powell ET 4th. Levels of medical care in the global war on terrorism. Am Acad Orthop Surg. 2006;14(10 Spec No):S7–9. https://doi.org/10.5435/00124635-200600001-00003.
37. Ground Surgical Team (GST). Air force tactics, techniques, and procedures 3–42.77. Published November 16, 2018. https://static.e-publishing.af.mil/production/1/af_sg/publication/afttp3-42.77/afttp3-42.77.pdf. Accessed 13 Aug 2024.
38. Battlefield Surgery: Special Operations Surgical Team. Air Force Special Tactics (24 SOW). https://www.airforcespecialtactics.af.mil/About/Mission/Battlefield-Surgery/. Accessed 12 Aug 2024.
39. Davis BJ III. Special operations: air force surgical teams are on the frontline of trauma care. Airman Magazine. Published February 15, 2019.

https://www.airmanmagazine.af.mil/Features/Display/Article/2599045/special-operations/. Accessed 12 Aug 2024.
40. United States Air Force Special Operations Surgical Teams. Air Force Recruiting Service. https://www.recruiting.af.mil/Portals/78/HP%2021-002%20Spec%20Ops%20Surgical%20Team%20Digital.pd. Accessed 12 Aug 2024.
41. Holstein P. Air force ramps up flying ICU teams. Air Force Medical Service. Published April 30, 2018. https://www.airforcemedicine.af.mil/News/Display/Article/1506500/air-force-ramps-up-flying-icu-teams/. Accessed 11 Aug 2024.
42. Carnell J. Aeromedical evacuation knows no bounds. Air Force Medical Service. Published December 27, 2019. https://www.airforce medicine.af.mil/News/Display/Article/2047116/aeromedical-evacuation-knows-no-bounds/. Accessed 14 Aug 2024.
43. Report to the Committees on Armed Services of the Senate and House of Representatives. Reports on composition of medical personnel of each military department and related matters. Published December 2023. https://health.mil/Reference-Center/Reports/2023/12/05/Composition-of-Medical-Personnel. Accessed 11 Aug 2024.
44. Air Force Medical Service. https://www.airforcemedicine. af.mil/Organizations/. Accessed 13 Aug 2024.
45. Military Demographics. https://www.afpc.af.mil/Portals/70/documents/DEMOGRAPHICS/MIL%20DEMOGRAPHICS.pdf?ver=Q-ejTBrAR4E4rbh6vailpA%3D%3D. Accessed 13 Aug 2024.
46. Bedi S. Air force medicine maintains medical mission supporting space force. Air Force Medical Service. Published March 3, 2021. https://www.airforcemedicine.af.mil/News/Display/Article/2523313/air-force-maintains-medical-mission-supporting-space-force/. Accessed 11 Sept 2024.
47. Paine LP. The sea and civilization: a maritime history of the world. 1st ed. New York, NY: Alfred A. Knopf; 2013.
48. Koutserimpas C, Samonis G. Machaon: the first trauma surgeon in Western history? J Wound Care. 2018;27(10):659–61. https://doi.org/10.12968/jowc.2018.27.10.659. PMID: 30332356
49. Robinson JO. The barber-surgeons of London. Arch Surg. 1984;119(10):1171–5. https://doi.org/10.1001/archsurg.1984.01390220053012. PMID: 6383267
50. Goethe H, Watson EN, Jones DT. Handbook of nautical medicine. Berlin: Springer; 1984.
51. Taylor JS. Military and naval medicine med in Roman and medieval times. Mil Surg. 1917;40:589–94.
52. Watt J. Some forgotten contributions of naval surgeons. J R Soc Med. 1985;78:753–62.
53. Watt J. The injuries of four centuries of naval warfare. Ann R Coll Surg Engl. 1975;57(1):3–24.

54. Gordon MB. Naval and maritime medicine during the American revolution. Ventnor: Ventnor Publishers; 1978.
55. Sobocinski AB. The formative years of the U.S. Navy Medicine Corps, 1798–1871. Naval History and Heritage Command. 2024.
56. Adams WT. Red rover: first hospital ship of the U.S. Navy Proc. 1968;94(11):789.
57. Mann WL. Medical tactics in naval warfare. Washington government printing office; 1926. p. 34–7.
58. Falciola V, Waisel DB. Surgical and anesthetic challenges aboard non-hospital ships in the Pacific during world war II. J Anesth Hist. 2018;4(4):214–21. https://doi.org/10.1016/j.janh.2018.07.007. Epub 2018 Aug 1. PMID: 30558764
59. McLaughlin CW. The treatment of major burns in naval warfare. Nebr State Med J. 1945;31:11–9.
60. Riske M. A history of hospital ships. Naval History and Heritage Command. Published August 23, 2017. Accessed 3 Sept 2024.
61. Lane DA. Hospital ship doctrine in the United States navy: the Halsey effect on scoop- and-sail tactics. Mil Med. 1997;162(6):388–95. PMID: 9183159
62. Tadlock MD, Hernandez AA, Miller BT. The ship's surgeon and surgery at sea: a brief history. In: Tadlock MD, Hernandez AA, editors. Expeditionary surgery at sea: a practical approach. Springer Nature; 2023.
63. Cressman RJ. Consolation (AH-15). Naval History and Heritage Command. Published April 6, 2020. Accessed 3 Oct 2024.
64. Hernandez A, Sobocinski A, Tadlock M. Anchors aweigh! The history of women surgeons at sea. J Am Coll Surg. 2024;238(5):814–20. https://doi.org/10.1097/XCS.0000000000001038.
65. Cubano MA, Luther JH, Antosek LE. First laparoscopic hernia repair onboard an aircraft carrier at sea. Mil Med. 1997;162(3):219–20. PMID: 9121672
66. Gregory JP. Sailors in olive drab. Naval History; 2023.
67. Bilski TR, Baker BC, Grove JR, Hinks RP, Harrison MJ, Sabra JP, Temerlin SM, Rhee P. Battlefield casualties treated at Camp Rhino, Afghanistan: lessons learned. J Trauma. 2003;54(5):814–21. https://doi.org/10.1097/01.TA.0000046627.87250.1D. PMID: 12777893
68. Bohman HR, Baker BC, Stevens RA. Professional note: forward resuscitative surgery in operation Iraqi freedom. Proceedings. 2004;130(2):1212.
69. Stevens RA, Bohman HR, Baker BC, Chambers LW. The U.S. Navy's forward resuscitative surgery system during operation Iraqi freedom. Mil Med. 2005;170(4):297–301. https://doi.org/10.7205/milmed.170.4.297. PMID: 15916298
70. Chambers LW, Green DJ, Gillingham BL, Sample K, Rhee P, Brown C, Brethauer S, Nelson T, Narine N, Baker B, Bohman HR. The experience of the US marine corps' surgical shock trauma platoon with 417 operative

combat casualties during a 12-month period of operation Iraqi freedom. J Trauma. 2006;60(6):1155–61; discussion 1161–4. PMID: 16766956. https://doi.org/10.1097/01.ta.0000220340.91356.7e.
71. Sallee DR, Love JW, Welling LE. The United States marine corps shock trauma platoon: the modern battlefield's emergency room. Prehosp Emerg Care. 2008;12(1):80–6. https://doi.org/10.1080/10903120701707997. PMID: 18189183
72. Sobocinski AB. Eleven years in Kandahar: the life and legacy of the NATO role III multinational medical unit, 2009–2020. Navy Medicine; 2020.
73. Adams KL. First robot-assisted surgery onboard USNS mercy: multinational surgeons. US 7th Fleet; 2018.
74. Roles of Care. Emergency war surgery. 5th ed. Borden Institute. p. 19–22.
75. Lowry DM, Johnston MG, Van Gent J, Tadlock MD, Edson TD. Overview of current maritime surgical platforms and operations environments: part 1—United States navy and marine corps. In: Tadlock MD, Hernandez AA, editors. Expeditionary surgery at sea: A practical approach. Springer Nature; 2023.
76. Required operational capabilities and projected operational environment for the role 2 light maneuver expeditionary resuscitative surgical system. OPNAV Instruction 3501.408. 2021.
77. Fontana G. NMFP augments casualty receiving treatment ship, enhances capabilities. U.S. Navy; 2023.
78. Naval operational medicine capabilities handbook. Department of the Navy Bureau of Medicine and Surgery. 2023.
79. SECNAV names navy's first-in-class expeditionary medical ship after National Naval Medical Center Bethesda. Navy Press Release. 2023.
80. Required operational capabilities and projected operational environment for the role 3 navy expeditionary medical facility. OPNAV Instruction 3501.176D. 2016.

3 The Evolution of Small Surgical Teams and Austere Resuscitative Surgical Care (ARSC) in the US Military

Paul B. Allen Sr., Mark Ervin,
Linda C. Benavides, Theodore D. Edson,
and Matthew D. Tadlock

Introduction

The history of surgery in austere settings by the US military dates back to the Revolutionary War [1]. The early days of battlefield surgery by the US military were rudimentary and fraught with poor outcomes and severe complications [2]. Morbidity and mortality rates were high due to a nascent knowledge of disease, human anatomy, and physiology, and the lack of available or effective treatments for those wounded in combat. In its early development, land-based battlefield surgery was located near the frontline but was moved to a geographic area where surgeons and medical personnel could safely sort and treat the wounded [2].

P. B. Allen Sr.
Department of Physician Assistant Studies, University of Texas Health Sciences Center, San Antonio, TX, USA

Oak Ridge Institute of Science and Education, Oak Ridge Associated University, Oak Ridge, TN, USA

M. Ervin
Oak Ridge Institute of Science and Education, Oak Ridge Associated University, Oak Ridge, TN, USA

A. T. Schlussel et al. (eds.), *The SAGES Manual for Navigating a Successful Military Surgical Career*,
https://doi.org/10.1007/978-3-031-88490-0_3

Within the naval forces, close ship-to-ship engagement, especially during boarding operations, meant that shipboard medical personnel were performing their craft at the point of injury (POI).

As our nation expanded, so too did the armed forces. Over 250 years, the US military transformed from a largely volunteer militia designed to protect the nation's borders into a modern expeditionary fighting force capable of deploying around the globe in support of the nation's objectives. By the end of the nineteenth century and the beginning of the twentieth century, the practice of medicine grew exponentially, and modern medical techniques were discovered and developed worldwide; the surgical care of combat wounded followed suit [3–5]. As the United States became involved in the first truly large-scale wars since the Civil War, forward surgical care rapidly advanced to meet the needs of globally deployed forces engaged in increasingly lethal kinetic activity [2]. To effect greater survival of combat casualties and decrease the morbidity associated with the weapons of modern warfare during World War I (WWI), World War II (WWII), the Korean War, and the Vietnam War, advances in technology, epidemiology, medical research, and experience with combat casualty care drove efforts to bring surgical intervention closer to the POI.

At the turn of the twenty-first century, the United States returned to expeditionary warfare on a relatively smaller scale,

L. C. Benavides
Committee on Surgical Combat Casualty Care,
DoD Center of Excellence for Trauma,
Joint Base San Antonio-Fort Sam Houston, TX, USA

Department of Surgery, Madigan Army Medical Center,
Joint Base Lewis-McChord, WA, USA

T. D. Edson
Department of Surgery, Naval Medical Center, San Diego, CA, USA

M. D. Tadlock (✉)
Committee on Surgical Combat Casualty Care,
DoD Center of Excellence for Trauma,
Joint Base San Antonio-Fort Sam Houston, TX, USA

Department of Surgery, Naval Medical Center, San Diego, CA, USA

Department of Surgery, Uniformed Services University of the Health Sciences,
Bethesda, MD, USA

finding itself evolved into the sustained counter-insurgency operations (COIN) that characterized the wars in Iraq, Afghanistan, and Syria during the Global War on Terror (GWOT). To meet the needs of an increasingly kinetic, geographically disparate battlefield, military medicine rapidly met the challenge (e.g., en route care, whole blood resuscitation, and Role 2 forward resuscitative care) to provide both far-forward surgical care and combat casualty care on a global scale. To save the lives of US and partner nation service members injured far from home, systems of care, technologies, and methods to effectively treat surgical combat casualties were developed, trialed, and depolyed [2].

While there are numerous examples of smaller surgical teams that are utilized by the US military and US Special Operations Command (USSOCOM) outside of doctrinal formations, this is not the focus of this chapter. Rather, this chapter will briefly summarize the evolution of forward surgical care in the conventional armed forces, from traditional field hospitals, with large footprints, providing treatment and convalescence for surgical casualties in safe areas near combat operations [6], to increasingly more mobile, though less capable, surgical hospital configurations in the Army, Navy, and Air Force [7], and ultimately to the modern concept of Austere Resuscitative Surgical Care (ARSC) designed to bring damage control resuscitation and surgery closer to POI [2]. We will also attempt to describe the challenges of meeting the requirements of far-forward ARSC teams in current conflicts and the anticipated challenges associated with future Large Scale Combat Operations (LSCO).

What Is Austere Resuscitative Surgical Care?

Prior to discussing the evolution of ARSC teams across the Services, the modern concept of ARSC and its evolution should be discussed first. ARSC capabilities fall within the spectrum of Forward Resuscitative Care, also known as Role 2 medical care. As defined by the most current version (2023) of Joint Publication 4–02, Joint Health Service Support (JP 4–02), "Role 2 medical personnel provide trauma management and emergency medical treatment, including continuation of resuscitation started in Role 1. Role 2 provides a greater capability to resuscitate patients than is available at Role 1 and may include damage-control surgery when augmented with a surgical capability" [8]. This definition has evolved over time as the doctrine has evolved and been updated. Within the spectrum of Role 2 care, previous versions of JP 4–02 also defined Role 2 Enhanced (R2E) as "basic secondary health care, built around primary surgery," including ward and intensive care beds; Role 2 Light Maneuver (R2LM) is defined as light and highly mobile medical unit "able to conduct advanced resuscitation procedures up to damage control surgery" that can set up as its own military treatment facility, in a "fixed building" of opportunity, or on a "naval platform" [8]. However, early on in GWOT, the 2006 edition of JP 4–02 did not formally refer to roles of care, but only forward resuscitative care and in-theater hospitalization equivalent to Role 2 and Role 3 care, respectively. To meet increasing demand to support COIN and the 2009 "Golden Hour" mandate during GWOT [9], the Services began developing smaller and smaller surgical teams in terms of both personnel, often single surgeon teams, and overall weight and cube of medical materials [10, 11]. However, the use of these teams was always predicated on robust and timely patient transport through the echelons of care—maintaining surgical team capability despite the risk of limited capacity. US military health service support (HSS) doctrine soon followed when the 2012 update of JP 4–02 formally adopted and defined the terms Role 1, Role 2, R2LM, Role 3, and Role 4. Despite the fact that JP 4–02 differentiated between R2E and R2LM at the time, the increasingly limited capability and capacity provided by small, single-surgeon teams were not defined [11]. As GWOT theaters of operation matured, conventional Role 2 capabilities became less mobile and stationary at forward operating bases and relied on a robust and responsive system of casualty movement after damage control resuscitation and surgery. Recognizing this, the Joint Trauma System (JTS) further refined the definition of small highly mobile teams as ARSC—an "advanced medical capability delivered by small teams with limited resources, often beyond traditional timelines of care, and bridges gaps in roles of care in order to enable forward military operations and mitigate risk to the force" [12].

US Army Experience

The Army Medical Department traces its lineage to its establishment by the Continental Congress in 1775 [1, 13]. As the United States was originally a colony of the British Empire, the practices of medicine and field medicine were largely influenced by their example, as many early colonial medical leaders had studied in England [1, 14]. It is important to note that at this time in history, the practice of medicine was distinct from surgery in that physicians were expected to treat hospitalized patients, whereas regimental surgeons were expected to treat soldiers in regimental hospitals who were sick or wounded in combat [2]. Furthermore, education requirements were higher for physicians, and most surgeons learned their trade through apprenticeships and often did not have a formal medical education [2]. As such, pay scales reflected a large difference in compensation between physicians and surgeons [13]. The state of medical care in the colonies was rudimentary at best, and the domain of combat surgical intervention was largely limited to amputations, trephination, and the treatment of the expected infectious complications that would inevitably follow [14]. Surgical disease was often treated medically due to both a rudimentary knowledge of pathophysiology, lack of anesthesia, and the associated morbidity of postoperative infectious complications in this pre-Listerian era. However, some advances were made as medicine moved away from the dogma of unproven medical theories, and practical lessons were learned by forward-deployed caregivers on the battlefield [15].

The practice of evacuating the wounded from regimental hospitals to larger hospitals was the norm, although this practice may have contributed to overall mortality due to the crowding that inevitably ensued [14]. In these early days, mobile "flying hospitals" were implemented to support forward military operations, and the larger general hospitals were located in safer locations [13, 15]. Although records are lacking for the number of casualties within militia formations, there have been estimates of roughly 7000 deaths attributed to combat, but almost twice as many additional deaths from nonbattle injury (DNBI) [2].

During the first half of the nineteenth century, the state of surgical care in the US Army saw little change through the War of 1812, the Mexican–American War, and the various "wars of westward expansion." DNBI still accounted for most of the morbidity and mortality during these conflicts, and the common practice in treating surgical casualties remained the transportation of those who survived their initial combat wounds to clearing stations and hospitals far from the area of combat. Casualties were collected either temporarily in tents or in fixed structures of opportunity behind the linear battle front [2]. However, major advances in the treatment of combat trauma did occur during the Napoleonic Wars. Considered the father of modern combat casualty care, French Surgeon Baron Dominique-Jean Larrey, developed and implemented many of the modern concepts that remain in practice today such as triage, POI care comprised of his "flying ambulances" with prototypical emergency medical technicians, and decreasing the time to a surgeon by placing surgical capabilities close to the front lines [16, 17]. Despite Larrey's advances in the late 1700s and early 1800s, these concepts were not widely disseminated or adopted in Western medicine.

Almost half a century after Larrey first developed the principles of triage, POI care, and forward surgical care, they were proven to be effective during the Crimean War (1853–1856), where rapid evacuation and close surgical support demonstrated significant improvements in battlefield morbidity and mortality [16]. Another advancement of the Crimean War was the use of chloroform during operations, allowing surgeons to work more deliberately. Very little regarding the movement of surgical care close to the POI had changed in the US Army during this timeframe, although techniques were improving. The US Army found itself vastly unprepared for what was to come during the Civil War, where techniques and outcomes saw only minimal improvement in combat casualty care. Although some medical and surgical advances occurred sporadically with the end result of decreasing morbidity and mortality as the war progressed [2].

The postwar period between the Civil War and WWI saw a revolution in medical care worldwide, beginning with Lister's work on antisepsis in 1867 [3]. While the influence of Larrey began to take hold in other nations [17], they were not incorporated within the US Army as the United States was involved in small-scale wars and conflicts. For example, during the incursion into Mexico in the early 1900s, the US Army was organized into a regimental system, and the only forward surgical capability was located in "dressing stations" designed to prepare wounded soldiers for evacuation to more definitive care in larger hospitals [2]. As this revolution in medicine and technology was taking place, medical support within the US Army began to accelerate and evolve significantly prior to WWI.

Prior to the US government's formal declaration of war, the experiences of American civilian surgical teams in WWI influenced the provision of forward surgical care in US military doctrine. Driven primarily by civilian volunteers and philanthropic efforts, civilian medical and surgical teams sponsored by major US academic medical institutions traveled to Europe to provide additional medical capabilities [2]. Surgical leaders such as Cushing and Crile were exposed to French mobile surgical hospitals and mobile surgical units (group complementaires), as well as British mobile surgical capabilities, during the war. Although attempts were made to move surgery closer to the POI, there was much disagreement regarding where best to place surgical assets: in safe areas or closer to the POI [2]. Over time, surgical hospitals on all sides tended to become large and static, located near points of embarkation for further evacuation to rear areas away from combat despite the original intent for mobility [2].

During WWII, the US Army recognized the need to provide smaller, more highly mobile surgical assets, although these facilities differed significantly between the European Theater of Operations (ETO) and the Pacific, China, Burma, India (PCBI) area of operations. In the ETO, surgical assets tended to be located in larger hospitals in rear areas [2]. Due to significant geographic challenges and thick jungle terrain or amphibious operations, it was recognized that a smaller, more mobile capability was needed in the PCBI [2]. Army doctrine and field manuals at the time began to change to meet this need for flexibility and by the end of the war, Field Manual 8–5, *Mobile Units of the Army Medical Department*, reflected the flexibility of one mobile surgical unit to be available for this purpose using a portable surgical hospital which could be placed less than one mile from the front lines, an area deemed safe yet close enough to provide effective care [2]. After action reviews at the time showed that once a mobile surgical unit was set up, they tended to become static [2]. This phenomenon was noted in subsequent wars, including GWOT. A notable development during WWII was the development of a forward surgical team delivered via parachute by British forces in North Africa, which was very successful in saving lives [18].

The Korean experience demonstrated a renewed effort to provide a truly mobile surgical hospital, not only in concept but in name. The "Mobile Army Surgical Hospital" or MASH has enjoyed widespread recognition largely due to the Hollywood portrayal. As noted above, despite its name, due to factors surrounding the static evolution of the conflict itself, these facilities became static and more permanent as the war progressed [2]. Another notable development, which somewhat changed the paradigm of proximity, was the use of helicopters to transport the wounded from the POI to surgical care.

The Vietnam War saw a significant increase in the reliance on helicopter medical evacuation, decreasing the time to surgical intervention. Like in previous wars, MASH units, Surgical Hospitals, Evacuation Hospitals, and Field Hospitals during this conflict became fixed and more permanent in nature with increasing medical capabilities as the war progressed. This phenomenon, coupled with expedient rotary evacuation and air superiority, was credited as one of the reasons for a significant reduction in mortality, providing casualties with access to the equivalent of a level one trauma center in theater [2].

Between the Vietnam War and the 1980s, surgical capability was located in Combat Support Hospitals (CSH) and MASH units [18]. However, major world events drove strategic thinking within the Army medical leadership, including the rise of trans-national terrorism and the Cold War great power competition. USSOCOM began to employ small surgical teams in the late 1970s. Medical personnel assigned to those formations or involved in their creation shared lessons learned during the real-world implementation of small surgical team concepts with Army Medical

Department leadership and the Army Surgeon General [19, 20]. The widespread conventional force experience with small surgical teams in the military was born out of the recognized lack of mobile surgical support during the invasion of Grenada in 1983, where surgical care was unavailable until after initial entry operations were complete, and similar lessons were shared by the British from the Falkland Islands campaign [2, 18]. Due to this identified capability gap, the army began developing small, highly mobile forward surgical detachments that could accompany combatants during initial entry operations throughout the 1980s and 1990s as a test and evaluation concept within the 18th Airborne Corps. The first employment of these new, smaller, highly mobile surgical detachments (termed Forward Surgical Teams or FSTs) was during the invasion of Panama in 1989 by the US Army [18]. This unit would later be formed into the first prototype FST, the 274th [2, 18]. These units were employed subsequently during Desert Shield and Desert Storm in the early 1990s [2]. Although highly mobile in the relative sense, these teams were still very large in terms of personnel (20 members) and equipment, requiring significant logistical support to be employed effectively.

By the early 2000s, these small, highly mobile surgical teams were organized across the US Army and subsequently deployed during Operation Enduring Freedom (OEF) and Operation Iraqi Freedom (OIF), supporting multiple different tactical formations across the service components in support of combat operations [2, 18]. Due to the operational constraints and terrain factors experienced in Afghanistan, the practice of splitting small forward surgical teams into even smaller teams, termed "split FSTs," began to occur in the US Army. This practice was employed to provide damage control resuscitation (DCR) and damage control surgery (DCS) to remote geographic areas far from the larger combat support hospitals [21]. In 2009, Secretary of Defense Robert Gates issued a directive to the Services mandating a standardized medical evacuation transport time from call to arrival at military treatment facilities of 60 min or less for US military casualties [22]. This "Golden Hour" mandate had the effect of further increasing the requirement for and reliance on FSTs distributed across the area of combat operations where US military forces were employed, creating overlapping evacuation and surgical team rings along all of Highway 1 in Afghanistan. As a result, the practice of split FSTs became codified in US Army doctrine but splits varied due to odd numbers of personnel on the FSTs (e.g., three general surgeons and one orthopedic surgeon or three medics and one emergency medicine nurse, etc.). Although not part of current US Army doctrine, the ongoing practice of using even smaller nondoctrinal surgical elements has continued to the present day, being employed as troop numbers decreased in Afghanistan to compensate for the no longer overlapping evacuation and surgical team rings. Nondoctrinal teams continue to be used during contingency operations in support of Special Operations Forces (SOF) or Globally Integrated Operations (GIO) across all the Services. Starting in 2018, the Army started the transition from FSTs to Forward Resuscitative Surgical Detachments (FRSDs), allowing for equal splits of ten and further splitting to a six-person surgical team and four-person resuscitative team. Current Army Doctrine codifies FRSDs support requirements, modularity, surgical capabilities, and patient hold expectations for the 20, 10, and 6-person (Fig. 3.1) surgical elements [23].

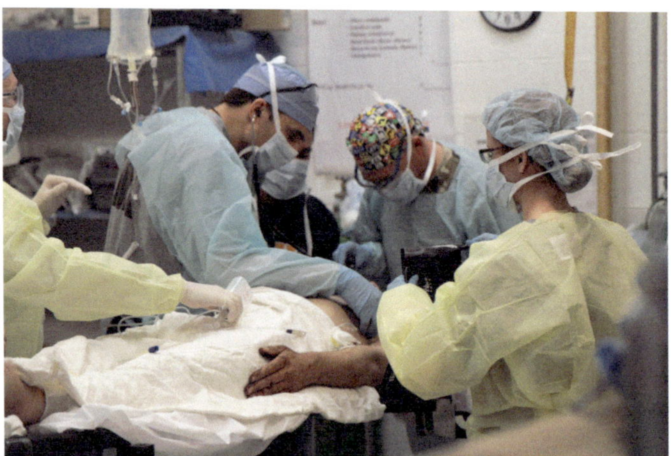

Fig. 3.1 Example of the six-person team in a building of opportunity is mobile but limited to no post-op holding capability. (Source: Photo courtesy of Linda C. Benavides MD)

US Navy and Marine Corps Experience

During the Revolutionary War, embarked on warships, the ship's surgeons and surgeon's mates of the Continental Navy were the first US military members to perform surgery at or near the POI during naval combat. This capability can be directly traced to the British Royal Navy and the navies of Europe during the Age of Sail (approximately 1600–1850) [24]. As warships traded cannon broadsides in the naval battles of the Revolutionary War, crews were at significant risk for injury or death. A direct hit from a cannonball or "wind of ball" near the torso would be instantly fatal. Ship's surgeons typically managed soft tissue wounds ravaged by splinters, shrapnel, or musket balls, treated burn injuries, and set fractures. The ship surgeon's armamentarium for what were often complex extremity wounds near the POI, included tourniquets, knives, and surgical saws to perform amputations. Though trephination was occasionally performed for head injuries, surgery was not performed for injuries of the chest and abdomen beyond attempts to remove shrapnel and other foreign bodies. In the dark and dank cockpit, located below the waterline on the orlop deck (the lowest deck in a ship), surgery was performed without anesthesia in the seated position [24–26]. These early examples of surgery at sea are included in the history of ARSC teams because the surgical teams were small, typically comprised of a single surgeon and two surgeon's mates, had limited surgical and medical supplies, and provided surgical care in harm's way at the POI. The Battle of Farmborough Head is typical of the casualty burden that characterized naval warfare during the Age of Sail. During the battle, the Bonhamme Richard, captained by John Paul Jones—"Father of the U.S. Navy," battled against the HMS Serapis, where 63 (18%) of Jones' crew were killed and 87 (25%) were wounded [26].

By the Civil War, US Navy combatant vessels were increasingly heavily armored with iron, and powered by steam, and surgeons continued to manage traumatic wounds at or near the POI. However, now maritime ARSC surgeons acquired another tool when anesthesia in the form of chloroform became available, further enabling improved forward surgical care at sea [24, 27].

The USS Red Rover, deployed with Union gunboats along the tributaries of the Mississippi during the Civil War in the brown water navy, foreshadowing how blue water naval vessels would provide forward surgical care during WWII. The ship had a formal operating room and wards, bringing surgical capability at or near the line of battle. Considered the first hospital ship in the US Navy, unlike its noncombatant successors, the USS Red Rover was armed with a 32-pounder gun and was fired upon and hit by Confederate forces [24, 28, 29].

By WWI, heavily armored battleships had elaborately equipped and staffed medical departments with formal spaces for an operating room, ward, pharmacy, and x-ray suite. This trend continued with the US Navy capital ships of WWII [24]. Military planners quickly realized that mobile forward surgical resuscitation capabilities were needed to manage the large numbers of anticipated combat casualties during amphibious assaults in both the European and Pacific theaters. To meet this need, Landing Ship Tanks (LST) and Auxiliary Personnel Attack (APA) combatant vessels were augmented with medical personnel and surgical teams. Eventually, some of these LSTs and APAs were converted to deliver surgical care far forward and move patients along a chain of evacuation. While the surgical teams on these ships could manage a significantly larger number of casualties compared to modern ARSC teams, they were often operating in danger secondary to how far forward they were deployed. As the war progressed in the PCBI theater, LSTs filled with casualties were under direct threat of Imperial Japan kamikaze attacks [30].

US Marine Corps (USMC) Medical Battalions made up of US Navy physicians, surgeons, and Corpsmen provided forward surgical care to Marines and Soldiers during the Pacific Island campaigns of WWII. However, further forward were the Battalion Aid Stations (BAS), led by nonsurgeon physicians, deployed to the frontline providing resuscitation and minor damage control surgical procedures near or at the POI subject to the same enemy threats as the marines they supported. Examples of procedures performed include resuscitation with reconstituted freeze-dried plasma, removal of foreign bodies and initial debridement of war wounds, ligation of bleeding extremity vessels, fracture stabilization, temporary closure of open chest wall and perineal wounds after washout, and completion of traumatic amputations [31]. The Korean and Vietnam Wars saw an increase in the deployment of field hospitals to support maneuver warfare in geographically defined areas of operation [10]. Concomitant with the development of ARSC capabilities by the US Army in the 1980s and 1990s [10], similar efforts were made by Navy Medicine personnel assigned to the USMC to enable its unique expeditionary maneuver warfare capabilities. While the contemporary USMC Role 2 comprised of a Shock Trauma Platoon (STP) and Forward Resuscitative Surgical System (FRSS) would not currently be classified as an R2LM or ARSC capability, its employment during the initial invasion of Iraq was an example of ARSC capabilities enabling maneuver warfare to support battalion and regiment sized units as US Marine's "streaked… toward Baghdad in the Corps' largest and most rapid overland combat operation." [32] Pioneered by Navy colorectal surgeon Captain (retired) Harold R. Bohman, the FRSS/STP was designed to perform resuscitative surgical and holding capability with a moderate capacity near the POI, with a minimal footprint, during expeditionary maneuver warfare [32, 33]. During the initial invasion of Iraq from March 21 through April 22, 2003, six FRSS/STP teams managed 338 combat casualties, of which 90 required surgery, with 97% leaving the FRSS alive and all US Marines who were treated in an FRSS surviving to evacuation [34]. These outcomes were dependent on the resupply of consumable and blood products and ongoing rapid throughput and evacuation of casualties to higher echelons of care after DCR/DCS [32, 34].

During the invasion, USMC surgical teams were rapidly mobile as they were trained to set up and receive casualties within an hour and rapidly disassemble and be ready to embark for transport within an hour as the Marines rapidly advanced [32]. Three teams were within 15 kilometers of direct action engagements, and the other three were staged more than 50 kilometers away from combat operations [32]. Over the course of the wars in Iraq and Afghanistan, as the battlespace became more defined and set, USMC Role 2 s were no longer required to support maneuver warfare and, like in previous wars, evolved into stationary surgical capabilities fixed on forward operating bases. While these teams continued to provide life-saving forward surgical care, the increasing size, footprint, capability, and capacity made them no longer rapidly mobile. This maturation of USMC forward surgical capabilities, coupled with the "Golden Hour" mandate, led to a significant decrease in Role 1 USMC BAS capabilities compared to the ARSC care they provided during WWII.

As the Army started developing conventional R2LM and ARSC capabilities to enable forward operations in the era of the "Golden Hour," so did the US Navy. Since approximately 2007, the US Navy experimented with multiple configurations of small conventional R2LM surgical teams to support land-based, shipboard, and from-the-sea operations under different names (e.g., DCS, NATT—Navy Adaptive Trauma Teams, and ERSS—Expeditionary Resuscitative Surgical System) [10, 35]. These efforts eventually coalesced into one ARSC capability—the ERSS—intended to task-organize to provide advanced resuscitative surgical care on land or sea including augmenting Role 1 capable surface (Fig. 3.2) or subsurface vessels. After years of experimentation, in 2021, the ERSS finally became a doctrinal US

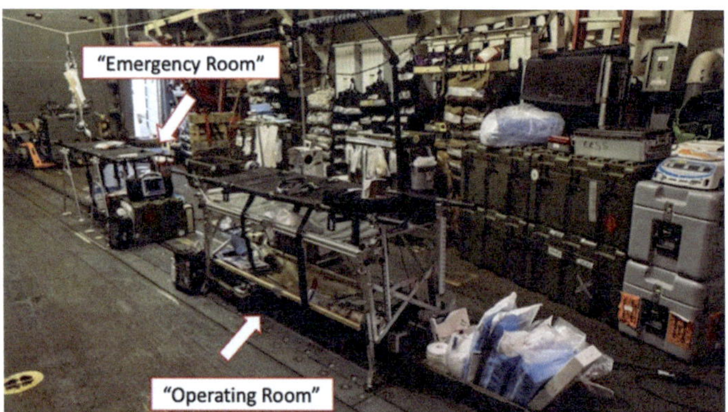

Fig. 3.2 Expeditionary Resuscitative Surgical System (ERSS) resuscitation/postoperative care area adjacent to the Operating Room (OR) area in a Destroyer (DDG) hangar bay, 2020. (Source: Photo courtesy of Matthew D. Tadlock, MD)

Navy capability [36, 37]. ERSS teams have successfully deployed and integrated with land-based units or embarked on a wide variety of US Naval warships to mitigate risk to the operational forces during contingency operations. However, like many other ARSC capabilities, there are no significant outcome data available to assess their effectiveness during current operations or during potential future LSCO [37].

US Air Force Experience

The origin story of the Air Force ARSC capabilities resulted from a perceived gap illustrated during the Beirut bombing in 1983. Air Force General and Trauma surgeon P. K. Carlton, Jr. (who would later rise to the rank of Lieutenant General and serve as the Air Force Surgeon General), based at Wiesbaden Air Base in Germany, was critical of the time interval between injury and trauma surgical care and sought out a new paradigm to accelerate the forward deployment of Air Force surgical capability. In 1984, he is credited with developing a 20-person, deployable surgical capability for US Air Forces—Europe (USAFE) named the Flying Ambulance Surgical Team (giving homage to Larrey's Flying Ambulances) [38]. General Carlton continued over the next decade to champion the development of small, austere surgical units. During his tour as commander of Wilford Hall Medical Center, he enlisted a cadre of innovative surgeons, physicians, nurses, and medics to create a hyper-mobile, lowest-possible footprint surgical capability. Conceptually, the intent was to design a small enough footprint that the surgical team and equipment would be able to be "squeezed" into the unfilled spaces on almost any Air Force cargo plane in the initial airlift salvo supporting any operation [39].

The team's work resulted in a five-person team consisting of a general/trauma surgeon, orthopedic surgeon, anesthesia provider, emergency medicine physician, and operating room (OR) technician. The Mobile Field Surgical Team (MFST) equipment could support up to ten damage control surgical procedures using supplies housed in five man-portable bags with a combined weight of less than 500 lbs. During design, the project team honed the tactics, techniques, procedures, and allowance standards during numerous isolated airfield operations. Ultimately, practiced MFST teams were able to obtain a "ready to receive casualty" status within 15 min of arrival to a shelter of opportunity and were able to repack the kit for movement in under an hour [38, 39]. In 1995, two MFSTs from Wilford Hall were deployed to Oklahoma City in response to the bombing of Murrah Federal Building. Later the same year, the MFST officially came online, and teams were established at multiple Air Force facilities. In what would later prove to be a critical decision, five MFSTs, based at Lackland and Keesler Air Force Bases (AFB), were aligned to primarily support USSOCOM missions [38, 39].

For the designers of the original MFST, it quickly became apparent that far-forward DCR/DCS results in stabilized (but not stable) patients that exceed the clinical capability of Aeromedical Evacuation (AE) crews [39]. As the MFSTs had minimal patient holding capability, the three-person Critical Care Aeromedical Transport Team (CCATT) was developed to augment traditional AE and allow for patient movement of stabilized post-DCR/DCS MFST patients. Over time, it became common to deploy CCATTs alongside MFSTs as an austere ICU/postoperative care team [40, 41]. This arrangement allowed for increased surgical throughput, an extension of holding times from 4 to 24 h, and a forward-deployed critical care team that could augment the first available AE platform air tasked to the casualty. For a brief time, this configuration was trialed as a separate deployment package known as the Small Portable Expeditionary Aeromedical Rapid Response (SPEARR) system and consisted of ten persons (MFST, CCATT, and an AE team), additional medical supplies, and a towable trailer [42].

In the early months of Operation Enduring Freedom (OEF) in 2001, several of the Special Operations Forces (SOF) tasked MFSTs deployed and provided life-saving surgical interventions long before more robust surgical capabilities were able to be established in the theater. The first successful DCS of the war was performed by a Keesler AFB MFST on a casualty suffering severe pelvic trauma who was then evacuated by collocated CCATT to Landstuhl Regional Medical Center (LRMC) for continuing stabilization [43]. As the deployed trauma capabilities expanded during the first years of both OEF and OIF, most of the critical MFST deployments ended, except for support to special operations missions functioning away from robust military bases. The increase in the special operations demand signal led to the Air Force Special Operations Command (AFSOC) taking direct control of five MFSTs (and five CCATTs) to provide direct support for USSOCOM missions. These teams developed habitual training relationships with other SOF forces, increased field skills training, and made modest modifications to the MFST allowance standard to better support SOF forces. Eventually, these teams would be renamed Special Operations Surgical Teams (SOST) and Special Operations Critical Care Evacuation Teams (SOCCET) [43].

During GWOT, casualty outcomes reviews from the JTS noted improved survival rates for injured service members evacuated by a British physician-led evacuation crew known as the Medical Emergency Response Team (MERT). This drove USAF Air Mobility Command (AMC) Surgeon Brigadier General Bart Iddins to direct the development of a new physician-led, three-person evacuation capability for Rotary and short-range fixed-wing evacuation called the Tactical Critical Care Evacuation Team (TCCET). The hallmark of this capability, first deployed in 2012, was to deliver advanced resuscitative care as far forward as the casualty collection point transfer to traditional rotary wing Medical Evacuation (MEDEVAC) platforms [44]. Two years later, AMC developed a two-person surgical augmentation to TCCET referred to as the TCCET-Enhanced (TCCET-E) (Fig. 3.3) to address gaps in surgical care response in theaters such as the Africa Combatant Command (AFRICOM) area of responsibility without a well-developed ground military trauma system. The TCCET-E could respond to the nearest airfield following a casualty-producing event and, as soon as the plane ramp dropped, provide resuscitative care and up to ten DCR/DCS cases on a static or inflight AE C-130 or C-17 using a five-bag allowance standard designed to accommodate the unique aerospace environment [12, 45].

In the last years of OEF, the reduction of ground medical facilities resulted in a greater need for fixed-winged evacuation of unstable and stabilized patients. As a significant subset of the

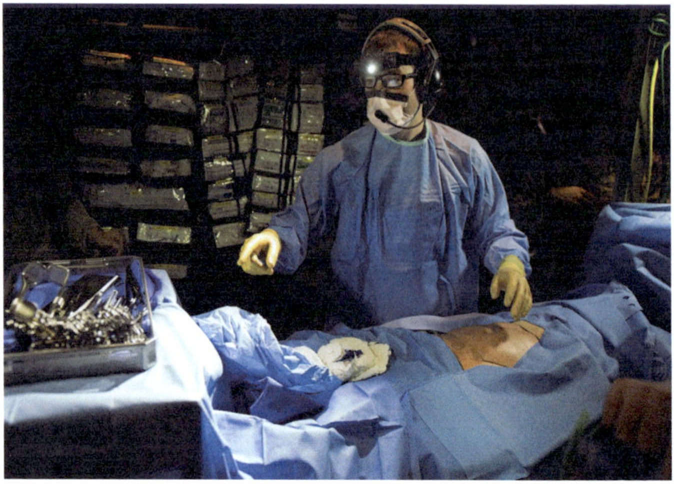

Fig. 3.3 Tactical Critical Care Evacuation Team-Enhanced performed a mock in-flight surgery during a training flight with the 86th Aeromedical Evacuation Squadron on March 26, 2015, above Ramstein Air Base, Germany. (Source Staff Sgt Sara Keller. Public Domain image, not in copyright. Available at: https://www.ramstein.af.mil/News/Photos/igphoto/2001041264/)

in-theater USAF CCATT missions began to resemble TCCET environments (but utilizing fixed-wing aircraft), AMC decided to merge the capabilities with CCATT training, expanding to cover core TCCET skill sets. By 2019, the CCATT austere evacuation mission was fully incorporated into the CCATT training, and the last TCCET deployments were completed by 2020 [46].

During the middle decade of OEF, the MFST was rarely used in its designed capacity, but as the war began to wind down, it was more commonly tasked. It was noted that the MFST package had not been revised significantly in the last decade, nor had JTS lessons learned been incorporated into the allowance standard or tactics, techniques, and procedures (TTPs). In 2016, AMC engaged with Air Combat Command (ACC) and AFSOC with a proposal to use the TCCET-E as a framework to refresh the MFST. The resultant package proposal would have renamed the TCCET-E as the Austere (or Air) Surgical Team (AST) and nominated the MFST replacement as the Ground Surgical Team (GST). Ultimately, it was decided that one capability would be created, the GST, for all Air Force missions and managed by ACC. Besides the conversion of the MFST allowance standard to a facsimile of the TCCET-E's kits, the most critical change was the development of a robust training pipeline for GST team members on the clinical, environmental, and operational aspects of austere surgery. In 2018, the six-person GST (a Medical Admin/Communicator was added to the original MFST cadre) was approved as the USAF's ARSC capability and the initial entry force of the EMEDS (Expeditionary Medical Support System) medical deployment system [12, 38, 47].

ARSC Capabilities During Large-Scale Combat Operations

The current environment in which the Services are working has been termed one of strategic competition. This phase does not rise to the level of open warfare, but national and strategic interests nevertheless are of major importance to US Foreign Policy. The US military is facing a period where it needs to be prepared to respond across a spectrum of operations including low-intensity conflict, peacetime great power competition below the level of war (Grey Zone Conflict), counterterrorism, counterproliferation, while simultaneously being able to rapidly respond to peer LSCO involving increasingly kinetic engagements that will strain capacity and capability of current units [8, 48]. All of these mission sets share the potential for delays in patient movement and disruption of en route care, especially when compared to the air superiority and rapid MEDEVAC paradigm that characterized OIF/OEF [48].

The Joint Chiefs of Staff outline their vision for the future in a dynamic environment through the "Joint Concept of Health Services" [8], as discussed above. Each branch of the military has issued service-specific directives regarding the future of HSS based on the concept of future operations. These documents communicate the anticipated need for smaller, more mobile units (e.g., small surgical teams) capable of performing their functions in dispersed formations that can be surged forward when necessary to support combat operations, then reassemble into larger groups as required by evolving tactical and strategic situations. This envisioned flexibility in capability and capacity to meet rapid re-deployment of HSS was exemplified during the Kabul International Airport attack in 2021, when multiple small surgical teams merged to conduct Mass Casualty (MASCAL) operations and later disbanded for the withdrawal from Afghanistan [49]. Similarly, the MASCAL response on the USS Bataan in 2017, where three single surgeon teams in conjunction with the ship's medical department successfully managed six severely injured casualties, required DCR/DCS with 60 units of blood products and multiple resuscitative procedures [50].

Recent conflicts have revealed the ability of potential adversaries to target company-sized or larger facilities and even smaller formations with significant radio frequency signatures. Medical capabilities across all Roles of Care (Role 1–4) are also being routinely targeted in the Russia–Ukraine War [51]. Therefore, medical capabilities, including ARSC teams, should anticipate being targeted in the future fight. To provide life-saving care and survive on the future battlefield, ARSC teams comprised of forward-deployed caregivers from conventional forces must have standardized team training focusing on austere clinical decision making, exposure to tactical and operational environments, and develop cohesive team dynamics and effective communication. Finally, it is ideal if they have the ability to integrate with their supported units before deployment as the ability to provide effective casualty care on the future battlefield should not be an isolated medical capability, but a command-directed unit capability.

A key concern in assessing casualty survival with smaller teams is the limited evidence on how small surgical units affect overall morbidity and mortality, particularly in operations that are projected to generate an increased number of casualties over a sustained period of time without the benefit of a robust chain of resupply and evacuation [11]. The ARSC team is designed to "bridge the gap" in scenarios where prolonged evacuation times negatively impact patient outcomes [12]. These teams are most effectively employed in areas of operation distant from traditional Role 2 surgical capabilities, providing wounded combatants with access to DCR/DCS when such resources would not ordinarily be available near the POI. The logistical requirements to bring those casualties out of harm's way and back to more definitive care still exist (as in the Revolutionary War), and the services are trying to address these potentialities with doctrine and practice guidelines focusing on evacuation, Role 1 prolonged casualty care, and prolonged Role 2 holding.

The need to provide far-forward care in the logistically stressed, geographically dispersed, contested environment serves as the primary consideration in planning for the use of an ARSC team. To achieve this projected need, the ARSC team's surgical resuscitation capability will require meticulous operational planning, thorough preparation, basic tactical proficiency, and special measures to mitigate the additional risks of operating in austere environments. The skills necessary for success during LSCO have evolved from those needed during GWOT, characterized by the robust and timely patient movement to more definitive surgical care. ARSC teams may need to be capable of providing more definitive surgical care and longer patient holding during LSCO. However, there will always be a need for an evacuation chain capable of moving patients to more definitive care capabilities outside the zones of engagement.

ARSC Team Resources and Essential References

Currently, each Service has its own platform-specific training courses. Based on authorities from the National Defense Authorization Act 2017, the Joint Requirements Oversight Council Memorandum (JROCM) 125–17, and the DoD Inspector General (IG) Audit "Audit of Training of Mobile Medical Teams in the US Indo-Pacific Command and US Africa Command Areas of Responsibility," the JTS Joint Trauma Education and Training (JTET) has created a modular ARSC curriculum designed for the Joint Force [52–54]. This Joint ARSC curriculum addresses current crisis and contingency operations and prepares small surgical teams for the potential of future LSCO. Not only does the curriculum include common curricular elements identified from standard courses across the Army, Air Force, Navy, and Marine Corps but also includes curricular elements to prepare teams for LSCO including exposure to operational and tactical environments, austere clinical decision making, austere critical care, definitive Role 2 surgery, effective communication, and the nonclinical skills required to be an effective team in austere and operational environments. What follows is not comprehensive but an essential list of references and resources [55].

- Austere Resuscitative and Surgical Care (ARSC) Clinical Practice Guideline [56]. October 30, 2019. https://jts.health.mil/index.cfm/PI_CPGs/cpgs
- Baker JB, Marc Northern MD, Frament C, Aaron Baker D, Remick K, Seery J, Stephens L, Shackelford S, Gurney J. Austere resuscitative and surgical care in support of forward military operations-joint trauma system position paper. Mil Med. 2020;186(1–2):12–17 [12].
- Committee on Surgical Combat Casualty Care Position State on Single Surgeon Teams. February 24, 2022 [57]. https://jts.health.mil/assets/docs/cosccc/CoSCCC_Position_Statement_on_Single_Surgeon_Teams.pdf
- Gurney JM, Jensen SD, Gavitt BJ, Edson TD, Brown SR, Cunningham CW, et al. Committee on surgical combat casualty care position statement on the use of single surgeon teams and invited commentaries [11]. J Trauma Acute Care Surg. 2022;93(2S):S6–S11.
- Austere Resuscitative Surgical Care Learning Objectives. July 22, 2024 [55]. https://deployedmedicine.allogy.net/learner/collections/featured/337246fc-fc70-488e-8304-4ed47e507449/contents/3996

Conclusion

Far-forward surgical care has always been required in war, either on land or sea. Throughout the history of the US military, forward surgical capabilities have had many labels, and in contemporary lexicon, it is often referred to as Role 2 Light Maneuver, but more commonly as ARSC—Austere Resuscitative Surgical Care. In the US military's recent past, ARSC capabilities have been successfully deployed and have saved lives all over the world, but given their small size in terms of personnel and materiel, ARSC capability and capacity are limited compared to larger forward surgical capabilities and dependent on a logistical chain providing patient movement and resupply. Despite these limitations, ARSC teams will likely be required during LSCO. To be successful and save lives on the battlefield requires adequate clinical and nonclinical training. The challenges ARSC teams face in balancing capability, capacity, and maneuverability have remained the same throughout history despite advances in medicine and are elegantly summarized by this quote from British World War II-era surgeon William Olgivie: "Good surgery must be done as far forward as possible. If it is too good, in the sense of too elaborately equipped, it will not be far enough forward, and if it is too far forward, it will not be good enough" [55].

References

1. Gillett M. The Army medical department 1775–1818. US Government Printing Office; 1981.
2. Steahly LP, Cannon DW. The evolution of forward surgery in the US Army: from the Revolutionary War to the combat operations of the 21st century. Borden Institute, US Army Medical Department Center and School, Health Readiness Center of Excellence; 2018:xiv, 476 pages.
3. Lister J. On the antiseptic principle in the practice of surgery, vol. 38. PF Collier and Son: Harvard Classics; 1867.
4. Lister J. On a new method of treating compound fracture, abscess with observations on the condition of suppuration. Lancet. 1867;89(2272):326–9.
5. Lister J. On the antiseptic principle in the practice of surgery. Br Med J. 1867;2(351):245–60.
6. Smith CM. United States Army in World War II, the Technical Services. The Medical Department: Hospitalization and Evacuation, Zone of the Interior. Center for Military History, Office of the Chief of Military History; 1989.
7. Cowdrey AE. The medics' war. US Army Center for Military History; 1987.

8. JP 4–02 Joint Health Services (Joint Forces Development) (2023, 29 August).
9. Kotwal RS, Howard JT, Orman JA, et al. The effect of a golden hour policy on the morbidity and mortality of combat casualties. JAMA Surg. 2016;151(1):15–24. https://doi.org/10.1001/jamasurg.2015.3104.
10. Bingham J, Satterly S, Eckert M. Austere resuscitative and surgical care in modern combat operations. Curr Trauma Rep. 2021;7(3):53–9. https://doi.org/10.1007/s40719-021-00214-0.
11. Gurney JM, Jensen SD, Gavitt BJ, et al. Committee on surgical combat casualty care position statement on the use of single surgeon teams and invited commentaries. J Trauma Acute Care Surg. 2022;93(2S):S6–S11. https://doi.org/10.1097/ta.0000000000003676.
12. Baker JB, Northern DM, Frament C, et al. Austere resuscitative and surgical care in support of forward military operations—joint trauma system position paper. Mil Med. 2021;186(1–2):12–7. https://doi.org/10.1093/milmed/usaa358.
13. Brown HE. The Medical Department of the Unites States Army from 1775 to 1783. Surgeon Generals Office; 1873.
14. Dunham GC. Medical Men in the American revolution 1775–1783. Medical Field Service School; 1931.
15. Eichner LG. The military practice of medicine during the revolutionary war. Winter 2004. HIstory Quarterly. Accessed 3 Oct 2024.
16. Manring MM, Hawk A, Calhoun JH, Andersen RC. Treatment of war wounds: a historical review. Clin Orthop Relat Res. 2009;467(8):2168–91. https://doi.org/10.1007/s11999-009-0738-5.
17. Ortiz JM. The revolutionary flying ambulance of Napoleon's surgeon. US Army Med Dept J. 1998;4:17–25.
18. Stinger H, Rush R. The army forward surgical team- update and lessons learned, 1997–2004. Mil Med. 2006;171(4):269–72.
19. Savory C. Forwward surgical support to special operations task forces in the late 1970s. In: Sr. PBA, editor. 08/13/2024.
20. Llewellyn C Genesis of forward surgical team concepts in the late 1970's historical recollection. In: Sr. PBA, editor. 2024.
21. Nessen SC, Cronk DR, Edens J, et al. US Army two-surgeon teams operating in remote Afghanistan—an evaluation of split-based Forward Surgical Team operations. J Trauma. 2009;66(4 Suppl):S37–47. https://doi.org/10.1097/TA.0b013e31819ce302.
22. Gates R. Memoirs of a secretary at war. Random House; 2014.
23. ATP 4-01.25. The medical detachment, forward resuscitative and surgical (U.S. Army Publishing Directorate). 2020.
24. Tadlock MD, Hernandez AA, Miller BT. The ship's surgeon and surgery at sea: a brief history. Expeditionary surgery at sea: a practical approach. Springer; 2023. p. 33–52.
25. Watt J. The injuries of four centuries of naval warfare. Ann R Coll Surg Engl. 1975;57(1):3–24.

26. Sobocinski A. Born in harm's way: the advent of navy medicine in the revolutionary war. October 12, 2022. https://www.navy.mil/Press-Office/News-Stories/Article/3186885/born-in-harms-way-the-advent-of-navy-medicine-in-the-revolutionary-war/. Accessed 12 Jan 2025.
27. Cutter L, Clarke T Jr. Anesthesia advances during the civil war. Mil Med. 2014;179(12):1503. https://doi.org/10.7205/MILMED-D-14-00344.
28. Adams WT. Red Rover: first hospital ship of the US Navy. 1968:149.
29. Red Rover. Naval history and heritage command. September 23, 2005. https://www.history.navy.mil/research/histories/ship-histories/danfs/r/red-rover.html. Accessed 13 Jan 2025.
30. History of the Medical Department of USS LST (H) 464. December 17, 1945. Bureau of Medicine and Surgery (BUMED) Archives.
31. Vedder JS. Surgeon on Iwo: up front with the 27th marines. Presidio Press; 1984.
32. Bohman H, Baker B, Stevens R. Forward resuscitative surgery in operation Iraqi freedom. US Naval Inst Proc. 2004;130(2):73–6.
33. Brethauer SA, Chao A, Chambers LW, et al. Invasion vs insurgency: US navy/marine corps forward surgical care during operation Iraqi freedom. Arch Surg. 2008;143(6):564–9. https://doi.org/10.1001/archsurg.143.6.564.
34. Chambers LW, Rhee P, Baker BC, et al. Initial experience of US marine corps forward resuscitative surgical system during operation Iraqi freedom. Arch Surg. 2005;140(1):26–32. https://doi.org/10.1001/archsurg.140.1.26.
35. The evolution of wartime surgery: the first official navy program for a light-maneuver, surgical team completes its first successful trial underway, augmenting Rushmore's Medical Department for Dawn Blitz 2017. October 28, 2017. https://www.dvidshub.net/news/253373/evolution-wartime-surgery-first-official-navy-program-light-maneuver-surgical-team-completes-its-first-successful. Accessed 14 Jan 2024.
36. OPNAV INSTRUCTION 3501.408. Required operational capabilities and projected operational environment for the role 2 light maneuver expeditionary resuscitative surgical system. June 14th, 2021. https://www.secnav.navy.mil/doni/Directives/03000%20Naval%20Operations%20and%20Readiness/03-500%20Training%20and%20Readiness%20Services/3501.408.pdf . Accessed 14 Jan 2025.
37. Lowry DM, Johnston MG, Van Gent J-M, Tadlock MD, Edson TD. Overview of current maritime surgical platforms and operational environments: part 1—United States navy and marine corps. Expeditionary surgery at sea: a practical approach. Springer; 2023. p. 3–21.
38. Smyth C. Air force tactics, techniques and procedures 3-42.77, Ground Surgical Team. 2018. https://static.e-publishing.af.mil/production/1/af_sg/publication/afttp3-42.77/afttp3-42.77.pdf. Accessed 31 Aug 2024.

39. Manifold C. Air force medical service concept of operations for the mobile field surgical team (MFST). September 10, 1999. https://www.google.com/url?sa=t&source=web&rct=j&opi=89978449&url=https://www.brooksidepress.org/Products/Military_OBGYN/Textbook/MilitaryOrganizations/AirForce/MobileFieldSurgicaTeam.doc&ved=2ahUKEwiJypXx84GLAxX1L9AFHWEDOpMQFnoECBcQAQ&usg=AOvVaw1owxm8X1_ocaheAAvHC-xl. Accessed 31 Aug 2024.
40. Carlton Jr PKLG. New millennium, new mind-set: the air force medical service in the air expeditionary era. Aerospace Power J. 2001;15(4):8–15.
41. Beninati W, Meyer MT, Carter TE. The critical care air transport program. Crit Care Med. 2008;36(7):S370–6.
42. Jenkins D. Air force medical service (AFMS) concept of operations for the small portable expeditionary aeromedical reapid response (SPEARR) team. May 12, 2000. https://www.brooksidepress.org/Products/Military_OBGYN/Textbook/MilitaryOrganizations/AirForce/spearr.pdf. Accessed 31 Aug 2024.
43. Ervin MD. Air force special operations command special operations surgical team (SOST) CONOPS. J Spec Op Med. 2008;8:68–75.
44. Drinnon, R. AMC aims to increase casualty survivability in Afghanistan. Air Mobilty Command Press Release. May 8, 2012. https://www.af.mil/News/Article-Display/Article/111216/amc-aims-to-increase-casualty-survivability-in-afghanistan/. Acessed 31 Aug 2024.
45. Svan J. New Air force concept for aeromedical evacuation to meet challenges in Africa. December 26, 2013. https://www.stripes.com/migration/new-air-force-concept-for-aeromedical-evacuation-to-meet-challenges-in-africa-1.259333. Accessed 31 Aug 2024.
46. Brown DJ, Jeffries J, Broderick J, et al. Divide and save: a critical care Air transport team case with prolonged field care. Mil Med. 2024:usae450.
47. Edmonds R, Hansen D. Aligning air force ground surgical team (GST) training with the deployment experience. Mil Med. 2023;188(5–6):997–1002.
48. Hoffman FG. Examining complex forms of conflict gray zone and hybrid challenges. J Complex Operations Prism. 2018;7(No 4):30-47.
49. Bozzay JD, Murphy TP, Baird MD, et al. The last days: the medical response of United States and allied military teams during the Afghanistan exodus. J Trauma Acute Care Surg. 2023;95(2S Suppl 1):S13–8. https://doi.org/10.1097/TA.0000000000004062.
50. Miller BT, Lin AH, Clark SC, Cap AP, Dubose JJ. Red tides: mass casualty and whole blood at sea. J Trauma Acute Care Surg. 2018;85(1S Suppl 2):S134–9. https://doi.org/10.1097/TA.0000000000001831.
51. Kekatos M. WHO records 1,940 health care attacks in Ukraine since war with Russia began. August 19, 2024. https://abcnews.go.com/International/records-1940-health-care-attacks-ukraine-war-russia/story?id=112944980#:~:text=During%20the%20course%20of%20the,now%20occurring%20nearly%20every%20day. Accessed 17 Jan 2024.

52. Joint Requirements Oversight Council Memorandum (JROCM) 125–17. Forward resuscitative care in support of dispersed operations DOTmLPF-P change recommendation. December 11, 2017.
53. Section 708 of the National Defense Authorization Act for Fiscal Year 2017 (Public Law 114–328): "Establishment of Joint Trauma Education and Training Directorate" Interim Report and Implementation Plan. February 14th, 2018. https://www.health.mil/Reference-Center/Reports/2018/02/14/Joint-Trauma-Education-and-Training-Directorate#:~:text=This%20interim%20report%20and%20implementation,(d)%20Personnel%20Management%20Plan. Accessed 2 Jan 2024.
54. Inspector General (IG) Audit "Audit of Training of Mobile Medical Teams in the U.S. Indo-Pacific Command and U.S. Africa Command Areas of Responsibility" (Report No. DODIG-2020-087) dated June 8, 2020. https://www.dodig.mil/reports.html/Article/2213982/audit-of-training-of-mobile-medical-teams-in-the-us-indo-pacific-command-and-us/. Accessed 1 Jan 2024.
55. Austere Resuscitative Surgical Care Learning Objectives. July 22, 2024. https://deployedmedicine.allogy.net/learner/collections/featured/337246fc-fc70-488e-8304-4ed47e507449/contents/3996. Accessed 14 Jan 2025.
56. Austere Resuscitative and Surgical Care (ARSC) Clinical Practice Guideline. October 30, 2019. https://jts.health.mil/index.cfm/PI_CPGs/cpgs. Accessed 14 Jan 2025.
57. Anonymous A, Anonymous A. Committee on surgical combat casualty care position: statement on single-surgeon teams. J Spec Oper Med Spring. 2022;22(1):144–5. https://doi.org/10.55460/SOZV-TQN9.

History of the Joint Trauma System

4

Jeffrey A. Bailey, Brian J. Gavitt, and Jennifer M. Gurney

Civilian Trauma Systems

In 1966, the National Academy of Sciences published a landmark article, "Accidental Death and Disability: The Neglected Disease of Modern Society" [1], that advocated for an organized approach to the treatment of seriously injured patients. A decade later, and led by surgeons who returned from the Vietnam War, the American College of Surgeons Committee on Trauma (ACSCOT) published "Optimal Hospital Resources for the Care of the Injured." This publication established criteria for hospitals to build the "ideal trauma center" and then sub-categorized trauma centers by capability as levels 1–4. Level 1 trauma centers offer the broadest

J. A. Bailey (✉)
Joint Trauma System, US Department of Defense, JBSA Fort Sam Houston, San Antonio, TX, USA

Section of Acute and Critical Care Surgery, Washington University in Saint Louis, Saint Louis, MO, USA
e-mail: jeffrey.a.bailey3.ctr@health.mil

B. J. Gavitt
Wright-Patterson Medical Center, Wright-Patterson AFB, OH, USA

J. M. Gurney
Joint Trauma System, US Department of Defense, JBSA Fort Sam Houston, TX, USA

A. T. Schlussel et al. (eds.), *The SAGES Manual for Navigating a Successful Military Surgical Career*,
https://doi.org/10.1007/978-3-031-88490-0_4

spectrum of clinical resources in addition to providing trauma education, research, and leadership in the community; level 1 trauma centers, then as now, are most often large academic health centers. Level 2–4 trauma centers offer progressively lower levels of complex trauma care, educational, or research responsibilities.

The trauma program is the operational hub of the trauma center and is led by a surgeon trauma medical director (TMD) and trauma program manager (TPM); these leaders are supported by a staff of trauma nurse coordinators (TNC) and trauma registrars. The trauma program focuses on optimizing trauma outcomes by leveraging data to drive performance improvement (PI). Critical sources of data to support performance improvement include electronic health records, trauma registries, trauma peer review, and systems of care reviews. Performance improvement activities inform evidence-based best practices, trauma education, community outreach and prevention, and trauma research to deliver measurable improvements in trauma outcomes.

The original "Optimal Resources" publication was followed by "Resources for Optimal Care of the Injured Patient" which focused on the larger ecosystem of collaborating hospitals, namely the "trauma *system*" (Table 4.1). This network of trauma centers is linked with an emergency medical system to support the full spectrum of trauma prevention, prehospital care, acute care, rehabilitation, education, and research. Subsequent updates expanded the network to include all treatment facilities and resources that may be engaged to provide trauma care to patients within a community (the *inclusive* trauma system). The ACSCOT also implemented a *verification program* for trauma centers (a *quality* program), while US state and regional governmental programs developed a complementary rubric for the *designation* of trauma centers (a *regulatory* program) [2]. Most recently ACSCOT implemented a consultation program available at the request of governmental or institutional "lead agents" (ex: State Departments of Health) to survey and make recommendations for implementation or improvements in state or regional trauma systems (Table 4.1). Thirty years after the original "optimal hospital resources" manual was published, data analysis showed a 25 percent reduction in trauma deaths where trauma systems were implemented [3].

Table 4.1 Recommended websites for a combat surgical deployment

Resources for optimal care of the injured patient	https://www.facs.org/quality-programs/trauma/quality/verification-review-and-consultation-program/standards/
Trauma systems consultation program	https://www.facs.org/quality-programs/trauma/systems/trauma-systems-consultation-program/
Clinical practice guidelines—joint trauma system	https://jts.health.mil/index.cfm/PI_CPGs/cpgs
Damage control resuscitation—joint trauma system	https://jts.health.mil/index.cfm/PI_CPGs/damage_control
Joint trauma system forms and after action report submissions	https://jts.health.mil/index.cfm/documents/forms_after_action

Joint Theater Trauma System and Joint Theater Trauma Registry

Although trauma systems had been implemented in the civilian health sector over the two decades that preceded the Global War on Terror, paradoxically this was not the case for the US military. The US Military entered the conflicts in Afghanistan and Iraq with robust trauma care capabilities—including delivery of ATLS predeployment training to military providers—but these capabilities were not fully integrated into a trauma system to ensure the right patient received the right care at the right place at the right time. Senior US military trauma surgeons recognized this gap and were directed to survey the combat theater of operations (akin to the ACSCOT trauma systems consultation) [4–7]. The initial recommendation was to implement a regional trauma system at the level of the US Army Medical Brigade supporting Operation Iraqi Freedom (OIF) in 2003. The US Central Command (CENTCOM) Surgeon agreed but directed that the regional system be implemented across the entire Combatant Command (CCMD) Area of Responsibility (AOR). The US CENTCOM "Joint Theater Trauma System" (JTTS) was established with the assignment of its first Trauma Medical Director in 2004. Subsequently, the US

CENTCOM JTTS team was expanded to include the TMD, TPM, TNC, and noncommissioned officers (NCOs) assigned to the office of the US CENTCOM Surgeon and detailed to theater. This organizational alignment allowed the JTTS team to pursue its mission of performance improvement in coordination with, but functionally independent of the in-theater chain of command (Table 4.1). This enabled its freedom to engage and travel across the in-theater continuum of care and engendered its impartiality which in turn enhanced a trusted relationship with trauma teams and their leadership. The JTTS produced a military "challenge coin" featuring the US CENTCOM emblem as well as the motto of "right patient, right time, right care, right place." The TMD gifted this coin to recognize trauma team members during travel in theater. The TMD, TPM, and Lead NCO occupied the JTTS primary offices (in Baghdad and later at Bagram Airfield) with teams of TNCs and NCOs embedded in Role 3 facilities. The last JTTS teams left Iraq with the transition of OIF to Operation New Dawn (OND) in 2010 and were consolidated in support of Operation Enduring Freedom (OEF) embedded at the Afghanistan Role 3 facilities at Bagram Airfield, Kandahar Airfield, Camp Bastion, and Camp Dwyer [5–7].

A "Joint Theater Trauma Registry" (JTTR) was developed and served as the backbone to guide evidence-based clinical best practices, inform military trauma education, augment prevention, identify clinical trauma care or system gaps, and prioritize requirements to drive combat casualty care research. The JTTR was implemented by the adaption of an off-the-shelf trauma registry customized to include combat casualty care relevant common data elements. The JTTR supported facility-based trauma record abstraction onto a Store and Forward Windows application and then exported to the central JTTR server hosted by Brooke Army Medical Center in San Antonio, TX. Record abstraction was initiated by JTTS TNC and NCOs embedded at the Role 3 facilities in Theater and then continued as casualties were evacuated across the global continuum of care to receiving facilities in Europe and the Continental US. Finally, a support element at the US Army Institute of Surgical Research completed record abstraction by a review of web-based DoD record repositories. This USAISR support element also assured data quality and monitored registrar performance through programmatic audits. As such *only records for casualties that arrived to a Role 3, where record abstraction was initiated (including abstraction of "forward" records that arrived to the Role 3 facilities with casualties) were included in the JTTR*. In the early experience, the in-theater teams and support element at USAISR were *both* commonly identified as "the JTTS." In addition to maintaining the registry at the USAISR, this element also performed and supported system "PI" through JTTR data analysis and reporting to inform combat casualty prevention and best trauma care practices. The USAISR JTTS also informed and participated in combat casualty care research and provided predeployment training to prepare JTTS teams for their mission and roles in theater. Members of the JTTS team from the USAISR then traveled with the deploying theater team to Landstuhl Regional Medical Center (LRMC) in Germany for additional training and orientation to the facility and its unique responsibilities as the first US receiving facility for casualties evacuated from theater [4–7].

Trauma Programs were established at Role 3 Facilities in theater and at the Role 4 receiving facilities which included LRMC in Germany and in the Continental US including, among others, Walter Reed Army Medical Center (AMC), the National Naval Medical Center at Bethesda (later Walter Reed National Military Medical Center), Brooke AMC, Wilford Hall Medical Center (USAF), and Naval Medical Center San Diego (NMCSD). In theater, excepting the facility-assigned Trauma Medical Director (if one were appointed), the trauma program was staffed by JTTS TNCs and NCOs detailed to the Role 3 facilities that, in addition to JTTR record abstraction, supported facility-level performance improvement projects that were also facilitated by the JTTS TMD, TPM, and PI staff at USAISR. As such, unlike its civilian counterpart, the in-theater trauma program was not wholly organic to the facility's organizational structure, but rather "inserted" into the facility by the detail of JTTS TNCs and NCOs. Recurring casualty reports (typically monthly) generated at the facility and theater level included casualty numbers, injury patterns, care, mortality, and morbidity. Theater-level reports were widely distributed both in and out of theater. Special reports were also produced for topics ranging from emerging injury patterns to focus on specific care capabilities such as out-of-hospital blood transfusion and resuscitation fluids and the use of tranexamic acid for shock resuscitation. Unlike theater, the Role 4 trauma programs were organic to the facility organization and, aside from the facility trauma medical directors, consisted primarily of civil service and contract staff. The PI programs at these facilities were robust (particularly so at LRMC) and operated independently with the use of the JTTR, and for facilities that participated as designated and/or verified trauma centers in local civilian trauma systems (BAMC, WHMC), also a civilian trauma registry [4–7].

As is the case in civilian trauma systems, PI was the primary function of the JTTS and the primary output JTTS PI was to develop, review, and update evidence-based clinical practice guidelines (CPG) to inform and guide combat casualty care (Table 4.1). The first intervention developed by the JTTS targeted hypothermia prevention in 2004. Another performance improvement project focused on the ratio of transfused blood components for patients in hemorrhagic shock and resulted in perhaps the most well-known CPG: Damage Control Resuscitation (DCR). The DCR CPG recommended a balanced ratio of Red Blood Cells, Plasma, and Platelets ("1:1:1") for hemorrhagic shock resuscitation "to restore homeostasis, prevent or mitigate the development of tissue hypoxia, oxygen debt, and burden of shock, as well as coagulopathy" owing to a demonstrated improvement in casualty survival (Table 4.1). In comparison to civilian trauma systems, the organizational construct of the JTTS enabled *system-level* PI *at its inception*. Soon after JTTS teleconferences, moderated by the in-theater JTTS TMD were implemented to support communication across the continuum and provide system-level care review, and to a lesser extent, inform facility-level peer review. The JTTS TMD and TPM traveled frequently in theater to communicate directly with JTTS team members and trauma care teams to obtain the "ground truth" and to support CPG utilization and, when necessary, review variances in practice to bring trauma teams into compliance—or consider in updates to CPGs [4–7].

Early in the JTTS experience, it was widely recognized there was a large blind spot: namely casualties who did not arrive alive at a Role 3 facility were not included in the registry. While a "store and forward" Role 2 registry application was fielded in theater and supported at USAISR, little systematic data for casualty care and outcomes forward of the Role 3 facilities were applied to support Role 2 PI programs. The blind spot was especially large for combat casualties who died on the battlefield or somewhere forward of Role 2 surgical care [4–6]. A landmark project that included clinical data in the Armed Forces Medical Examiner registry documented, that as in prior conflicts, the vast majority (in this case 90%) died "on the battlefield" and that the majority of those "preventable" deaths were associated with hemorrhage (primarily truncal followed by junctional and to a lesser extent extremity) [8]. This enhanced system-level focus on prehospital care and supported the addition of a prehospital element, including a prehospital medical director to the JTTS team [4–7]. The original members of the team (TNC and NCOs) had been fielded to support reporting on the Secretary of Defense "Golden Hour" mandate in 2009 [6, 9]. Owing to the complexities and geography of the battlespace of OEF, it was noted that evacuation times from the point of injury were extended in comparison with those of Operation Iraqi Freedom. Convinced that this had an impact on casualty survival and outcomes, Secretary Gates directed that prehospital helicopter evacuation missions of critically injured combat casualties more than 60 min be reviewed and reported weekly. A support element at the USAISR was implemented to collect classified evacuation data to support weekly SECDEF reporting on compliance with what became known as the Golden Hour Mandate. The output from analysis of this data composite established that survival was negatively impacted for prehospital evacuations of critically injured combat casualties more than 60 min. In addition, the impact of en route advanced resuscitation practices, including blood product DCR, during the evacuation from the point of injury and in theater interfacility transport was associated with improved survival. These findings validated the "Golden Hour" and drove improvements in the en route care capabilities assigned to tactical evacuation platforms including advanced care providers [9].

Joint Trauma System and DoD Trauma Registry

As the conflict in Iraq wound down, concern began to mount that the JTTS, a regional trauma system funded as a contingency, would be lost to future generations. Although for its first decade, identified as a Joint *Theater* Trauma System, the "system" had transcended the "theater" as trauma PI—supported through abstraction of clinical data accumulated across a global continuum into the "JTTR"—was implemented. As such the "JTTS" at the USAISR was redesignated as the "Joint Trauma System" (JTS) to differentiate itself from the US CENTCOM JTTS. In partnership with ACSCOT, the JTS published the "Joint Trauma System: Development, Conceptual Framework, and Optimal Elements" manual to document its history, organizational structure, and primary functions that support the global DoD Trauma System in January 2012. In addition, in October 2011, the JTTR was redesignated as the "DoD Trauma Registry" (DoDTR) to reflect the global reach of its processes and contents. This was in fact beyond a change in terminology—major software enhancements allowed the program to operate globally and solely on a web-based real-time platform implemented in October 2011 [5, 6].

Well before in-theater JTTS teams in 2014, and through a series of invited theater trauma system reports— including civilian trauma leaders, Defense Health Board publications, and senior leadership engagement—support was engendered to institutionalize and fund the JTS as an enduring DoD-level organization [10–14]. In 2016 the "Joint Trauma System" (JTS) was formally established in DoD policy and US Government Law. A DoD Instruction was published assigning the JTS responsibilities to the maintenance of a global trauma care capability in support of the full range of military operation [15]. In addition, Section 707 of the 2017 National Defense Authorization Act (NDAA) established that a "JTS" with the responsibilities to serve as the reference body for trauma care, to establish standards of trauma care, coordinate the translation of research, and incorporate lessons learned from civilian partnerships [16]. In accordance with the DoD implementation plan Report to Congress (RTC IP), the JTS was established by the organizational realignment of the JTS elements at the USAISR from the US Army to the Defense Health Agency [17]. To support the ability of the JTS to meet its responsibilities, as specified in the RTC IP an organizational assessment was conducted to determine its ideal structure and required resources. This assessment was delivered to the DHA Director in October 2018; its recommendations continue to be evaluated and implemented.

The primary function of the JTS remains PI effected through the continuous "operational cycle" of data abstraction, data analysis, and PI outputs that support the "practice of bold and responsible battlefield medicine" (Fig. 4.1). In June of 2016—50 years following the publication of the landmark article, "Accidental Death and Disability: The Neglected Disease of Modern Society," the National Academy of Science, Engineering and Medicine published "A National Trauma Care System: Integrating Military and Civilian Trauma Care Systems to Achieve Zero Preventable Death." Among its recommendations is: "The Secretary of Defense should direct the DHA Director to expand and stabilize

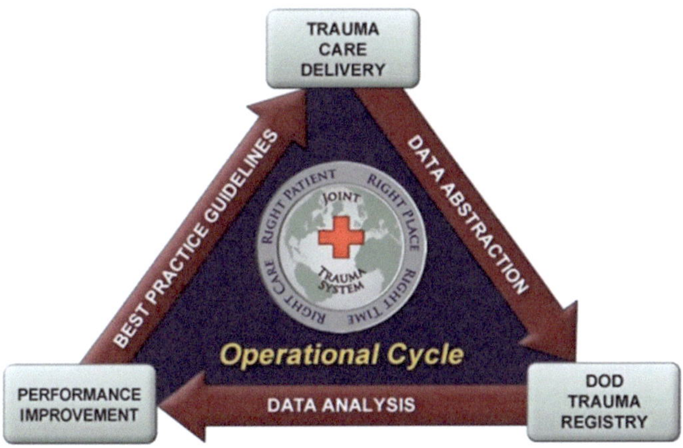

Fig. 4.1 Joint Trauma System Operational Cycle from *Out of the Crucible: How the US Military Transformed Combat Casualty Care in Iraq and Afghanistan* (Borden Institute | U.S. Army Medical Center of Excellence)

long term support for the Joint Trauma System so its functionality can be improved and utilized across all combatant commands, giving actors in the system access to timely evidence, data, educational opportunities, research, and performance improvement activities" [18].

References

1. Accidental death and disability: The neglected disease of modern society. Washington, DC: National Academy of Sciences; 1966.
2. Putting the Pieces Together: A National Effort to Complete the U.S. Trauma System. American College of Surgeons. Putting the Pieces Together: A National Effort to Complete the U.S. Trauma System | ACS (facs.org)
3. MacKenzie EJ, Rivara FP, Jurkovich GJ, Nathens AB, Frey KP, Egleston BL, Salkever DS, Scharfstein DO. A national evaluation of the effect of trauma-center care on mortality. N Engl J Med. 2006;354(4):366–78. https://doi.org/10.1056/NEJMsa052049. PMID: 16436768
4. Out of the Crucible: How the US Military Transformed Combat Casualty Care in Iraq and Afghanistan (Borden Institute | U.S. Army Medical Center of Excellence).
5. Spott MA, Kurkowski CR, Stockinger Z. The joint trauma system: history in the making, military medicine. Mil Med. 2018;183(suppl_2):4–7. https://doi.org/10.1093/milmed/usy166.
6. Bailey J, et al. Joint trauma system: development, conceptual framework, and optimal elements. U.S. Department of Defense, U.S. Army Institute for Surgical Research; 2012. (Joint_Trauma_System_final_clean2.pdf (health.mil)
7. Eastridge B, et al. Trauma system development in a theater of war: experiences from operation Iraqi freedom and operation enduring freedom. J Trauma. 2006;61(6):1366–73.
8. Eastridge B, et al. Death on the battlefield (2001–2011): implications for the future of combat casualty care. J Trauma Acute Care Surg. 2010;73(6 Suppl.5):S431–7.
9. Kowtal R, et al. The effect of a golden hour policy on the morbidity and mortality of combat casualties. JAMA Surg. 2016;151(1):15–24.
10. Defense Health Board. Combat trauma lessons learned from military operations of 2001–2013. 9 March 2015.
11. Trunkey D, et al. Military trauma system review US Central Command. Afghan-Trauma System-Review-18-Mar-2010.pdf (army.mil).
12. Rotondo M, et al. The United States Military Joint Trauma System Assessment. A Report Commissioned by the US Central Command

Surgeon, Sponsored by Air Force Central Command, 2011. US-Military-Joint-Theater-Trauma-System-Assessment-2011.pdf (health.mil)
13. Kotwal RS, Butler FK, Edgar EP, Shackelford SA, Bennett DR, Bailey JA. Saving lives on the battlefield: a joint trauma system review of pre-hospital trauma care in combined joint operating area – Afghanistan. J Spec Oper Med. 2013;13(1):77–80.
14. Sauer SW, Robinson JB, Smith MP, et al. Saving lives on the battlefield (part II) one year later: a joint theater trauma system and joint trauma system review of prehospital trauma care in combined joint operations area Afghanistan (CJOA-A) final report, 30 may 2014. J Spec Oper Med. 2015;15(2):25–41.
15. DoD Instruction 6040.47 (DoD Instruction 6040.47, "Joint Trauma System," September 28, 2016; Incorporating Change 2 on June 14, 2022 (whs.mil)
16. National Defense Authorization Act Fiscal Year 2017 (PUBL328.PS (congress.gov)).
17. US Government Accountability Office. New trauma care system: DOD should fully incorporate leading practices into its planning for effective implementation. March 2018. (GAO-18-300, NEW TRAUMA CARE SYSTEM: DOD Should Fully Incorporate Leading Practices into Its Planning for Effective Implementation).
18. Berwick D, et al. A national trauma care system: integrating military and civilian trauma systems to achieve zero preventable deaths after injury. National Academy of Sciences, Engineering, and Medicine; 2016.

Further Reading

American College of Surgeons National Surgical Quality Improvement Program (ACS NSQIP | ACS (facs.org)

Bailey JA, Morrision JJ, Rasmussen TE. Trauma systems development in Afghanistan—lessons for civilian systems? Curr Opin Crit Care. 2013;19(6)

Bailey J, Trexler S, Murdock A, Hoyt D. Verification and regionalization of trauma systems: the impact of these efforts on trauma care in the US. Surg Clin North Am. 2012;92(4):1009–24.

Blackbourne L, et al. Military medical revolution: military trauma system. J Trauma Acute Care Surg. 2012;73(6 Suppl.5):S388–94.

Bridges E, et al. Advancing critical care. AACN Adv Crit Care. 2010;21(3):260–76.

Concept of Operations (CONOPS) for the Joint Theater Trauma Registry (JTTR). U.S. Army Institute of Surgical Research; August 2008.

Eastridge B, et al. Impact of joint theater trauma system initiatives on battle-field injury outcomes. Am J Surg. 2009;198(6):852–7.

Eastridge B, et al. Implementation and dissemination of a military trauma system: utilizing medical lessons learned from the battlefield. Army Institute of Surgical Research; 2010.
Eastridge B, et al. Utilizing a trauma systems approach to benchmark and improve combat casualty care. J Trauma. 2010;69(Suppl. 1):S5–9.
Mabry R, et al. Impact of critical care-trained flight paramedics on casualty survival during helicopter evacuation in the current war in Afghanistan. J Trauma Acute Care Surg. 2012;73(2 Suppl. 1):S32–7.
National Academy of Sciences (US) and National Research Council (US) Committee on Trauma; National Academy of Sciences (US) and National Research Council (US) Committee on Shock. Washington, DC: National Academies Press (US); 1966.
Palm K, et al. Evaluation of military trauma system practices related to damage-control resuscitation. J Trauma Acute Care Surg. 2012;73(6 Suppl. 5):S459–64.
Resources for Optimal Care of the Injured Patient. American College of Surgeons. 2022. (Resources for Optimal Care of the Injured Patient | ACS (facs.org)
Shackelford SA, Del Junco DJ, Powell-Dunford N, et al. Association of prehospital blood product transfusion during medical evacuation of combat casualties in Afghanistan with acute and 30-day survival. JAMA. 2017;318(16):1581–91.

5 Journey from Cadet to Surgeon

Micaela Cuneo, Robert W. Krell, and Margaret E. Gallagher

Overview

Though graduates from the United States Military Academy at West Point (USMA), Naval Academy (USNA), and Air Force Academy (USAFA) account for less than 10% of military medical students entering residency training annually, they comprise a higher proportion of senior and career military physicians. There are well-established medical school pipelines for cadets at each service academy. The rigors of service academy life provide excellent conditioning for the demands of medical school and residency training. The qualities and attributes that contributed to cadets' success at Service Academies closely align with the American Association of Medical Colleges (AAMC) core competencies: ethical responsibility, capacity for improvement, reliability and dependability, critical thinking, and scientific inquiry to name a few.

M. Cuneo · R. W. Krell
Brooke Army Medical Center, Fort Sam Houston, TX, USA
e-mail: Micaela.r.cuneo.mil@health.mil; robert.w.krell.mil@health.mil

M. E. Gallagher (✉)
Blanchfield Army Community Hospital, Fort Campbell, KY, USA
e-mail: margaret.e.gallagher23.mil@health.mil

A. T. Schlussel et al. (eds.), *The SAGES Manual for Navigating a Successful Military Surgical Career*,
https://doi.org/10.1007/978-3-031-88490-0_5

Service Academy Premedical Curricula and Medical Training Allotments

Service academies' core curricula are generally broader than those at most civilian colleges and universities, with required engineering, leadership, and physical education courses that are not mandated or even found in most civilian premedical programs. Table 5.1 shows samples of required courses at each respective service academy. Within their majors, cadets can select additional courses and choose core courses that are more applicable to a premedical track.

While there is no official premedical major, most cadets with medical school aspirations major in biology, chemistry, or behavioral sciences. At USMA most cadets going to medical school are

Table 5.1 Comparison of core curriculum at USMA, USNA, and USAFA

	USMA	USNA	USAFA
First year courses	Math 1 Calc 1 Chem 1 Phys 1 Eng Comp/Eng Lit Psych 1 History of the Army American History	Chemistry 1/2 Calculus 1/2 Literature 1/2 American Naval History US Government Leadership 110 Fundamentals of Seamanship For Lang 1/2	Econ 201 Comp Sci 110 Math 141/142 Chem 100 For Lang 1/2 Officership 100 English 111 Behavioral Science 110 History 100
Second year courses	Philosophy Statistics Chem 2/Phys 2 Poly Sci Econ Lang 1/2	Calculus 3 Math IV (major specific) General Physics 1/2 For Lang 3/4 Leadership 203 His 215 Basic Navigation Navigation and Piloting	Law 220 Engineering Mechanics 220 Physics 110/215 Chem 200 Bio 215/315 History 300 Officership 200 Philos 310 Pol Sci 211 MSS (Military Strategic Studies) 251

(continued)

Table 5.1 (continued)

	USMA	USNA	USAFA
Third year courses	Leadership 1 Military Arts Cyber	ECE 310/312 Principles of Propulsion Naval Weapons Systems Control Systems Laboratory EE 301/331 His 216 Hum 1 Leadership 310 Advanced Navigation Maritime Warfare	Statistics Aeronautical Engr 315 Beh Sci 360 National Character and Leadership Symposium lecture series Officership 300 History 345 Pol Sci 302
Fourth year courses	MX400 Constitutional and Military Law	Introduction to Aeronautics Principles of Ship Performance Hum 2 Law for the Junior Officer Junior Officer Practicum	Astronautical Engr 310 Electrical and Computer Engr 315 Engl 411 MSS 444

Life Science majors. Cadets in other majors (e.g., engineering, military strategic studies, humanities) will have to take more courses outside their core and major curricula to meet medical school admission requirements than cadets majoring in biology or chemistry. Though that approach may entail more credit hours by graduation, it also can be favorably viewed by admissions committees seeking to maintain diversity in backgrounds and experiences in their medical school classes. Service academies also offer minor focus areas, of which the most commonly obtained are in foreign languages. There are also minors offered in nuclear weapons and strategy, religion, philosophy, and others related to both the humanities and STEM areas. Courses to fulfill major requirements are typically started in the second year and start to take up a larger portion of the academic load in the third and fourth years.

As evidenced by these curriculum guidelines, there are many more required engineering courses at a service academy than there are at civilian universities. There are also eight semesters of required physical education courses which factor into a cadet's final GPA. These can both skew the GPA, but many medical schools understand the unique circumstances of service academy cadets. For example, a 3.5 GPA at a service academy may be viewed differently than a 3.5 GPA at a civilian university because of the required athletic and military courses.

Most medical schools value a broad-based academic program. As an example, at USMA the Core Academic Program comprises 67% of the overall academic experience, but this contributes to forming well-rounded graduates able to succeed in Medical school and beyond.

Selection Criteria

The Department of Defense allocates funds for training hundreds of medical students annually to meet service-specific physician needs. Each service academy is allotted a certain number of training slots (typically less than 10% of the total number of positions). Cadets desiring medical training will be awarded those training slots if they show adequate potential for success as physicians. For example, USAFA typically allocates 18 Medical Service Corps positions for medical school annually. At USMA up to 2% (usually 10–20 cadets) of the graduating class were historically allowed to enter medical school directly after graduation if endorsed by the USMA Medical Program Advisory Committee (MPAC). In 2024 the Army G-1 asked West Point to raise the percentage from a maximum of 2% to a goal of 3%, so these numbers may change in the future.

In line with national trends, more medical school applicants and matriculants from service academies are women. As an example, in the most recent 5 years, there have been more women than men matriculating to medical school from USAFA, although there are still more men applying to medical school. From 2014 to 2023, there were 162 applicants (88 men, 74 women) and 138 matriculants (79 men, 59 women).

Cadets have two options for attending medical school: either attending the Uniformed Services University of Health Sciences (USU) as active-duty officers or attending civilian medical school as inactive reservists under their service's Health Professions Scholarship Program (HPSP). Selection for either USU or HPSP requires meeting Medical Corps academic and standardized testing standards, including a GPA greater than 3.2 and an MCAT score greater than 500 (with at least a 124 in each MCAT section). If one of these scores is below the minimum cutoff, the applicant may request a waiver and provide additional evidence demonstrating their commitment to a medical career. From 2019 to 2023, the average GPA and MCAT scores for USAFA medical school matriculants were 3.69 and 508.

Apart from selection for a training slot, the applicant must be competitive at the schools to which they apply. See Tables 5.2 and 5.3 for an aggregate of USAFA cadets' GPA and MCAT scores as well as examples of entry class GPA and MCAT scores for schools that accepted West Point cadet applicants from 2021 to 2023.

In general, the application process has become more holistic; leadership experience and extracurricular activities are given more weight, and cadets are encouraged to become well-rounded leaders of character with demonstrated interest in the medical professions. It is expected that cadets will show interest in health professions by shadowing physicians and seeking opportunities to gain experience that will help them in medical school and beyond. If a prospective applicant has no shadowing experience or it is clear that they are "getting into it for the wrong reasons," they do not receive full points for that portion of the review. A goal of

Table 5.2 Average GPA and MCAT score of USAFA medical school applicants and matriculants from 2019 to 2023

	Average GPA	Average MCAT
Applicants (2019–2023)	3.647	506.364
Matriculants (2019–2023)	3.69	508.0395

Table 5.3 Average GPA and average MCAT for schools that accepted West Point cadets during the years 2021–2023

School	Average GPA	Average MCAT
Vanderbilt	3.94	521
Harvard	3.94	520
Yale	3.93	521
University of Virginia	3.93	520
Nebraska (UNMC)	3.90	513
Stanford	3.89	519
Case Western	3.86	519
University of Arizona-Phoenix	3.84	515
UCLA	3.84	516
Texas A&M	3.84	513
Medical University of South Carolina	3.83	510
Brown	3.83	517
LSU-New Orleans	3.82	509
USC-Greenville	3.81	509
Penn State	3.81	512
Tufts	3.78	515
Dartmouth	3.77	516
Wake Forest	3.76	513
Uniformed Services University	3.76	510
Drexel	3.75	512
Medical College of Wisconsin	3.73	511
Washington State University	3.67	510
University of Texas-Houston	3.66	505
Rocky Vista University	3.55	506

200 h of healthcare volunteer work and shadowing is targeted. The application process and timeline at USMA and USNA are very similar. The interview with the selection board is one of the most important factors, along with GPA, BCPM (biology, chemistry, physics, math) GPA, and MCAT. Volunteer work, community service, research, and clinical exposure are also encouraged. At West Point, every cadet applying to medical school has undergraduate research experience. USAFA has opportunities for cadets to participate in research throughout their cadet time. There is also a 6-week dedicated summer program that allows cadets to

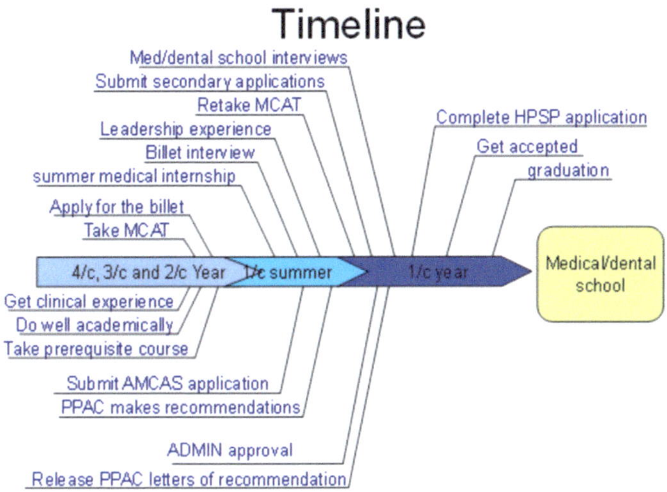

Fig. 5.1 Timeline of application requirements from USNA. https://www.usna.edu/ChemDept/ChemMajor/med-corps-info.php

partner with civilian universities and other Air Force bases for research projects.

Figure 5.1 shows a brief timeline of events and application requirements to follow for a successful HPSP application.

Applying to Medical School as an Active Duty Officer

Many service academy graduates apply to USU or compete for HPSP scholarships while on active duty. In fact, the number of USMA grads who attend med school after a period of active Army service approaches or even exceeds those who go directly. There are benefits to the leadership experience junior officership provides prior to going to medical school, but it is advisable to take the prerequisite courses while a cadet since it can be difficult to find time to take additional college-level courses while on active duty.

Medical School: Military Obligations and Medical Training

Different from their nonmedical school-bound classmates, cadets selected for medical school will be commissioned as Second Lieutenants in the Medical Services Corps (MSC, for Army and Air Force) or Ensigns in the Medical Corps (Navy) for medical school, whether in an active duty capacity (USU) or in the reserves (HPSP students in civilian programs). The current policy maintains medical students in the O-1 pay grade throughout their schooling. While in training, students are required to adhere to military policies and protocols in addition to their medical training requirements. For students at the USU, this is ingrained in their daily lives as active-duty members. For HPSP students, their military duties are limited to annual/semi-annual Active Duty Tours (ADTs) throughout their schooling (typically 1 per academic year, but the absolute number of ADTs covered varies by year) that they can use to attend courses, such as the basic officer leader course (BOLC) in the Army, or to do scheduled audition/interview rotations.

Distinct from their nonmedical classmates, medical students will bypass the O-2 (First Lieutenant/Lieutenant Junior Grade) pay grade during school and get recommissioned as an O-3 (Captain/Lieutenant) in the Medical Corps upon medical school graduation.

Somewhat distinct from civilian medical students, military medical students are required to spend time annually on active duty (ADT) performing either military training or on a service rotation. Each service requires and funds the number of ADT opportunities differently. Most students have the opportunity to complete (ADT) rotations, though the number of service-funded ADT opportunities varies by service and year. These ADT rotations are as important as interview rotations. On occasion, and if the student deems it important enough, the student may fund their own ADT as long as their medical school schedule permits. These rotations are set up differently for USU students, who are also still completing required rotations at MTFs. Most HPSP students use their ADT to perform audition rotations at military training programs (see below).

Audition Rotations

Audition rotations allow residency programs to see potential applicants for weeks in an "extended interview" while allowing the applicant extended time to see the program's culture and setting in more detail. Audition rotations are similar to students' home institution sub-internships and are especially important for military residency programs in how they rank applicants. The overall purpose of the audition rotation at military training programs is the same as for civilians: to see whether the student is a good fit for the program and vice versa. Formal interviews are also conducted while students are on site, but the entire month spent working with residents and faculty ends up being an important factor in the program's rank list of applicants. Most military general surgery programs open applications for audition rotations in the winter prior to that academic year. Applicants are typically required to send a CV, personal statement, and board scores.

USU students or students with no home institution residency program should plan to ask for letters of recommendations in their early ADT rotations. The best way to do this is to find a faculty member you work with frequently and let them know you would like to ask them for a letter of recommendation. Ask them what you can do to ensure it will be a strong letter, and follow up at the end of the rotation. These letters can carry a significant amount of weight in the military match, as many of the faculty at MTFs know and have trained with each other.

The Match

The Joint Services Graduate Medical Education Selection Board (JSGMESB, also called the military match) selection process starts earlier than, and the timeline overlaps with, the civilian match. The application platform for the military match is the

Medical Operational Data System (MODS); the platform for the civilian match is the electronic residency application service (ERAS). HPSP and USU students are encouraged to participate in both match processes and must do so simultaneously given the overlapping timelines. Both require a CV, personal statement, letters of recommendation, and medical licensing exam (Step or COMLEX) results. If the applicant attends a civilian medical school via HPSP, they should generally plan to ask for letters of recommendation from surgical mentors they have worked with as third- and fourth-year medical students. These letters of recommendation do not need to be from a military surgeon. Most programs also require either a department chair or program director (PD) letter, and medical schools often have meetings or sessions to discuss career interests and prospective programs with the chair or PD.

Air Force and Navy applicants can apply to military general surgery residencies and also have two options for civilian training: civilian deferred vs civilian sponsored, while Army applicants, in general, must be in a Tri-Service residency spot at a dedicated civilian hospital (see below) or at a military residency. Military residency programs entail a "double life" of military service obligations and surgical training subject to the same ACGME requirements as any other accredited surgery residency. In addition to surgical training, military residents are expected to comply with all service- and DoD-relevant regulations. If matched to a military position, the resident will be Active Duty during residency and will have to complete requirements like service-specific physical fitness tests. They will also receive O-3 pay in addition to Basic Allowance for Housing (BAH) and Basic Allowance for Subsistence (BAS). Most programs have partnerships with nearby civilian institutions, so residents will still have the opportunity to train in a civilian setting.

In a civilian deferred residency, the resident is an inactive reservist and considered (and paid and received benefits) the same as their institution's civilian residents. Military obligations are administered and accounted for via a branch-specific civilian training organization (e.g., the Air Force Institute of Technology's Civilian Institutions Program) and the resident has several annual "check-in" requirements. Residents are eligible to apply for fellowship training the same as those in military residencies (via the JSGMESB), or submit preferences for their first assignment during their Chief Resident year. Deferred residency training does not incur an additional duty service obligation (ADSO), but the resident also does not accrue time in service toward retirement and their eventual military pay while in residency. In a civilian-sponsored residency, the resident works at a civilian hospital, but their salary is paid by the Department of Defense and they are considered active-duty service members. This means they will have time added to the ADSO, but they are also accruing time in service.

More recently, certain civilian programs have established partnerships with the DoD, reserving 1–2 residency spots in each class for military applicants (so-called Tri-Service spots). These residency spots are considered civilian-sponsored training, meaning the residents will be paid and receive military benefits as an O-3. They are also required to fulfill active duty requirements such as PT tests, urinalysis, and other mandatory requirements. There may be an option for applicants to match directly into integrated vascular or plastic surgery residency programs through ERAS, also considered civilian-sponsored training.

Residency

After matching, residents spend the next 5–7 years in surgical training. All ACGME-accredited residency programs must fulfill core and surgery-specific requirements, leading to minor variations across the country in residency structure. Both military and civilian residencies vary in whether they offer dedicated research time, for how many residents, for how long, and when research time starts. In general, surgery programs offering dedicated research time offer 1 or 2 years, starting after the 2nd or 3rd clinical year. There are advantages and drawbacks to every research time structure. In general, research time is encouraged (or mandatory depending on the program) to make residents more competitive for fellowship and to be well-rounded surgeons. For military residents, and especially former cadets, research and fellowship must be considered carefully because of their implications for additional service commitment and future military career plans. If in military or sponsored training, each year of research entails an additional year of service commitment.

In addition to ACGME requirements, military training programs offer military-specific training opportunities for each service, ranging from didactics focused on military-specific topics to formal combat medicine/surgery coursework and fieldwork. Faculty have direct experience with military life and obligations like deployments. Though this enriches military residency programs' training experience, there are no data whether it prepares military residents better for service as military surgeons. In military residency programs, former cadets often assume peer leadership roles given their prior experience with cloistered military life and help their less-experienced colleagues adjust to military lifestyle demands.

General Surgery Residency is among the most challenging undertakings a person can do. In addition to the physical demands of working up to 80 h weekly as well as the intake and development of medical and surgical knowledge along with technical skills, the duration of training means that major life events are likely to happen during one's training. Cadets have likened residency training to their most challenging experiences at the academies and often state residency was harder given its duration and the stakes inherent in surgical patient care (frequently life and death). Depression and suicidal ideation are common in surgical residency training. Fortunately, there has been increasing emphasis on surgical trainee stresses and vulnerabilities as well as increasing support resources available. For military residents in particular, their "dual life" offers multiple avenues for support through both ACGME, surgery residency program, and their military service branch.

Fellowship Training

One of the joys of surgery residency training is identifying and nurturing an interest in a particular surgical field. Additional training in a subspecialty fellowship permits one to focus on their passion and, particularly for military residents, has profound career implications. Military residents, and especially service academy graduates, are highly regarded in fellowship application pools and benefit both from their military experience and fellowship directors' senses of patriotism and philanthropy.

Like residency, potential fellowship applicants must go through the dual process of the JSGMESB and civilian match. Except for trauma/critical care and, to a lesser extent, vascular surgery, surgical fellowship training occurs in civilian programs. The number of fellowships available or offered in the military varies yearly and is based on service-specific needs estimations. The fellowship offerings for a given match cycle are released in the summer prior to the application cycle. Historically the military values trauma surgery/critical care given its obvious operational applicability, but also sponsors subspecialty training in diverse fields as they enrich both the military training environment and trauma missions with their skill sets.

Fellowship training has profound implications for a surgeon's military career. First, it lengthens the surgeon's service commitment. Also, subspecialty training reduces the pool of available service locations given the structural support required for subspecialist practice. For example, as of this writing, Air Force surgical oncologists can work in only four military hospitals nationwide. While this restricts work placement options, it can also permit longer service in a particular area without needing to move like general surgeons. More importantly, it allows the surgeon to focus on an area they have passion for during a busy military career with expectations for local command and hospital committee work, military-specific obligations in garrison, and deployment.

Life Beyond Surgical Training

Working as an attending surgeon is the culmination of over a decade of undergraduate, medical, and residency training and is among the most fulfilling life experiences. Passing the American Board of Surgery Certifying Examination consistently ranks as a top pride-inducing experience for military surgeons. In-garrison surgical work is varied and depends on the surgeon, their local military treatment facility, and opportunities for work outside the MTF (either through memoranda of understanding with civilian hospitals or through moonlighting/Off-Duty Employment [ODE]). Like other servicemembers, surgeons are expected to progress through different leadership roles. Unlike other servicemembers, there are varying tracks through which a surgeon may progress: leadership/command, clinical expert/master clinician, or educator. Proper mentorship and an open attitude are necessary qualities to progress in any field. The importance of mentors and sponsors early in one's career cannot be overstated. Thankfully, the small community of active-duty military surgeons and the broader community of former military surgeons and their specialty organizations (e.g., the Excelsior Surgical Society and American College of Surgeons) help facilitate these relationships.

With rare exceptions, military surgeons are expected to deploy and provide surgical support to combat operations worldwide, with specific assignments varying by service branch and primary duty station. Deployments can be physically and emotionally taxing experiences but also can be fulfilling and life enriching. Life as a cadet, in general, prepares one well for the tolls of deployment, both from the early exposure to the military lifestyle as well as early installation of service core values. Service academy graduates are generally looked upon to supply leadership roles (for better or worse) given nonmedical personnel and leadership's biases regarding them and these roles should not be taken lightly.

Conclusion

The service academy cadet experience leads to success as a military surgeon. There are many leadership opportunities that service academy graduates often pursue. Not only can a military surgeon excel as a surgeon/clinically, but they are also known to excel in operational, administrative, and command positions. The military offers the opportunity to move between these career paths. Though in the military for many years due to long service obligations, there are endless opportunities and limitless success.

Acknowledgments Thank you to COL (ret) Alan Beitler, MD, Health Professions Advisor in the Office of the Dean, United States Military Academy, West Point, NY and Katherine Bates, PhD, Health Professions Advisor, United States Air Force Academy, Colorado Springs, CO.

Undergraduate Medical Education

6

Danielle B. Holt, M. H. Remondelli, M. M. Shields, M. J. Bradley, and E. A. Elster

Introduction

There are two main pathways in undergraduate medical education (UME) for individuals aspiring to become military physicians: the Uniformed Services University (USU) School of Medicine (SOM)

D. B. Holt (✉)
Office of Admissions, Uniformed Services University, Bethesda, MD, USA

Department of Surgery, Uniformed Services University, Bethesda, MD, USA
e-mail: danielle.holt@usuhs.edu

M. H. Remondelli
School of Medicine, Uniformed Services University, Bethesda, MD, USA

M. M. Shields · M. J. Bradley
Department of Surgery, Uniformed Services University, Bethesda, MD, USA

E. A. Elster
Department of Surgery, Uniformed Services University, Bethesda, MD, USA

School of Medicine, Uniformed Services University, Bethesda, MD, USA

A. T. Schlussel et al. (eds.), *The SAGES Manual for Navigating a Successful Military Surgical Career*,
https://doi.org/10.1007/978-3-031-88490-0_6

and the Health Professions Scholarship Program (HPSP) for the Air Force, Army, and Navy. The Navy also offers the Health Services Collegiate Program (HSCP), which provides a partial stipend and benefits as a civilian direct accessions program with a service obligation. Between twenty and twenty-five percent of Military Health System (MHS) physicians are graduates of USU, while HPSP graduates make up the remainder [1]. Medical students at USU pay no tuition and receive full pay and benefits as an active duty second lieutenant or ensign in exchange for 7 years of military service following residency completion. USU graduates comprise a higher proportion of senior and career military physicians within the MHS, with approximately one-third of leaders in the most senior ranks being USU graduates with nearly three-quarters of USU graduates remaining in public medical service at the local, state, or federal level after completion of their service obligation [2]. HPSP offers two, three, and 4-year scholarships that cover tuition and a living stipend with corresponding service obligations of 2, 3, and 4 years after residency training. Military physicians who enter via HPSP generally serve a total of 7–10 years depending on their selected residency, whereas many USU graduates will more often serve past their service obligation to retirement at 20 or more years. Surgical faculty also have the opportunity to participate in UME as well as pursue faculty development, certificate, and dual degree programs at USU.

Uniformed Services University School of Medicine

The only medical school owned and operated by the U.S. government, USU was founded in 1972 when Congress enacted the Uniformed Services Health Professions Revitalization Act, officially authorizing the establishment of the Uniformed Services University of the Health Sciences and the Armed Forces Health Professions Scholarship Program [3]. The Health Professions Revitalization Act envisioned USU as the "West Point" for physicians to address concerns over physician shortages following the expiration of the "doctor draft," which began during the Korean

War and ended after the Vietnam War. Located in Bethesda, MD, USU shares a campus with Walter Reed National Military Medical Center (WRNMMC) and is adjacent to the National Institute of Health. USU is accredited by the Middle States Commission on Higher Education and by the Liaison Committee on Medical Education (LCME).

USU SOM's goal is to recruit medical students with demonstrated potential for and commitment to long-term careers as medical corps officers while providing a comprehensive medical education to train the next generation of military physicians [4]. Known as "America's Medical School," USU provides medical education in a joint interagency environment. With a current class size of approximately 180 students, USU educates over 60 students in the Army along with 50 students in the Navy and Air Force within the Department of Defense, as well as 5 students in the Public Health Service under the Department of Health and Human Services, and 5 students in the Coast Guard as part of the Department of Homeland Security beginning in 2021. Both civilian and military applicants complete an application through the American Medical College Application Service (AMCAS). In 2024, USU began a binding Early Decision Program for applicants. Approximately 2,500 students apply every year for rolling admission, with an average GPA of 3.7 and an MCAT score of 510. A minimum cumulative GPA of 3.0 and an MCAT score of 496 are required for consideration at USU. Approximately 40% of USU students have prior or current military experience including attending a service academy or participation in the Reserve Officers Training Corps (ROTC), with the majority of students entering as civilians. Applicants must be US citizens and meet commissioning standards in their respective service to include a Defense Medical Readiness Board (DoDMERB) physical and medical accession standards described in DoD Instruction 6130.03.

Graduate Degrees and Certificates

The SOM is one of four schools at USU in addition to the Graduate School of Nursing, the Postgraduate Dental College, and the

College of Allied Health Sciences. The SOM also includes the Graduate Education Office (GEO), which has programs in biomedical sciences, psychology, and public health. Medical students can pursue a dual MD/PhD degree through applications to the SOM and GEO. The physician-scientist program trains 2 to 3 students through a rigorous combined curriculum over 7 to 8 years in the following disciplines: emerging infectious diseases (MD/PhDEID), molecular and cell biology (MD/PhDMCB), neuroscience (MD/PhDNES), and public health (MD/PhDPH).

Surgical faculty can pursue graduate degrees to include a Master's or PhD in Health Professions Education, Master of Public Health, or Master of Health Administration and Policy. The Center for Health Professions Education also offers distance-learning certificate programs that can build toward a master's or doctorate degree. Additional certificate programs include the Global Health Graduate Certificate Program and Training in Tropical Medicine and Traveler's Health. The SOM provides a pathway program for enlisted service members to become physicians called the Enlisted to Medical Degree Preparatory Program (EMDP2). EMDP2 is a tuition-free, 2-year, post-baccalaureate program where students serve on active duty while completing their required premedical coursework, with 15–20 students matriculating to the SOM every year.

Military Unique Curriculum

Since the University's founding, the School of Medicine has provided a curriculum that prepares students for their dual professions as physicians and military officers. USU's curriculum includes military unique training, focusing on areas such as disaster and humanitarian response, tropical medicine, global health, preventive medicine, and health systems science [5]. USU prepares students for the unique challenges they may face by incorporating key elements of military medical practice and leadership throughout the 4-year curriculum, including four medical field practicum exercises. USU, with its early clerkship introduction, unique military medicine curriculum, and hands-on field exercises, positions it as the leadership academy for training the next generation of military physicians to care for those in harm's way.

USU combines a medical school curriculum with a military-unique curriculum known as "Molecules to Military Medicine" or M2MM (Fig. 6.1). The curriculum utilizes an organ system-based approach that enables students to learn and apply the fundamentals of basic and clinical sciences with over 700 hours of military unique curriculum and 100 hours of leadership didactics and exercises. The M2MM curriculum is divided into three major segments: preclerkship, core clerkship, and postclerkship. Students complete the 16-month preclerkship period and begin working with patients early in their medical education for the year-long clerkship period, followed by a 15-month postclerkship period that includes advanced clinical rotations. Students receive dedicated hands-on instruction in the transition to clerkship and residency. During clerkships, USU medical students rotate across the United States with over 5,900 military and civilian faculty at 23 military treatment facilities (MTFs) within the MHS. USU students rotate locally with the collection of Graduate Medical Education programs in the National Capital Consortium, including WRNMMC, Alexander T. Augusta Military Medical Center at Fort Belvoir, VA, and Malcolm Grow Medical Clinics and Surgery Center at Joint Base Andrews, MD.

The military medical practice and leadership (MMPL) track represents the core of the military unique curriculum taught longitudinally during the preclerkship period. The MMPL track includes topics in professionalism, medical intelligence, health service support, medical planning and logistics, the military decision-making process, and stability operations through combat medical skills (CMS) labs teaching skills in point-of-care ultrasound, prehospital trauma life support, and tactical combat casualty care. Students engage in two field exercises, a full day of field training, and a military history "staff ride" at Antietam National Battlefield. Advanced combat medical experience, or ACME, is one of the field practicums that evaluates forward resuscitative care skills taught during CMS among teams of 2–5 students. During the summer between first and second year, USU SOM students also have

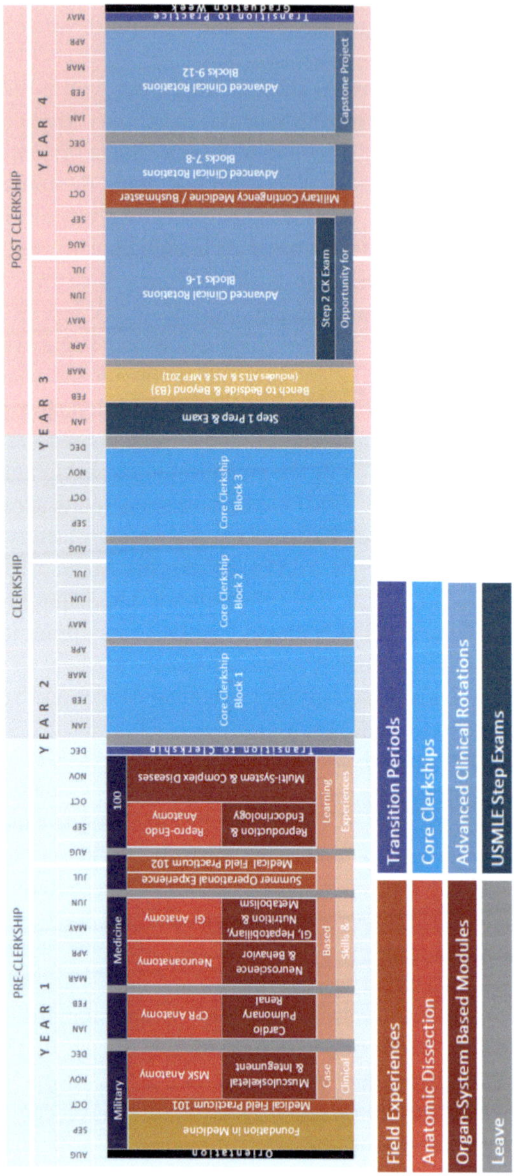

Fig. 6.1 Molecules to military medicine (M2MM) 4-year curriculum

the opportunity to take part in Summer Operational Experiences (SOEs), which increase familiarity with the medical departments' capabilities and service-specific operational environments. Examples of SOEs include the Operational Ultrasound Course, Aerospace Medicine Primary Course, Navy Shipboard Experience, Special Operations Combat Medical Sergeants Sustainment Course, and the Ranger Medic Assessment and Validation Course. Students can also pursue military training such as Airborne School, Air Assault School, Rappel Master, FRIES/SPIES Masters, Sapper School, and the Expert Field Medical Badge.

The postclerkship period consists of two medical field practicums, Operation Gunpowder and Operational Bushmaster. Operation Gunpowder places postclerkship students into leadership positions in teams of 6–8 individuals to demonstrate competency in performing tactical field care, forward resuscitative care, prolonged casualty care, and casualty evacuation over 2 days. Most notably, Operation Bushmaster is the culminating medical field practicum and one of the distinctive features of attending USU. In this 5-day mock deployment activity at Fort Indiantown Gap, Pennsylvania, students test their cumulative medical knowledge and skills following more than 3 years of the military-specific curriculum. Joined by faculty, colleagues from the Graduate School of Nursing, and international partners, students learn to respond to leadership and ethical challenges while providing combat casualty care in mock resource-limited and isolated locations. In demanding operating conditions, students rotate through the roles of combat medic, battalion surgeon, behavioral health, security, and medical logistics personnel, relying on their extensive preparation to provide combat casualty care in a dynamic environment. Bushmaster simultaneously provides both an incredibly challenging and rewarding experience offered nowhere else in American medical education.

Ultimately, the military unique curriculum prepares graduates with leadership skills specific to military medical providers, including mass casualty scenarios, disaster management, and decision-making in resource-limited environments. Throughout their educational experience, each USU student is assessed through Knowledge, Skill, and Ability (KSA) metrics to ensure they can function as a Joint Expeditionary Medical Officer (JEMO) upon graduation, regardless of their future specialty [6]. Studies indicate that USU's leadership and operational medicine training equips graduates with superior confidence and skills for successfully navigating their initial deployment [7]. USU graduates also report feeling better prepared for residency and military cultures compared to their HPSP peers [8]. As a result, 97.8% of the USU class of 2024 medical students agreed with the statement "overall, I am satisfied with the quality of my medical education" compared to 89.9% of all medical students nationally in the American Association of Medical Colleges (AAMC) medical school Graduation Questionnaire.

Longitudinal Coaching and Assessment Program

Students at USU receive longitudinal academic coaching and individualized assessment to support professional identity formation as military physicians. With 12 faculty coaching sessions throughout their four years at USU, students learn to reflect on their experiences, set goals, problem-solve, and develop action plans. National faculty coaches are available at various MTFs to provide support to students while on rotations away from USU. Faculty coaches receive over 20 hours of structured faculty development education and training in academic coaching. As USU moves toward competency-based medical education, students also have access to individual dashboards of preclinical and clinical performance to assess their progress.

Research

Research at USU spans over 15 multi-disciplinary centers that are military-relevant and DoD-focused (Table 6.1). Centers include research in combat casualty care, traumatic brain injury and regenerative medicine, behavioral health, advanced biotechnology and bioprinting, infectious diseases and immunity, cancer, human performance optimization, preventive medicine and public health, precision and personalized medicine, disaster and humani-

Table 6.1 Uniformed services university research centers

• Armed Forces Radiobiology Research Institute (AFRRI)
• Center for Deployment Psychology (CDP)
• Center for Global Health Engagement (CGHE)
• Consortium for Health and Military Performance (CHAMP)
• Center for Health Professions Education (CHPE)
• Center for Health Services Research (CHSR)
• Center for Military Precision Medicine (CMPH)
• Center for Rehabilitation Sciences Research (CRSR)
• Center for the Study of Traumatic Stress (CSTS)
• DoD Medical Ethics Center
• Defense and Veterans Center for Integrative Pain Management (DVCIPM)
• Infectious Disease Clinical Research Program (IDCRP)
• Military Traumatic Brain Injury Initiative (MTBI2)
• National Center for Disaster Medicine and Public Health (NCDMPH)
• John P. Murtha Cancer Center Research Program (MCCRP)
• Surgical Critical Care Initiative (SC2i)
• Val G. Hemming Simulation Center (SIMCEN)

tarian assistance medicine, women's health, and global surgery. According to the 2023 National Center for Science and Engineering Statistics Higher Education Research and Development Survey, USU ranks among the top 5% of institutions with over $403 million in federal research and development funding [9]. Medical students at USU have the opportunity to participate in an elective capstone research program. Students can devote up to 3 months to their faculty-led capstone research project during the post-clerkship period, which ranges from traditional basic science projects to integrative, operational, or translational clinical projects. Over 80% of medical students complete a research capstone project during their time at USU.

Surgical Faculty

There are a variety of job opportunities available to military surgeons after the completion of residency. Assignments include operational engagements attached to various deployable surgical teams, CONUS and OCONUS billets, and positions in more traditional community-based and academic-based military treatment facilities (MTFs) working with both UME and GME cadre. However, typically, positions at the teaching MTFs are staffed with surgeons with a few years of experience as a general surgeon after graduation and/or with subspecialty, fellowship training.

Academic promotion in the military follows a very similar pattern to civilian academic centers, which may not coincide with military promotion. Items to consider for academic promotion include contributions in one, or more, of the following three pillars: education, research, and clinical leadership. Educational contributions include participation in teaching both students and residents, enrollment in faculty development courses, and contributing to resident and student educational curricula (teaching and leading courses and developing curriculum). Building a research portfolio can include contributing to basic science, translational, and clinical research. Documentation of your scientific efforts, primarily through peer-reviewed publications, is a requirement. Submitting proposals and obtaining research funding is also important. There are many opportunities to chair clinical committees within the hospital or to lead your department as the chief or department head. Additionally, surgeons should be board-certified and in good clinical standing. A surgeon can focus on one or contribute to multiple pillars.

Academic appointments are obtained through the Uniformed Services University. USU School of Medicine Instruction 1100A describes the policies and procedures for faculty evaluation and academic promotion. The Department of Surgery can guide a surgeon through the professorial process. The Department can also assist with grant writing and funding for research proposals. In addition, the University offers many opportunities to participate in faculty development to support the growth of the surgeon as an educator.

Health Professional Scholarship Program (HPSP)

The Health Professions Scholarship Program (HPSP) is a competitive program offered by the Army, Navy, and Air Force that provides scholarships to medical students in exchange for a commitment to serve in the military after graduation. HPSP recipients receive full tuition coverage for up to 4 years, a monthly stipend, and funding for books and equipment, as well as pay for 45 days while on active duty for training to rotate at MTFs while in medical school. As part of the scholarship program, students fulfill a service obligation in their respective service following completion of surgical residency. Minimum academic requirements include a cumulative GPA of 3.0 and an MCAT score of 500, with at least 124 in each section. Applicants interested in HPSP apply through a healthcare recruiter through an application separate from applying to medical school. Approximately 200 scholarships are awarded yearly, with the most in the Army, followed by the Navy, and the fewest in the Air Force. Applicants must be U.S. citizens and meet commissioning requirements, including a physical examination through Military Entrance Processing Station (MEPS) or DoDMERB.

Military Benefits

USU and HPSP offer military benefits that allow students to focus on their medical education while minimizing debt. According to the AAMC, the average medical student graduates with $200,000 in debt [10]. USU students serve in an active duty status in contrast to HPSP students who serve in a reserve status with a corresponding difference in service obligation of 7 vs. 4 years. USU is tuition-free with books and instruments furnished either without charge or on a loan basis. While enrolled in the School of Medicine, students serve as active duty commissioned officers in grade O-1 (i.e., second lieutenant in the Army or Air Force, ensign

Table 6.2 Combined compensation for commissioned officers in grade O-1 at USU

Pay type	With dependents	No dependents
Annual base pay	$45,914.40	$45,914.40
BAH	$35,316.00	$32,832.00
BAS	$3,803.76	$3,803.76
Total (annual gross pay)	$85,034.16	$82,550.16

in the Navy, Coast Guard, or Public Health Service) with full pay and allowances for that grade. Base Pay, which is taxable, is based on years of service. Basic Housing Allowance (BAH) is calculated based on rent or mortgage payment amount, service member's primary duty station location, and dependent status. This allowance is provided to all service members who reside off-base and is nontaxable. Additionally, all officers receive the same set amount for Basic Allowance for Subsistence (BAS), which is also nontaxable. USU students who have prior service retain their base pay of the highest obtained rank but receive BAH and BAS at the O-1 rate. Table 6.2 depicts the annual pay for a USU student with no prior service as of January 2024.

As active duty officers, USU students receive 30 days of leave per year. USU students are also eligible for other military benefits, including the use of the commissary (military supermarket) and post exchange (military department store). Certain legal services, such as advice on income tax matters and executing personal wills, are free. Students are eligible for low-cost life insurance and are provided comprehensive medical and dental care at no charge. Medical care is provided through the military health program, TRICARE. Dependents of USU students are entitled to the same benefits as dependents of other active-duty personnel. The University also has its own campus health service, the University Family Health Center (UFHC), which is available to students and their families for medical care and counseling.

Both the Uniformed Services University and HPSP offer pathways to military medicine. Students should research both options carefully to determine which pathway is best suited for them. Table 6.3 provides a side-by-side comparison of USU and HPSP.

Table 6.3 Side-by-side comparison of UME pathways

	USU	HPSP
Application process	AMCAS application, school code 821: choose service branch if accepted to USU	Apply through service-specific medical recruiting district
Tuition	Tuition-free until graduation or disenrollment	Full tuition paid by HPSP (maximum 4 years); no payment when not enrolled full-time
Books/ instruments	Provided at no charge	Fees and charges for books and equipment vary by institution
Computers	Learning Resource Center offers computers for student use; students may also purchase their own laptops	Most institutions offer computers for student use; students may also purchase their own laptops
Pay	Full O-1 pay, with or without dependents, plus BAH and BAS	Monthly stipend of $2,728 for 10.5 months; 45 days of O-1 active duty pay + BAH and BAS (partial if government housing is provided)
Service obligation	7 years of Active Duty following GME. IRR obligation (up to 6 years) for less than 10 years of Active Duty service. GME does not count toward service obligation	4 years Active Duty following GME. IRR obligation for less than 10 years of Active Duty service. GME does not count toward service obligation. Service obligation increases to 5, 6, or 7 years for students who participate in 5-, 6-, or 7-year GME
Benefits	Active Duty benefits for self and dependents, including low-cost life insurance, free and convenient health care for self and dependents, and unlimited commissary and base exchange privileges	Active Duty benefits for self only during 45-day Active Duty periods. Limited base exchange and commissary privileges when not on Active Duty

(continued)

Table 6.3 (continued)

	USU	HPSP
GME deferments	Eligible for 1-year and full deferments	Eligible for 1-year and full deferments
Career planning	Structured coaching program offers 1:1 coaching throughout 4 years of medical school. Faculty serve as military mentors and students are offered opportunities to participate in operational activities and specialized training	Access to HPSP liaison or Professional School Liaison Officer. Operational opportunities are limited

Conclusion

The Uniformed Services University and the Health Professions Scholarship Program offer distinct UME pathways for aspiring military physicians. USU provides a fully immersive military experience with students serving on active duty and receiving a comprehensive medical education, while HPSP offers a civilian medical school education with military benefits (Table 6.4). Receiving their education in a joint environment prepares USU graduates for successful military medical careers. Through its military unique curriculum, longitudinal coaching and assessment, and research, USU's School of Medicine supports the development and sustainment of medical and operational training throughout the lifecycle of a military physician from UME to GME and CME. Surgical faculty have opportunities for teaching, research, faculty development, certificate, degree programs, and academic promotion. Both USU and HPSP provide unique opportunities for military service and medical education to "learn to care for those in harm's way."

Table 6.4 UME references and websites

USU SOM Admissions	https://medschool.usuhs.edu/admissions
Army HPSP	https://recruiting.army.mil/MRB_Physicians/
Navy HPSP	https://www.med.navy.mil/Accessions/Health-Professions-Scholarship-Program-HPSP-and-Financial-Assistance-Program-FAP/
Air Force HPSP	https://www.airforcemedicine.af.mil/Organizations/Physician-Education-Branch/Medical-School-Scholarships/
USU Research Centers	https://www.usuhs.edu/research/centers
USU Faculty Affairs	https://medschool.usuhs.edu/about/faculty-affairs
USU Department of Surgery	https://medschool.usuhs.edu/sur
USU Center for Health Professions Education	https://chpe.usuhs.edu/

References

1. USU School of Medicine Annual Report 2023. https://medschool.usuhs.edu/sites/default/files/media/documents/school_of_medicine_annual_report_2023_compressed.pdf. Accessed 11 July 24.
2. DeZee KJ, Durning SJ, Dong T, Artino AR Jr, Gilliland WR, Waechter DM, McManigle JE, Saguil A, Cruess DF, Boulet JR. Where are they now? USU School of Medicine graduates after their military obligation is complete. Mil Med. 2012;177(9 Suppl):68–71.
3. Gardner JW, Harmon S, Stavish PJ. The Uniformed Services University of the Health Sciences, F. Edward Hébert School of Medicine: status of the Federal Medical School after 25 years. Mil Med. 1998;163(5):288–94.
4. Waechter DM, Gilliland WR, Laughlin LW, The F. Edward Hébert School of Medicine model: tuition-free medical school in exchange for public service. Acad Med. 2010;85(11):1683.
5. Pock AR, Witkop CT, Reamy BV, Servey JT, Williams PM, Bunin JL. F. Edward Hébert School of Medicine, Uniformed Services University of the Health Sciences. Acad Med. 2020;95(9S A Snapshot of Medical Student Education in the United States and Canada: Reports From 145 Schools):S211–5.
6. Henderson J, Pock A, Elster E. Development of the joint expeditionary medical officer. Mil Med. 2024:usae481. https://doi.org/10.1093/milmed/usae481.

7. Cole R, Dong T, Rudinsky SL, Tilley L, Reamy BV, Durning SJ. A comparison of uniformed services university and health professions scholarship program graduates' first deployment readiness. Mil Med. 2024;189(5–6):e1190–5.
8. Cole R, Durning SJ, Reamy BV, Stewart HC, Williamson SS, Rudinsky SL. A comparison of HPSP and USU graduates' preparation for residency. Mil Med. 2023;188(Suppl 2):98–105.
9. National Center for Science and Engineering Statistics (NCSES). Higher education research and development: fiscal year 2022. NSF 24–308. Alexandria, VA: National Science Foundation; 2023. https://ncses.nsf.gov/surveys/higher-education-research-development/2022
10. https://students-residents.aamc.org/advocacy/student-debt-ensuring-medical-school-remains-affordable. Accessed 22 Sept 2024.

Graduate Medical Education 7

Matthew Bradley, Jason Babcock,
and M. Keith Sellers

What Is the Process for Applying for a Military Residency?

The military application process is done through a military-network website called the Military Operational Data System (MODS), accessible using ".mil" addresses and only through on-base computers or secure remote-access networks for those stationed in civilian locations. It is mandatory to fill out an application and submit a rank list of programs, which may include listing a civilian deferment or civilian-sponsored position (more on this below), depending on your preference and/or service requirements. Documents for submitting your MODS package include your Curriculum Vitae, medical school transcripts, STEP/COMPLEX I and II scores, and letters of recommendation.

M. Bradley
Walter Reed National Military Medical Center, Uniformed Services University of the Health Sciences, Bethesda, MD, USA

J. Babcock
David Grant Medical Center, Fairfield, CA, USA

M. K. Sellers (✉)
Walter Reed National Military Medical Center, Bethesda, MD, USA

A. T. Schlussel et al. (eds.), *The SAGES Manual for Navigating a Successful Military Surgical Career*,
https://doi.org/10.1007/978-3-031-88490-0_7

One of the most important aspects of your application process is your active-duty tours (ADTs), done during your fourth-year of medical school. These are away rotations that you will do at military treatment facilities (MTFs). These should be considered "audition" rotations and should be performed at military residency programs where you are interested in matching. As a general rule, audition rotations are much more important in the military than in the civilian match. The smaller number of applicants and residency sites makes this an essential part of the military match process. It is unusual for a top military site to match an applicant who did not rotate there as a student. It is important to make a self-assessment and review the programs before deciding on which locations to rotate. There are many online communities, particularly on social media, where one can inquire about specific programs. You should be mindful of the information you receive from online networking and do your best to verify via a more senior student, resident, faculty, or former military surgeon you trust to help make your decision. These ADTs function essentially as month-long interviews. You will get to experience a program daily, performing at a sub-internship (Sub-I) level, while a program gets to know you. In general, these ADTs are organized and funded through temporary duty (TDY) orders generated from your military command, so you get two of these between July and early October of fourth year. Currently, the Army uses one of these funded rotations to send students to basic officer training in San Antonio. Therefore, the Army will pay for only one rotation at an MTF. Students will have to use their own funds for any additional rotations. Since your application is due mid-October (usually October 15th unless it lands on a weekend day), you should ensure you are not starting a rotation after October 15th. Most medical students begin the process of deciding their desired ADTs in the second half of third year of medical school and reach out to those programs' coordinators to schedule rotation dates. This should allow time to coordinate between your medical school schedule, the schedule of the desired program, and TDY orders through your command for travel and lodging. It should be noted that while your rank list and the MODS system closes in October, the military match results are not released until mid-December every year.

As mentioned above, ranking programs in MODS includes the option of training at an MTF or training within a civilian institution. Options to train in a civilian institution include civilian deferment and civilian sponsored. In the Navy, the civilian-deferment pathway is called Navy Active Duty Delay for Specialist (NADDS), and the civilian-sponsored program is called Full-Time Outservice (FTOS). If you are anticipating ranking these particular options in MODS, then you should also be completing the civilian application process called the Electronic Residency Application Service (ERAS). Much of the required materials will overlap but will come with application fees. The ERAS application process occurs over a longer period, with application submissions beginning in September of fourth year of medical school and ending in May the following calendar year. If you rank a civilian-deferred program or a civilian-sponsored program in MODS in October and you are selected for a civilian program by the military in December, you will also need to be approved by the associated civilian residency program through ERAS. Thus, students who anticipate including a civilian-deferred or civilian-sponsored program on their rank list must start the ERAS process concurrently. Registration for the civilian match typically opens in mid-September and schools upload applicant data in early October. Interview offers for civilian programs are typically generated in late October, with interview dates spanning from early November to January. Thus, it is important to work on this pathway prior to the military match in December. It is important to understand that an ERAS application must be submitted in a timely fashion. Civilian programs have many candidates to filter through and may not see or consider a late entry even if it is from a qualified applicant.

Just like the civilian residency match, applying to a surgical specialty in the military usually means a static number of residency positions for a fluid and often larger number of applicants, regardless of the branch of service. This means whether Army, Navy, or Air Force, there is a chance an applicant will not match their specialty. We will discuss more about this below.

What Are the Different Types of Military Residencies? Are They All Active-Duty?

Full Time In-Service (FTIS)

For all training in residency programs at military treatment facilities (MTF), you are officially on active-duty military orders, which you will receive from your respective branch of service. This type of training is called full time in-service (FTIS) training. This means your salary comes from the military according to your rank, which in most cases is higher than civilian resident salaries. Your default daily attire is(are) your military uniform(s), and your appearance like hair and jewelry will need to follow military regulations. While most of the time you are focused on being a resident and wearing scrubs, the amount of time you wear the uniform varies based on your program requirements (i.e., wearing a military uniform as a dress code for academic duties and/or clinic). Being on active duty at an MTF also means you will need to satisfy nonphysician military obligations, such as annual online training, random drug screenings, height and weight recording, and physical fitness tests.

There are several Air Force FTIS military training programs that are integrated or combined with local civilian institutions. This means you are part of a civilian residency with a mix of military and civilian residents and rotate at several hospitals in a given geographical area. In these programs, unless you are at your military hospital, you look like the civilians around you, meaning no military uniform. You have a few extra duties that you can read below, but on a day-to-day basis, you are just another resident.

The three Navy and six Army FTIS training programs are not integrated or combined with a civilian institution, so the military hospital you are assigned to is the main site of your residency. However, you will likely complete away rotations to other facilities, often civilian facilities, to supplement your residency education. For example, military hospitals see pediatric dependents, but you will likely rotate through a designated children's hospital at some point in residency to fully experience pediatric care related to your specialty. Since you will spend a greater amount of time at a military site, you will be more entrenched in military processes, customs and courtesies, and in military surgical training.

Full Time Out-Service (FTOS) or Civilian Sponsored

Another residency option is commissioning on to active-duty service but training at a civilian residency. This is known as full time out-service (FTOS) training in the Navy, or Civilian Sponsored in the Army and Air Force. Your salary comes from the military, but your residency location is 100% in a civilian program. You will be attached to a nearby military unit, usually a reserve unit, for paperwork and administrative functions. There are five dedicated tri-service and two Army-only FTOS/civilian-sponsored positions available for medical students. The tri-service positions are also available to Army, Navy, and Air Force preliminary ("pre-lim") interns, Transitional Year interns, and General Medical Officers ("GMO"-physicians who completed an internship and are working as general physicians for various military units). These civilian programs put aside active-duty slots that get filled through the military match pathway in December. It should be noted that the civilian institution gets the final approval of the military applicant so it is possible for any one of these civilian positions to go unfilled.

In the Navy, there are other FTOS positions offered to preliminary interns and GMOs. These spots are unrelated to the aforementioned FTOS positions. That is, these additional FTOS spots are not prearranged categorical positions with civilian institutions. Therefore, prospective residents would need to apply and match through ERAS if wishing to pursue one of these FTOS positions. The number of these FTOS offerings is usually in the single digits per year, typically around five.

Civilian Sponsored

Some services allow for training at a civilian residency while not on "active-duty" status. You are a civilian for your time in residency. This would mean that you will be in a special category of military service, not active duty or reserves, without the military responsibilities of the FTIS or FTOS programs. However, the military will be responsible for your salary and other benefits, hence the term "sponsored." These positions are not set aside by civilian programs as "active-duty slots" like FTOS positions. Hence, if you rank a civilian-sponsored position in MODS and you are selected for that position, you would then be responsible for being accepted into a civilian residency through ERAS. Once you complete your residency, you will be expected to return to military service as active duty and complete your service obligation. It's important to know that because the military is paying for your residency, but you are not serving as an active-duty military resident at a military facility, this will accrue additional years of service to your service obligation.

Civilian Deferment or Navy Active Duty Delay for Specialist (NADDS)

Some services allow for training at a civilian residency (again, if successfully matched on ERAS) where your service obligation is considered "deferred." During your deferment, you are temporarily released from active duty and placed in the Individual Ready Reserves (IRR) so the civilian residency will be responsible for your salary and any other benefits. Since you are supported by the civilian program and not by the military during residency, this does not add on additional years to your service obligation. Once you complete your residency, you will be expected to return to military service as active duty and complete your original obligated years of service. Residents in the Navy NADDS program will also need to maintain a yearly officer evaluation form called a Fitness Report, or FitRep.

Preliminary Interns, Transitional Year Interns, and General Medical Officers

If you do not match to your selected specialty, the supervisors of the military match process will work with you to place you in a pre-liminary (pre-lim) internship in surgery or a transitional year

(TY) position. The TY year typically involves rotating through a broader range of disciplines and specialties, organized by your own program director within Graduate Medical Education (GME). After completing a pre-lim or TY intern year, you may reapply for your desired specialty and repeat the application and interview process, this time with more experience, but without the opportunity to complete away rotations at desired programs. If an applicant does not match their specialty after prelim year, the Air Force and the Navy require a minimum two years of service as a General Medical Officer (GMO).

It is important to remember that regardless of your training status, your daily focus is on being a surgical resident, learning and providing patient care.

Are There Different Educational or Training Opportunities During Military Residency?

In general, the answer is no. There are requirements by the Accreditation Council for Graduate Medical Education (ACGME) and American Board of Surgery that residents and programs need to meet (e.g., total case numbers and defined category cases), thus prohibiting programs from creating drastically different training tracks within their residency programs. All residents in a program must get about the same training. There are a few opportunities for unique rotations, such as an intensive care unit (ICU) rotation at Landstuhl, Germany. Some programs incorporate a research year into their program, typically between post-graduate year two (PGY2) and PGY3 or between PGY3 and PGY4. There are several unique research opportunities within the military, particularly regarding global health, such as participating in research with the military hospital in Qatar. During your research year, there are opportunities to obtain an advanced degree (Master in Health Professions Education or Master in Public Health) within the military at the Uniformed Services University, which is free and without additional military commitment. Alternatively, you may be eligible to attend civilian graduate education courses and secure a scholarship from a civilian institution.

What Additional Responsibilities/Benefits Come with Being an Active-Duty Military Resident?

In addition to being a resident, you are also an active-duty member of the United States Military. This does come with extra responsibilities. This includes physical fitness: you must take and pass physical fitness (PT) tests. Height and weight measurements are taken to maintain standards of body composition, and given the diversity within body mass index (BMI), supplementary measures can be used such as waist circumference measurement or other methods of body fat determination. If these standards are repeatedly not met, it can hinder military rank promotion. Also, there are random drug screenings for all active-duty members. These happen at least once a year. The military needs 100% accountability for you at all times, so when you take a vacation (called "leave" in the military), you must get permission from both your program leadership and your military administrative chain of command. If you simply leave the area (i.e., >250 mile radius of your duty station) without permission, this is considered being absent without leave (AWOL), which can have negative consequences for both your program and chain of command. The military also provides an annual dental exam, hearing exam, and periodic health assessment (PHA) to ensure you are up to date on items such as immunizations and any age-appropriate laboratory analyses like cholesterol levels. Finally, there will be mandatory online or computer-based training (CBT) that will need to be completed throughout the year.

There are also benefits that go with these responsibilities. These benefits are largely twofold; first, is that you are nearly always paid more than your civilian counterparts. You have your base pay, based on your military rank (grade O-3 after medical school graduation, often promoted to O-4 after 6 years of active duty), and then you get a bonus for having a medical license starting your second year of residency. On top of these payments is your BAH, or basic allowance for housing (tax-free), which varies depending on your residency's geographic area, and your BAS, basic allowance for subsistence. On average, this results in $30,000–$40,000 more in your annual salary than civilian or nonactive-duty residents. You are eligible for other military benefits like any active-duty service member, such as a Veterans Affairs (VA) housing loan, GI Bill benefits, health insurance through Tricare, pay-in life insurance, and pay-in savings/retirement financial planning. The second category of benefit is that you are accruing active-duty time toward retirement while you are a resident, so if you plan to stay on active duty for 20 years (the earliest amount of time to receive a pension), then your residency years count toward that.

How Does the Lifestyle of Being a Military Resident Compare to That of a Civilian?

The differences between military and civilian residency depend largely on your residency. The more integrated a military residency is with a civilian program, the less of a difference exists. On one extreme, in a fully civilian-integrated program, there is little to tell a civilian or active-duty resident apart on a day-to-day basis. On the other extreme, in standalone military residencies, the residents work at military treatment facilities (MTFs) and so, depending on the military installation, may be required to wear their uniforms on a daily basis, especially when arriving and departing work. Regardless, the focus is still on training and patient care. It should be noted that while it is not an official policy, active-duty residents have not been included in the pool of deployable surgeons. However, deploying residents could be possible if the needs of the military should require it.

How Will My Opportunities Be Different After Completing a Military Residency?

You will still be eligible to apply for a fellowship after residency. However, this opportunity has to be in step with the needs of the military at that time. For example, if you are in the Army and want to do a 2-year Pediatric Surgery fellowship, the Army would have to anticipate needing another Pediatric Surgeon in 2 years time. So, in your second-to-last year of residency, the Army would have to approve your ability to apply for your desired fellowship, and then you would still have to be accepted to a fellowship program. There are only two surgical fellowship programs within the military (Vascular Surgery at Walter Reed and Trauma/Critical Care at Brooke Army Medical Center), so again, a civilian application process would need to be completed. In general, training at a civilian program would be similar to an FTOS residency position, in that you would be active duty, supported by the military, but working at a civilian center full time. This would again accrue additional years of service obligation. Generally, a one-year fellowship accrues two more years of service, and a two-year fellowship accrues three more years of service.

However, if you do not want to go into fellowship, or your branch of service does not anticipate a need for another fellowship-trained surgeon at the time you are completing residency, you will complete the board-certification process for your residency and then be assigned a duty station based on the needs of the military (and your input). You will be eligible for deployment. You will be assigned to a military unit that could range from a large military hospital in the United States to a small medical facility anywhere across the world. This may provide more exposure to non-medical military activity and opportunities for additional non-medical military training if desired (as long as that training matches the needs and resources available). Every year, the approval process repeats for fellowship opportunities, and seniority is weighed alongside many other factors, thus giving you another chance for approval to apply for the fellowship.

Once graduated from residency, it is important to note that you will be considered a *military* and *medical* leader. This comes with the honor and duty of being an officer of significant ranking in a military unit. Non-medical military members expect you to act with the military experience of any other O-3 or O-4 officer, while medical military members may look to you as the most senior medical provider for hundreds of miles. If you are one of two surgeons in the country on deployment, you may be the chief of the surgery department soon after graduating residency. These unique challenges (while better informed by an active-duty residency) can be daunting but also incredibly rewarding for personal growth and fulfillment. In addition, when you feel it is time to complete your military service, these experiences will be unlike your civilian counterparts and can elevate your patient care for the rest of your surgical career.

Graduate medical education points-of-contact and other related information		Health.mil/Military-Health-Topics/DHA-GME		
		Army	Navy	Air force
Applying for military residency	Match timeline	Fourth Year of Medical School – Sub-Internship Audition Rotations at MTFs July–October – ERAS Application Early September – MODS Application Due October 15 (MODS site opens July 1) – Military Match Day released on a middle Wednesday in December – Civilian Match Day March 15		
	Distribution of programs	FTIS—6 programs	FTIS—3 programs	FTIS—5 programs
		FTOS—5 tri-service, 2 Army-Only	FTOS—5 tri-service FTOS—pre-lim, GMO only	FTOS—5 tri-service
		Civilian sponsored—rare	Civilian sponsored—rare	Civilian Sponsored—rare
		Civilian deferred - rare	Civilian deferred—common every year	Civilian Deferred—common every year
	Military hospitals available for residency and location	**Tripler Army Medical Center:** Honolulu, HI **Madigan Army Medical Center** (Joint-Base Lewis-McChord): Tacoma, WA **Womack Army Medical Center** (Fort Liberty): Fayetteville, NC **William Beaumont Army Medical Center** (Fort Bliss): El Paso, TX **San Antonio Military Medical Center/Brooke Army Medical Center** (Joint Base San Antonio-Fort Sam Houston): San Antonio, TX **Eisenhower Army Medical Center** (Fort Eisenhower): Augusta, GA **Walter Reed National Military Medical Center**/National Capital Consortium: Bethesda, MD	**Naval Medical Center San Diego**: San Diego, CA **Naval Medical Center Portsmouth**: Portsmouth, VA **Walter Reed National Military Medical Center/** National Capital Consortium: Bethesda, MD	**University of Mississippi/Keesler Medical Center**: Biloxi, MS **University of Nevada Las Vegas/Mike O'Callaghan Medical Center** (Nellis Air Force Base (AFB)): Las Vegas, NV **Wright State University/Wright-Patterson Medical Center**: Dayton, OH **University of California, Davis/David Grant Medical Center** (Travis AFB): Fairfield, CA **San Antonio Military Medical Center/Brooke Army Medical Center** (Joint Base San Antonio-Fort Sam Houston): San Antonio, TX

(continued)

Graduate medical education points-of-contact and other related information		Health.mil/Military-Health-Topics/DHA-GME		
		Army	Navy	Air force
Education components of GME	Yearly fellowship spots at military hospitals—FTIS (remainder are FTOS)	**Trauma**—San Antonio Military Medical Center/Brooke Army Medical Center (Joint Base San Antonio-Fort Sam Houston) **Vascular**—Walter Reed National Military Medical Center/ National Capital Consortium	**Vascular**—Walter Reed National Military Medical Center/National Capital Consortium	**Trauma**—San Antonio Military Medical Center/ Brooke Army Medical Center (Joint Base San Antonio-Fort Sam Houston)
Additional responsibil-ities of military residency	Physical requirements + initial medical clearance	Height/Weight/Tape Chart Branch-Specific Physical Fitness Test—Minimum Standards Random Urinalysis Drug Screening (~every 2 months) Annual Periodic Health Assessment (PHA) with General Practitioner Annual Hearing and Dental Screenings		
	Additional training requirements	Annual Online HIPAA and Cyber Security Awareness Training Sexual Harassment/Assault Response and Prevention (SHARP) In-Person Training Other assigned trainings can be location dependent		
	Evaluation/ promotion timeline	O-1 >> O-3 After Med School O-3 >> O-4 ~6 years of service after O-3 promotion O-4 >> O-5 Variable ("in-promotional-zone" 6 years after O-4 promotion) O-5 >> O-6 Variable ("in-zone" 6 years after O-5 promotion)		
	Annual report needed for promotion	Officer Evaluation Report (OER)	Fitness Report (FitRep)	Annual Training Evaluations

Financial/ logistical differences between military and civilian residency	Signing bonus	Retention bonus after initially completing service obligation (Further information regarding DoD and branch-specific special pay are publicly available online)		
	Expected officer salary	By rank and time in service (also publicly available online)		
	Salary bonuses/ increases	After 2 years as a physician (obtaining medical license)	After 2 years as a physician (obtaining medical license)	Annual After Board Certification
	Basic allowance for housing	Tax-Free "Income"—a significant source of salary, putting the remainder of salary in a lower tax bracket		
	Retirement planning	Thrift Savings Plan Retirement Pension after 20 years (50% of salary at time of retirement)		
	Life insurance	Pay-in for up to $500,000 maximum policy		
	Disability insurance	Limited plans while active-duty military, but still available through private insurance companies		
	Healthcare	Tricare select/prime		
	Additional benefits	Medical licensing fees paid-for GI Bill VA Home Loan		

Part II

The Organizations

8 Defense Health Agency

Brian C. Lein

The Defense Health Agency's (DHA) role in the delivery of healthcare in our military hospitals has changed significantly over the last 20 years. It will be very important for you to understand the authorities and responsibilities of the DHA as you progress in your military and medical career. Prior to 2012, the DHA did not exist, and military service medical departments were responsible for the oversight of the delivery of healthcare, the medical budget, and every other aspect of healthcare and readiness. Since the end of World War II, over 17 different studies have looked at improvements in the oversight and management of the complex military medical system. In 2013, Department of Defense Directive 5136.13, DHA, was published, standing up the DHA. This initial

B. C. Lein (✉)
USUHS Department of Surgery, F Edward Hebert School of Medicine, Bethesda, MD, USA
e-mail: brian.c.lein.civ@health.mil

A. T. Schlussel et al. (eds.), *The SAGES Manual for Navigating a Successful Military Surgical Career*,
https://doi.org/10.1007/978-3-031-88490-0_8

oversight was limited in scope, responsibility, and authority and prompted further analysis, which culminated in the landmark decision codified in the National Defense Authorization Act of 2017.

This act of Congress significantly and fundamentally changed the oversight of military healthcare, directing that the role and responsibility of all healthcare delivery in our hospitals and clinics belong to the DHA. From 2017 to 2023, it took tremendous effort to complete the transition of these oversight functions from the military service medical departments to the DHA.

The DHA is run by a military Director and has four main sections: Healthcare Administration, Joint staff function for operations and plans J-3/5/7, Support and Component Acquisition Executive, and Resources and Personnel Integration. The DHA is a joint, integrated Combat Support Agency (CSA) that enables the Army, Navy, and Air Force medical services to supply a medically ready force and ready medical force to Combatant Commands in both peacetime and wartime.

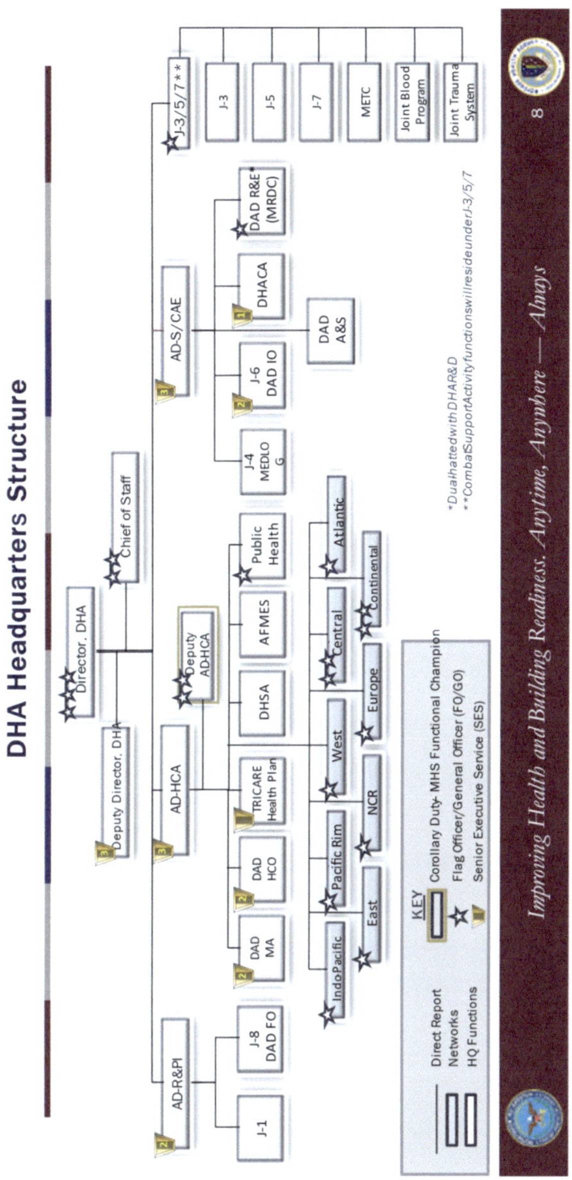
DHA Headquarters Structure
Director, DHA
Deputy Director, DHA
Chief of Staff
AD-R&PI
AD-HCA
Deputy AD-HCA
AD-S/CAE
J-3/5/7**
J-1
J-8 DAD FO
DAD MA
DAD HCO
TRICARE Health Plan
DHSA
AFMES
Public Health
J-4 MEDLOG
J-6 DAD IO
DHACA
DAD R&E* (MRDC)
DAD A&S
J-3
J-5
J-7
METC
Joint Blood Program
Joint Trauma System
IndoPacific
East
Pacific Rim
NCR
West
Europe
Central
Continental
Atlantic
Direct Report
Networks
HQ Functions
KEY
Corollary Duty- MHS Functional Champion
Flag Officer/General Officer (FO/GO)
Senior Executive Service (SES)
*DualhattedwithDHAR&D
**CombatSupportActivityfunctionswillresideunderJ-3/5/7
Improving Health and Building Readiness. Anytime, Anywhere — Always
8

Mission: The DHA supports our Nation by improving health and building readiness—making extraordinary experiences ordinary and exceptional outcomes routine.

Vision: Unrelenting pursuit of excellence as we care for our joint force and those that we are privileged to serve. Anytime, Anywhere—Always.

It is an integrated model of healthcare delivery and one of the most complex worldwide healthcare organizations. The oversight of the hospitals and clinics is directed through the network structure. Nine networks run the day-to-day execution of healthcare delivery and oversight. These nine networks are led by Flag and General Officers from the Army, Navy, and Air Force who are responsible for their service commands missions, as well as the direction and oversight delegated from the DHA Director for the healthcare delivery at each hospital and clinic. The following sections will further define the roles and responsibilities as they directly or indirectly impact your profession. The picture below provides a broad view of the magnitude of responsibilities of the DHA.

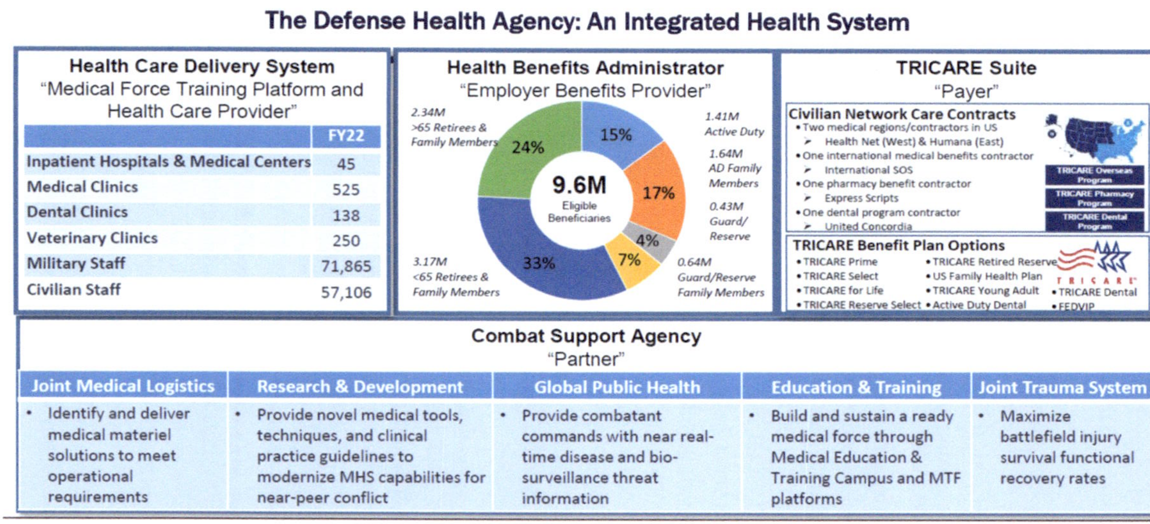
The Defense Health Agency: An Integrated Health System
Health Care Delivery System
"Medical Force Training Platform and Health Care Provider"
FY22
Inpatient Hospitals & Medical Centers 45
Medical Clinics 525
Dental Clinics 138
Veterinary Clinics 250
Military Staff 71,865
Civilian Staff 57,106
Health Benefits Administrator
"Employer Benefits Provider"
9.6M
Eligible Beneficiaries
2.34M >65 Retirees & Family Members 24%
1.41M Active Duty 15%
1.64M AD Family Members 17%
0.43M Guard/ Reserve 4%
0.64M Guard/Reserve Family Members 7%
3.17M <65 Retirees & Family Members 33%
TRICARE Suite
"Payer"
Civilian Network Care Contracts
• Two medical regions/contractors in US
➢ Health Net (West) & Humana (East)
• One international medical benefits contractor
➢ International SOS
• One pharmacy benefit contractor
➢ Express Scripts
• One dental program contractor
➢ United Concordia
TRICARE Overseas Program
TRICARE Pharmacy Program
TRICARE Dental Program
TRICARE Benefit Plan Options
• TRICARE Prime
• TRICARE Select
• TRICARE for Life
• TRICARE Reserve Select
• TRICARE Retired Reserve
• US Family Health Plan
• TRICARE Young Adult
• Active Duty Dental
• TRICARE Dental
• FEDVIP
TRICARE
Combat Support Agency
"Partner"
Joint Medical Logistics
• Identify and deliver medical materiel solutions to meet operational requirements
Research & Development
• Provide novel medical tools, techniques, and clinical practice guidelines to modernize MHS capabilities for near-peer conflict
Global Public Health
• Provide combatant commands with near real-time disease and bio-surveillance threat information
Education & Training
• Build and sustain a ready medical force through Medical Education & Training Campus and MTF platforms
Joint Trauma System
• Maximize battlefield injury survival functional recovery rates

Deputy Assistant Director for Medical Affairs

The Deputy Assistant Director for Medical Affairs (DAD MA) also serves in the role of Chief Medical Officer for the Military Health System. This office is responsible for policies and oversight of quality, safety, credentialing and privileging, as well as oversight of the Clinical Quality Management, Impaired Provider Program, and reporting of adverse actions to appropriate agencies.

All of our hospitals and clinics require continuous accreditation by the Joint Commission. Additionally, all of our facilities that perform surgical care are required to partake in the National Surgical Quality Improvement Program by the American College of Surgeons. All obstetric care is also required to be overseen by the National Perinatal Information Center. And our hospitals are required to undergo certification for other external national accreditations, including Leapfrog, ACS Committee on Trauma, and College of American Pathologists, to just name a few. Our facilities are among the most inspected in the United States because of these rigorous oversight programs.

Additionally, Medical Affairs is responsible for practice guidelines and parameters for each specialty. Relying on military experts in each specialty, the Medical Affairs team continually updates practice guidelines through published memoranda and weekly updates at the hospital and clinic levels. As you develop in your military and medical career, you will likely be asked to assist in the development of these guidelines as well as provide expert guidance on quality and safety oversight.

Medical Affairs is also responsible for the oversight of all Graduate Medical Education within the DHA. With over 100 residencies and fellowships in over 15 hospitals, DHA runs one of the largest GME programs in the nation. The DHA GME website https://www.health.mil/Military-Health-Topics/DHA-GME allows you to search residencies and fellowships by location and by branch of service. While the military services determine the number and type of physicians necessary for training, the oversight and development of all GME rest with Medical Affairs.

Healthcare Operations

The Deputy Assistant Director for Healthcare Operations (HCO) will have a profound impact on how you will be delivering healthcare. HCO develops standards for all aspects of how you will interact with your patients. Various policies define how standardized templates for clinical practice, both inpatient and outpatient, are used. These standards are based upon the experience and input of your current military leaders in your clinical communities and validated against best practices in civilian healthcare.

Over the last several years, the MHS has fully fielded an Electronic Health Record, MHS GENESIS, at every one of our hospitals and clinics. MHS GENESIS currently captures all inpatient, outpatient, virtual, and emergent encounters within our facilities. Over the next 3–5 years, HCO will be driving standardization of workflows and documentation and optimizing support for everything from appointing and coding to guideline development. Your expertise will be relied upon extensively as we build out the capability of this system-developing clinical pathways, standardizing surgical workflows, standardizing the vast majority of OR, clinic and inpatient coding, and aligning work to cost centers within your clinics will be invaluable.

HCO is leading the effort to develop a virtual digital interface with our patients. As we evolve from a sole face-to-face disease management healthcare delivery model to one focused on improving the health and wellness of our patients, the process and schedule of patient and provider interactions will change drastically. Working with our civilian healthcare partners, we will learn from those on the cutting edge of healthcare delivery to markedly change our current model of healthcare delivery.

Additionally, HCO oversees all aspects of our pharmacy benefits. Working with Medical Affairs, HCO is working to standardize the management of our formulary, the process for adding new drugs for our patients, and the operation of our inpatient, outpatient, and mail order pharmacies.

TRICARE Health Plan

TRICARE is similar to an insurance program in civilian healthcare. It is an entitlement of our 9.6 million beneficiaries around the world. This plan covers four main areas: healthcare delivery via TRICARE Health Plans, both in the United States and overseas, a TRICARE Dental Plan, and a TRICARE Pharmacy Plan. It is well beyond the scope of this chapter to go into depth on the coverage and benefits associated with these plans. The TRICARE website is the best source of information for you and your patients (https://www.tricare.mil/) and will be invaluable throughout your military career. The team of professionals at DHA oversees all aspects of these plans and works with your hospitals, physicians, and individual patients on the delivery of this entitlement.

Support

The responsibilities of the Assistant Director for Support are critical to daily operations in your hospitals and clinics. The oversight of all contracting actions and agreements, medical logistics, IT Support, and Medical Education and Training occurs within AD-S and will impact all aspects of your work. Over the past 3 years, a standardized approach to contracting support at all hospitals and clinics has been developed. This effort at standardization and centralization, where appropriate, has saved hundreds of millions of dollars, as well as eliminated duplicative and underperforming contracts. This section provides assistance to find the best practices and methods for contracting for routine and emergent personnel, equipment, and logistical support. All contracting is now overseen by contract specialists and captured in a centralized database for review and optimization.

Every agreement between your hospital and the community, whether it's with your military installation, agreements with downtown hospitals, or nursing, medical or dental schools, or any other programs of mutual support are overseen by the contract agreement's office. This office ensures we are keeping within the legal and ethical relationships of the Department of Defense, as well as providing standardized templates to expedite these agreements, where optimal. Your local MTF will be responsible for developing and coordinating any off-duty employment contracts, along with your initial point of contact for any support you will need for contracts and agreements. In most MTFs, this function falls within the responsibility of the Deputy for Administration.

Over the past decade, significant improvements in medical logistical support have been made possible by the increased oversight of medical logistics equipment. These sections oversee almost every purchase of equipment, medical supplies, and maintenance at your hospital. These support offices rely on you as clinicians to decide the best devices to purchase and then work to standardize the purchase, connectivity, and use within our hospitals. As much as possible, using the same radiologic, laboratory, communications, and patient treatment equipment standardizes care, eliminates duplication, and makes it easier for repair, replacement, and life cycle management of these costly devices.

Your IT support for all software, hardware, connectivity, and applications has been one of the most recognized accomplishments within the DHA. Elevating all hospitals and clinics to one standard of connectivity; using similar systems architectures across our hundreds of hospitals and clinics; purchasing and standardizing everything from computers, phone systems, Digital Patient Monitoring devices, and hundreds of other software systems has simplified how you will access all patient systems. Each hospital has its own IT support that can provide direct support at your worksite. This directorate is also instrumental in ensuring all of our software and hardware devices are cyber-secure and can be connected to our vast network of systems, so the data are readily available to both the provider and the patient.

The Research and Engineering directorate is responsible for the oversight of over $2 billion in research funding, as well as the oversight of labs across the United States and overseas. This robust clinical and bench research directorate guides requirement-driven, military-relevant research. It is responsible for material and clinical solutions that have proven fundamental in saving lives both on the battlefield as well as in our hospitals and clinics. Research on trauma, infectious diseases, brain injury, PTSD, cancer, prolonged casualty care on the battlefield, rehabilitation, vaccines, chemical and biologic weapons treatment and prophylaxis, radiation injury, and treatment are among the hundreds of research protocols actively ongoing throughout the Department of Defense. This directorate also works with other federal agencies and civilian universities and academic centers to partner in much of this groundbreaking research. For general surgeons, this will be very useful for identifying where grant and research money will be available for key interest areas. Medical Research and Development Command, USUHS, and direct congressional funding (Congressionally Directed Medical Research Program/CDMRP) are all sources of funds for research opportunities. Each currently has its own pathway for applications and oversight. Additionally, your parent MTF also has some R&D money, especially if you are at a teaching facility, to use for education and development of the residents/students.

J3/5/7

The role of this directorate is to coordinate all actions and taskings, requests for information, and support across the DHA, between DHA and the Services, DHA and the Department of Defense, and DHA and the subordinate networks and solo organizations. It has a staff of medical planners and coordinators who are responsible for getting answers quickly and getting needed support across the entire MHS. These actions are executed through the J3 in conjunction with the Defense Health Support Activities which work directly with the networks and combatant command liaison officers (LNO). This 24/7/365 operations function responds to routine and crisis efforts and is responsible for coordinating the effort across the DHA headquarters to support urgent and routine demands.

Also included in this directorate is the J5, a robust analytics and evaluation team. This organization is responsible for internal and external requests for analysis of our data, including hospital or clinic information, COVID response data, financial data, etc.

Requests for and support of data are all controlled centrally managed and analyzed through this team of professionals.

Finally, the last section in the J3/5/7 is the J7 or the Education and Training Directorate. Prior to 2017, all classes and training required for persons in leadership positions were provided by the Services, often in conjunction with precommand service courses. These responsibilities have now been transferred to the DHA. Classes for Group Practice Managers, Chief Medical, Dental, and Nursing Officers, and predirectorship training are all scheduled and developed by the DHA in the Education and Training Division. Over the next 3–5 years, additional classes will be developed for personnel in multiple levels of management within our hospitals and clinics. These courses will be advertised and available through Joint Knowledge Online or through the DHA Academy, which will be the central clearinghouse for all courses. Additionally, our education and training section oversees the Medical Education and Training Campus, responsible for the training of most of our enlisted specialties, which is located at Joint Base San Antonio and other training campuses across the United States.

Resources and Personnel Integration

This directorate is responsible for three major areas affecting the daily work in our hospitals and clinics—budget and finance (J8), personnel (J1), and facilities. The J8 is responsible for the daily oversight of the budgetary process. Your MTF director annually submits the budgetary requirements for your hospital or clinic, which includes the funding for civilian personnel, contracts, medical logistics, pharmacy, travel, equipment, and supplies. Additionally, this budget request also includes the expected workload, such as patients seen, operative cases done, babies delivered, prescriptions filled, and laboratory and radiology studies completed. This complex budget process is agreed upon, goals are established, and budget execution and workload production are measured monthly. Quarterly and midyear adjustments are made to ensure solvency at the MTF level. Unexpected bills, such as unexpected staff departures due to deployments or infrastructure crises due to natural disasters, are resolved at the Network and DHA level. Additionally, the J8 is responsible for developing the long-term budget strategy for the DHA (explained later), building a five-year budgetary forecast (POM—Program Objective Memorandum) for all hospitals, clinics, research, Public Health, etc. to align the future budgetary process with strategic goals established by the Director and the Office of Secretary of Defense. This is a gross oversimplification of the expansive role and responsibility of the J8. However, your daily responsibility for stewardship of resources and accountability of time, workload, and healthcare delivery are critical to the accuracy of data used to determine the funding for your hospital or clinic and all facilities within the MHS.

The role of the J1 is to develop and execute policies to manage the military and civilian workforce. As of today, over 140,000 people work in the MHS across the United States and dozens of countries around the globe. The policies that address all aspects of the workplace—recruiting, hiring, onboarding, retention, union management, conflict resolution, Equal Opportunity, awards and recognitions, ratings, evaluations, and the myriad of other personnel functions—are coordinated through this directorate. Each hospital has a manpower and personnel staff section that can assist you with any personnel issues. The other critical function of the J1 is the Human Capital Development Strategy. The J1, in coordination with the J8, the military services, and Healthcare Operations, hosts an annual summit to build the framework for staffing our hospitals, especially as it relates to the alignment of military medical personnel. This process starts by gathering many different data points and requirements including the patient population and service readiness requirements; evaluation of the capability of the surrounding civilian healthcare system to absorb workload; and our training requirements for GME, enlisted training, Healthcare Professional Nursing and Admin training, to build the personnel requirements for each hospital and clinic. Together with the military services, we also identify the expected needs of installation comments. Using all this information, we build and publish the Human Capital Development Plan (HCDP), which aligns military staff to hospitals and clinics based on need. The HCDP derives its source documents from the Defense Health Agency for the overall staffing model (Joint Table of Distribution/JTD). Each service medical personnel office is responsible for providing the numbers and types of physicians, nurses, etc., available for inventory to manage this process.

The Facilities Engineering branch is responsible for all aspects of facility management within the DHA. DHA is responsible for over 10,000 buildings across the globe. Daily operations, safety upgrades, new design builds, emergency repairs and maintenance, and Sustainment, Restoration, and Modernization (SRM) are centrally managed by this section. Your local facilities manager is critical to this process by ensuring the status and quality of the building and all utilities, facilitating the daily upkeep, and projecting new needs and repairs are all done at the local level and then fed into a system that tracks every facility in the DHA inventory.

As you can see, the R&PI directorate has a daily impact on your ability to work and the care your patients receive. While much is controlled centrally, understanding who oversees the budget, personnel, and facility at your local hospital or clinic will be critical for your success and will ensure you can optimize the healthcare you deliver.

Strategic Plan

Both the below Military Health System (MHS) and DHA strategy are living documents and currently under review as we continue to modernize and improve our vision. The ones below are current as of the time the chapter was written, but will likely be historical by the time of publication. However, the links provided will present the most updated strategies for your use. Two very important documents have been published—The MHS Strategic Plan and the DHA Strategic Plan. These documents are available on DHA Sharepoint sites as well as on Health.mil websites. Both of these documents lay out where we are going as healthcare providers, the status of our healthcare system, areas of focus and directed improvement, and opportunities for rapid innovation. The MHS Strategy is strongly based on the National

Defense Strategy and the National Military Strategy. The DHA Strategic Plan is nested within the goals and objectives of the MHS Strategy. The diagram below is a representative pictorial of the guiding principles—People, Service, and Health—which are the pillars of the strategy and align with our national goals of building and maintaining a medically ready force and a ready medical force and focusing on healthcare delivery. The Assistant Secretary of Defense for Health Affairs has stated the strategic goals as taking care of our people, stabilizing and modernizing our military health system, and integrating our capabilities. It will be imperative for all of us to understand how we individually contribute to the success of each of these strategic goals. Each goal has measures and key areas that we will be responsible for within our hospitals and clinics. The details of all of the initiatives supporting this plan are beyond the scope of this chapter, but for more details, I recommend you read through the strategy document as part of your onboarding into the MHS.

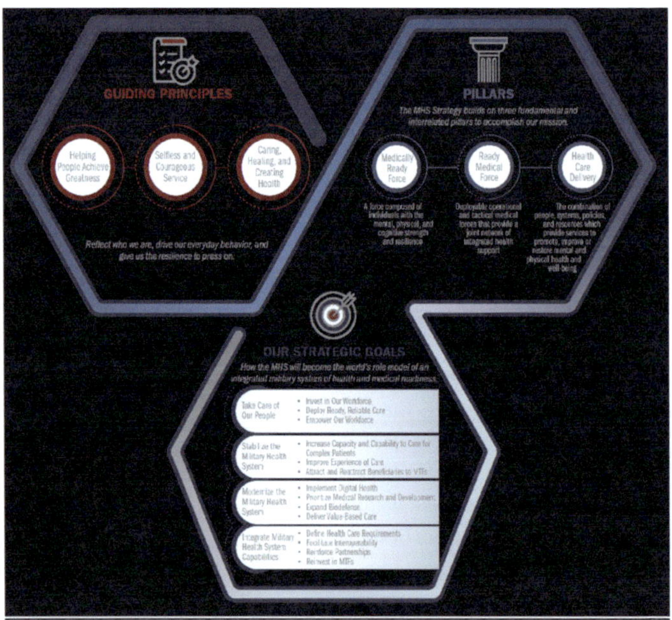

We are all in a critical period of healthcare delivery, and the DHA is representative of the larger US healthcare challenge facing our nation. Despite a national expenditure of over 4.7 trillion dollars in 2023, we still face health inequities; hundreds of thousands of personnel shortages in physicians, nurses, and ancillary staff; worsening lifestyle choices with increasing obesity; maternal and fetal mortality; and other worrisome signs of a healthcare crisis in our nation.

To ensure that our 140,000 civilians and hundreds of hospitals and clinics are aligned appropriately and maintain the focus on providing quality healthcare to all our beneficiaries, the DHA developed a Strategic Plan. This plan links the priorities of the Department of Defense with our requirements of taking care of 9.6 million beneficiaries and managing the budget of over $54 billion and a workforce of over 140,000. Attached below is the framework of the Strategic Plan for the DHA, and the full document link is included in the references.

This plan focuses on three major areas: Healthcare Delivery, Enterprise Support, and Combat Support. Major initiatives are aligned to each major focus area. Your hospital or clinic will be responsible for supporting many of these initiatives. Our goal is to rapidly drive these initiatives to completion to improve health and maintain our training base. During all these efforts, we must ensure we are meeting our number one priority, which is to ensure we have the skills and capabilities to respond to crises worldwide and receive our wounded, ill, or injured servicemembers and return them to their home station as expeditiously as possible.

A major key to this strategy is the development of a digital patient strategy. These digital first and digital front door initiatives will fundamentally change the way we interact with our patients as well as how the patients will interact with us as providers. Immediate access to personal medical information, evidence-based interventions instead of face-to-face meetings, improved provider-to-provider communication algorithms, and getting care to the patient when and where THEY are, rather than directing clinic- and hospital-based care, will drive major changes in how we care for, track, and ultimately improve the lives of our beneficiaries.

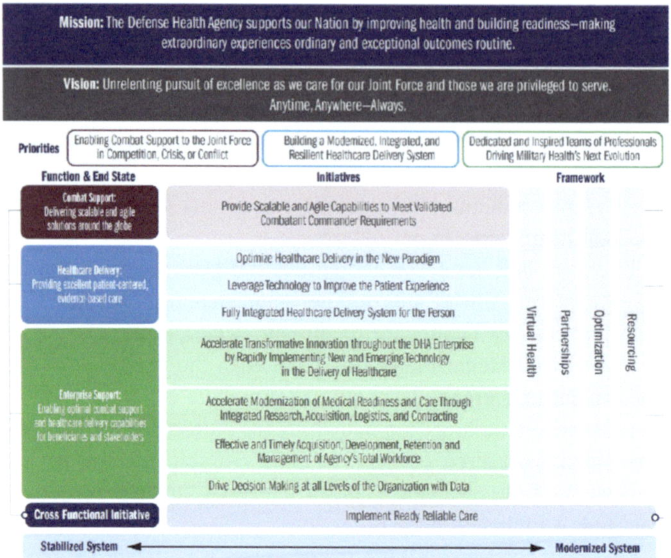

Conclusion

Your ability to provide state-of-the-art care to your patients is critically linked to the roles and responsibilities of the DHA. Every aspect of healthcare delivery will be supported by the entire leadership of the DHA. In the previous sections, the overview demonstrates the areas of the DHA that will be most important to you as you come to work each day. An organization is only as successful as the people who work in it, the resources they receive, and the information to which they have timely access. Leaders at your hospital or clinic will be able to provide much more in-depth discussions on any of the areas outlined above. I also encourage you to use the resources attached and linked to help you become more knowledgeable or reach out to your leadership or the leadership at DHA with any questions or recommendations. Thank you for volunteering to be part of the most significant healthcare organization in the country; an organization that has the solemn responsibility of caring for our nation's finest—the servicemembers who serve, their family members, and those who have served.

Military Health System Website References:

https://www.health.mil/About-MHS/OASDHA/Defense-Health-Agency
https://www.health.mil/About-MHS/OASDHA/Defense-Health-Agency/DHA-Strategic-Plan
https://www.health.mil/About-MHS/Our-Strategy
https://www.health.mil/About-MHS/Military-Medical-History/Historical-Timelines/History-of-the-DHA
https://www.health.mil/Reference-Center/Presentations/2022/11/03/DHA-101-Organizational-Structure

Bibliography

1. DHA Administrative Instruction Number 5136.01. DHA terms of reference. November 24, 2021. https://health.mil/Reference-Center/DHA-Publications/2021/11/24/DHA-AI-5136-01.
2. DHA Stakeholder Report 2021. https://www.health.mil. Reports 2022/11/15
3. Report to the Armed Services Committees of the Senate and House of Representatives. Final Plan to Implement Section 1073c of Title 10, United States Code. https://www.health.mil/Reference-Center/Reports/2017/03/31/Plan-to-Implement-Section-1073c-of-Title-10-United-States-Code
4. DHA Strategic Plan Fiscal Year 23–28. https://www.health.mil/About-MHS/OASDHA/Defense-Health-Agency/DHA-Strategic-Plan
5. Military Health System Strategy Fiscal Years 2024–2029.

9 Navigating an Army Career

Joel Brockmeyer and Danielle B. Holt

Introduction

Navigating a career as an Army surgeon requires a strong understanding of both the profession of surgery and that of a military officer. Ultimately, all Army surgeons must be prepared to deploy to deliver lifesaving surgical care in a variety of environments with a mix of equipment, supplies, and expertise. Heraclitus, as quoted by Plato in the Cratylus, sums up this challenge by stating that you could not step twice into the same river, and that change is the only constant [1]. This is especially true of the current world of Army surgery. In this chapter, we will discuss the milestones of an Army surgery career and ways to pursue opportunities as a surgeon and military officer.

As a value-based organization, surgery in the US Army differs from the civilian sector in the primary commitment to care for the readiness of service members both at home and abroad. The oath

J. Brockmeyer (✉)
Department of Surgery, D.D. Eisenhower Army Medical Center, Fort Eisenhower, GA, USA
e-mail: joel.r.brockmeyer.mil@health.mil

D. B. Holt
Uniformed Services University, Bethesda, MD, USA
e-mail: danielle.holt@usuhs.edu

A. T. Schlussel et al. (eds.), *The SAGES Manual for Navigating a Successful Military Surgical Career*,
https://doi.org/10.1007/978-3-031-88490-0_9

of office for an Army officer uniquely differs from the enlisted oath in that allegiance is sworn to the Constitution and a set of ideals rather than to an individual or a commander. Framed within the context of the Army values, including loyalty, duty, respect, selfless service, honor, integrity, and personal courage, military surgeons consider how medical care impacts the service member and provides counsel to commanders. For service members, both the timing and nature of surgical care can ultimately impact their ability to serve, requiring shared decision-making with the patient. For commanders, surgeons serve as medical subject matter experts communicating the capabilities that can be safely performed to what standard of care, the risks, and the capacity of surgical care depending upon resourcing. As an Army surgeon, you will often be entrusted with significant decisions at earlier points in your career than in the civilian sector. You will be asked to make increasingly difficult decisions with incomplete information, remembering to seek not only clinical guidance but also military guidance through regulations, policies, instructions, and legal advice within the framework of the commander's intent and the Army values. Managing and setting up your Army career for success begins as soon as you enter the Army, be it in medical school, surgery residency, or as a direct commission after surgical training. Finding a mentor is important both as you join the Army and as you navigate the advancement of your surgical and military career. During medical school, you should focus on being as academically prepared as possible while cultivating surgical relationships. The Association of American Medical Colleges (AAMC) has numerous resources at https://careersinmedicine.aamc.org on choosing a career and specialty in surgery. Applying for an Army residency is run through the Office of the Surgeon General (OTSG) via the Medical Operational Data System (MODS) website, https://education.mods.army.mil/meded. The website will help to determine your active-duty service obligation (ADSO) for residencies and any other commitments you have made, such as ROTC, service academy attendance, or HPSP. All military residency graduate medical education (GME) training programs fall under the Defense Health Agency which also has resources for comparing programs at https://www.health.mil/Military-Health-Topics/DHA-GME.

Finding Surgical Advisors, Mentors, Coaches, and Sponsors

As you progress throughout your career, forming professional relationships with surgeons in a variety of positions will help clarify your goals and identify pathways for attainment. Advisors generally give formal career-specific advice, whereas mentors tend to know you more personally and can help identify strengths and weaknesses or offer support during challenging times [2]. These roles differ from that of a coach who helps you personally determine the best course forward for a focused problem and a sponsor who recommends or nominates you for an award or position. One individual may fill multiple roles. Increasingly, mentoring has expanded to include peers and networks of mentors because one individual will not be able to meet all needs throughout one's career. Finding a mentor in the Army differs in that rank, profession, and clinical experience should be taken into account. The mentoring process requires identifying shared interests, goals, strengths, and needs; setting ground rules and mutual expectations; planning meetings with clear agendas; defining goals and ways to track progress; and having ongoing bidirectional feedback [3].

Establishing mentorship relationships can occur both formally and informally. Residency and fellowship faculty often develop informal mentorship through longitudinal relationships. While on rotations, Army residents should directly approach attendings and ask to serve as mentors. Professional societies with a military focus offer opportunities for mentorship outside of supervisors and military chains of command. Through the American College of Surgeons, Excelsior Surgical Society provides annual registration to set up Army surgery residents with attendings.

In addition to surgical mentors, military mentors can be found through Army and joint training exercises and courses. Army surgeons may be nominated for the Junior Leaders Course (O3), and Iron Majors Course as well as the Healthcare Management Course, Intermediate Executive Skills Course (O4-O5), or Capstone (O6) Courses offered by the Joint Medical

Executive Skills Institute [4]. Female Army surgeons also may be nominated to the Military Health System Female Physician Leadership Course. Attending Army Professional Military Education (PME) to include the US Army Medical Center of Excellence Basic Officer Leader Course and Captains Career Course, the Command and General Staff College (Intermediate Level Education), and the US Army War College (Senior Service College) also can be good opportunities to expand your network of potential mentors.

Work-Life Integration

Being a surgeon in the Army presents both the challenges of a surgical lifestyle compounded by deployments, training, and moving with the military. Previous studies have shown that about half of physicians report lower work-life satisfaction compared to other workers in the United States [5]. The Army provides multiple benefits that allow for improved work-life integration compared to civilian practice. Physicians receive 30 days of paid leave per year. Military discounts and subsidized lodging allow for cost-effective travel. Multiple reduced-cost hotels exist exclusively for military members such as the Shades of Green resort at the Walt Disney World Resort in Lake Buena Vista, FL, the Hale Koa hotel on Waikiki Beach, HI, or the Edelweiss Lodge and Resort in the Alps, Germany. Current military, veterans, and Gold Star Families receive free entrance to all national parks either via the National Park Service free annual Military Pass or lifetime Military Pass which can be obtained at entrance stations [6].

Army Morale, Welfare, and Recreation (MWR) falls under the G9 of the Installation Management Command and oversees several programs and services designed for providing recreation and community integration for service members (Table 9.1) [7]. Local MWR offices provide reduced-rate tickets to most major theme parks and tourist venues in the U.S. Administered by MWR, Army Community Services (ACS) an provide assistance with spouse relocation and employment after a permanent change of station (PCS). The Exceptional Family Member Program

Table 9.1 Helpful links for your career

HRC	https://www.hrc.army.mil	Access for information on promotions and permanent change of station (PCS). Requires CAC for login
AIM	https://aim.hrc.army.mil	Current AIM marketplace for job applications and relocation
IPPS-A	https://ipps-a.army.mil	System that will replace AIM and currently used for leave, awards, and personnel actions. Requires CAC for login
MWR	https://www.armymwr.com	System with access to information and resorts and resources for families
MODS	https://education.mods.army.mil/meded	Website for residency and fellowship applications
ESS	https://www.facs.org/for-medical-professionals/membership-community/military-health-system-strategic-partnership/ess/	Website for military surgical society with options for mentorship
SAGES	https://www.militarysurgeons.org	Website for military surgical society with options for mentorship

HRC Human Resources Command, *CAC* Common Access Card, *IPPS-A* Integrated Personnel and Pay System-Army, *MODS* Medical Operational Data System, *ESS* Excelsior Surgical Society, *SAGES* Society of American Gastrointestinal and Endoscopic Surgeons

(EFMP) assists family members with healthcare conditions that require specific treatments or specialty care not available at every MTF by targeting assignment locations to ensure access to care. Parental and sick leave policies also provide significant support if you decide to join the military as a surgeon. Effective in 2022, the Military Parental Leave Program allows 12 weeks of non-chargeable leave following medical convalescent leave for service members who have a child from birth, adoption, or long-term foster care. Army Directive 2022–06, Parenthood, Pregnancy, and Postpartum, applies to birth mothers and fathers, same-sex couples, adoptive parents, foster parents, and surrogate parents and represents one of the most comprehensive family leave policies available in the U.S. Convalescent leave is medical leave for injury or illness, typically six weeks following childbirth. Service members also are authorized for emergency leave up to 30 days for family emergencies, serious illness, or death of household or immediate family members.

Choosing a Career Path

Flexibility in career paths and practice models provides some of the largest benefits in choosing military service as a surgeon. Military surgeons can pursue a range of positions as community-based clinical surgeons, academic faculty, research, physician executive leadership and command, and operationally focused roles. Most commonly, general surgeons with additional fellowship training will be assigned to platforms with graduate medical education. Academic faculty leadership positions include program and assistant program directors of both the general surgery residency or transitional internships, fellowship directors, and chief of graduate medical education also known as the Designated Institutional Official (DIO). Hospital administrative and leadership roles include chiefs of surgical specialties, general surgery clinic and service chiefs depending on the size of the facility, and department of surgery chief which may or may not include oversight of the operating room unless the facility is large enough for a deputy commander for surgical services (DCSS), or director of surgical services (DSS) typically seen at large teaching facilities. You can lead a primarily research-focused career while assigned at Uniformed Services University (USU) or places such as the Institute for Surgical Research (ISR). If you are serving in a primarily clinical role, your position will be coded by the Human Resources Command (HRC) as a 61 J area of concentration (AOC). The first time you can be considered for command assessment in a command (05A AOC which is AMEDD immaterial) billet is as a major (promotable) and requires completion of professional military education (PME) which will be discussed in the following sections. Lastly, operational physicians are referred to as "surgeons" although the positions can be any specialty and are the primary medical advisors to the commander of the unit. Battalion, brigade, division, and corps surgeons will commonly be staffed with primary care, pediatrics, and emergency medicine physicians; however, general surgeons can fill in these 60A roles.

Your primary focus after completion of general surgery training should be developing clinical competence and building a practice in your chosen field. When deciding on whether to pursue a fellowship, understand that it will limit your assignment locations to hospitals that support that subspecialty. Although completing a fellowship while on active duty does incur an additional active-duty service obligation, military applicants have a competitive advantage for fellowships partially because the Army funds their salary. Fellowships available to Army general surgeons include trauma/critical care, surgical oncology, colorectal surgery, minimally invasive surgery/bariatrics, plastic surgery, vascular surgery, cardiothoracic surgery, and pediatric surgery. The Army runs fellowships in trauma/critical care and burns in San Antonio and vascular surgery in Bethesda. Application for a military-sponsored fellowship occurs the year prior to the civilian fellowship application cycle. The Joint Graduate Medical Education Selection Board (JGMESB) makes selections for fellowships based on the specialty needs of the Army and an order of merit selection list to include recommendations from program directors, academic scholarship, and for those not applying directly following residency clinical experience to include deployments. Fellowship applications are submitted through the MODS website (https://education.mods.army.mil/meded).

Some fellowships allow for unique military-civilian partnership opportunities for skills sustainment such as the Army Military-Civilian Trauma Team Training (AMCT3) program. Primarily for trauma surgeons, AMCT3 embeds surgical teams at trauma centers for skills maintenance. AMCT3 programs are currently located at Cooper University Health Care, Oregon Health and Sciences University, Harborview Medical Center, Vanderbilt University Medical Center, Grady Memorial Hospital, University of North Carolina at Chapel Hill Medical

Center, University of Chicago Medical Center, and the Medical College of Wisconsin [8].

The decision to pursue a fellowship and timing for training depends on a variety of personal and professional factors. When deciding whether to pursue additional training, fellowship-trained general surgeons will primarily be located at GME training platforms. Although Army general surgeons may have lower case volume in comparison to their civilian counterparts because of military requirements, you have the opportunity to pursue a variety of leadership opportunities at earlier stages of your career. Unlike the civilian sector, surgical practice in the military depends on readiness, not relative value units (RVUs), meaning fewer administrative hurdles for reimbursement and prior authorization. When considering whether to apply for a fellowship while in the Army or after completion of your service obligation, the likelihood of matching is often higher while in service and you are guaranteed a stable income that is higher than that of a civilian fellow. If you wait to apply until the end of your Army commitment and you do not match a fellowship, you will need to find another job for at least a year; whereas if you are on active duty, you remain employed and can reapply the following year. The benefit of completing a fellowship as a civilian is post-fellowship case volume and stability while establishing your surgical practice.

Military Educational Requirements

Army surgeons commit themselves to two professions both as a physician and military officer. Professional military education (PME) provides the foundational education and training to understand the role of the Army officer at increasing levels of responsibility in the tactical, operational, and strategic environments. PME is required for medical officer accessions and for promotion to higher grades. While Army promotions are discussed elsewhere, promotion boards are designated either fully qualified or best qualified in the number of officers selected. Fully qualified means officers who meet the minimum requirements of the board for promotion will be advanced to the next grade. Best-qualified boards will only select officers for promotion who have met all the requirements for the next grade. A Medical Corps officer should plan to complete PME depending on their Active-Duty Service Obligation (ADSO), career plans, and ultimate military ambitions. Leadership roles at the organizational and strategic level will generally require the corresponding PME. Remember that your career goals may change, so planning to attend PME is recommended to broaden career opportunities including potential for promotion.

PME consists of five courses for an Army officer to attend throughout their career. Initially, new officers attend Basic Officer Leadership Course-A (BOLC-A). For new Army surgeons, this course can be completed in multiple ways. During their undergraduate education, some Army surgeons will have completed the Reserve Officer Training Corps (ROTC) curriculum. Others may have attended the US Military Academy, also known as West Point. Still others may have previously served as Army officers or enlisted personnel prior to medical school. Since most Army surgeons enter directly through the Health Professions Scholarship Program (HPSP), the Direct Commission Course (DCC) is completed first while in medical school. All Army Officers then attend Basic Officer Leadership Course-B (BOLC-B). BOLC-B is a branch-specific technical training course. The general goals of BOLC-B are to prepare officers to perform in their specific jobs and to understand the basics of supply, maintenance, personal and organizational equipment accountability, and leadership.[350-1] Uniformed Services University students complete a 4-week DCC prior to medical school and do not attend BOLC because of the military-unique curriculum provided throughout their 4 years of medical school.

After BOLC, Army officers complete mid-grade level education which corresponds to the Captains' Career Course (CCC) for Medical Corps officers. Most Army surgeons will need to complete this course as their active duty service obligation (ADSO) will usually take them to the rank of Lieutenant Colonel (LTC), and CCC is required for promotion to that rank. CCC has varied in length and short courses (4 weeks) are available in addition to the traditional 9-week course. If possible, taking the short course CCC during the research year of your residency will allow completion of the course during the typical timeframe for promotion. Otherwise, most Army surgeons will complete CCC as Majors following completion of training which can put you at a disadvantage for promotion particularly if you are unable to complete CCC until after fellowship training. CCC is followed by Command and General Staff College (CGSC) also known as Intermediate Level Education (ILE) and Senior Service Education (SSE) also known as Army War College (AWC) [9]. Completion of ILE is desired for promotion to colonel and for pursuing leadership roles such as deputy commander roles in the MTFs or staff officer positions such as division surgeons. Selection for ILE occurs through a competitive board process similar to promotion boards and can be completed in-residence either via a 10-month course which includes a PCS to Fort Leavenworth where you can elect to pursue a Master in Military Art and Science, a 14-week satellite course which is completed TDY, distance learning which includes 3 phases, or a hybrid course that includes the ILE common core (CC) with each phase as a 2-week in-person option and the advanced operations course (AOC) through distance learning utilized by the Army Reserves. Surgeons generally complete ILE via satellite or distance learning commonly when deployed as majors and lieutenant colonels to build or maintain clinical practice at their home station. Senior service college is similarly selected by a competitive board process with 1-year in-residence options and fellowships as well as a 2-year distance learning option through the Army War College at Carlisle Barracks that includes completion of a Master of Strategic Studies. SSC is required for strategic assignments and promotion to general officer.

Post-Training Assignments (Operational/Clinical)

After completing training, be it residency or fellowship, it is time to begin practice as an Army surgeon. During the final year of residency or fellowship, you will work with the general surgery consultant to the Surgeon General who will determine your assignment. As of 2024, the consultant team centrally manages Army general surgeons for their first assignment with follow-on assignments managed by a matching system modeled from the residency match called the Assignment Interactive Module (AIM) marketplace (https://aim.hrc.army.mil) which will be replaced by the Integrated Personnel and Pay System-Army (IPPS-A). The IPPS-A is already in use for filing leaves, awards, and tracking other personnel actions (https://ipps-a.army.mil). Currently, the Army evaluates and reviews assignments every 3 years, allowing for a PCS if desired. Recently, Medical Corps leadership announced that the 3-year reviews designated as the year/month available to move (YMAV) would not be mandatory unless you desire to move increasing stability for Army surgeons. For surgeons who have just completed their residency or fellowship or surgeons brand new to the service as direct accessions, the first assignment can vary and depend on specialty and seniority. Surgeons who have completed fellowship training will most often be assigned to medical centers (MEDCEN) that support surgical graduate medical education (GME). The Army has seven MEDCENs with general surgery GME programs: Walter Reed National Military Medical Center (WRNMMC) in Bethesda, MD; San Antonio Military Medical Center (SAMMC) in San Antonio, TX; Madigan Army Medical Center (MAMC) in Tacoma, WA; Tripler Army Medical Center (TAMC) in Honolulu, HI; William Beaumont Army Medical Center (WBAMC) in El Paso, TX; Eisenhower Army Medical Center (EAMC) in Augusta, GA; and Womack Army Medical Center (WAMC) in Fayetteville, NC. Other MEDCENs without independent GME programs include Alexander T. Augusta Military Medical Center at Fort Belvoir, VA (WRNMMC residents rotate), Carl R. Darnall Army Medical Center (SAMMC residents rotate), at Fort Hood, TX, and Landstuhl Regional Medical Center (multiple GME programs rotate), Landstuhl, Germany. Surgeons without fellowship training are more likely to be assigned to community hospitals called Medical Department Activities (MEDDAC) which serve the installation soldiers and similarly do not have surgical residency programs. MEDCENs and MEDDACs without their own GME surgical programs have opportunities for teaching and may include other GME programs, such as family medicine or emergency medicine, students from the Army Interservice Physician Assistant Program (IPAP) program, or medics from operational units. All of these MTFs fall under the Defense Health Agency (DHA).

DHA MTFs may also have agreements with surrounding government or civilian medical facilities to expand the care opportunities for their patients and surgeons. External resources sharing agreements (ERSA) utilize a local civilian hospital for surgeons to practice outside of the MTF providing a capability or capacity not provided at the MTF such as access to a surgical robot. For instance, you could see a patient in your MTF clinic and perform the surgery at the ERSA hospital to ensure faster access to care. Veteran Affairs (VA) Sharing Agreements allow surgeons from the MTF to provide care at the VA or for VA patients at the MTF with opportunities to apply for Joint Incentive Funds (JIF) for care that is beneficial to the DoD and the VA (https://www.va.gov/VADODHEALTH/Joint_Incentive_Fund_JIF.asp). Other options for patient care, skills maintenance, or education and training are coordinated by the DHA Agreements and Partnerships Management Office (APMO) and include memorandums of agreement (MOA), memorandums of understanding (MOU), and training agreements (TAA) that allow surgeons to work at civilian hospitals. Training agreements that have been approved by the DHA Office of General Council can be found at the APMO SharePoint site, https://info.health.mil/staff/cae/sa/SitePages/Home.aspx.

Army surgeons can be assigned to operational roles in addition to a clinical role at the MTF. Being assigned to the MTF is considered a TDA or table of distribution and allowances position that does not deploy as an operational unit compared to an MTOE or modified table or organization and equipment assignment that does. Examples of MTOE assignments could include the officer-in-charge of a forward resuscitative surgical detachment (FRSD), a 20-person team that provides forward damage control, and resuscitation or the deputy commander for clinical services (DCCS) of a field hospital. Operational assignments will typically be coded as a 60A or medical corps officer regardless of specialty. With operational assignments, you will generally serve in a staff officer position as the subject matter expert for medical readiness and will participate in collective unit training events and field exercises. No matter whether you choose an operational or clinical assignment, general surgeons are often part of the teams that ensure surgical care and enhance morale for our forward-deployed elements (Fig. 9.1). Deployments are the highest priority mission and the raison d'être or justification for the Army to maintain active-duty surgeons. Combat and non-combat deployments make an Army surgeon uniquely able to provide combat casualty care in austere environments unlike their civilian counterparts (Fig. 9.2). Despite personal hardships, many surgeons describe their deployments as the most meaningful aspect of their time in service (Fig. 9.3). Proactively work with the surgical consultant to coordinate taskers and deployments around major life events where

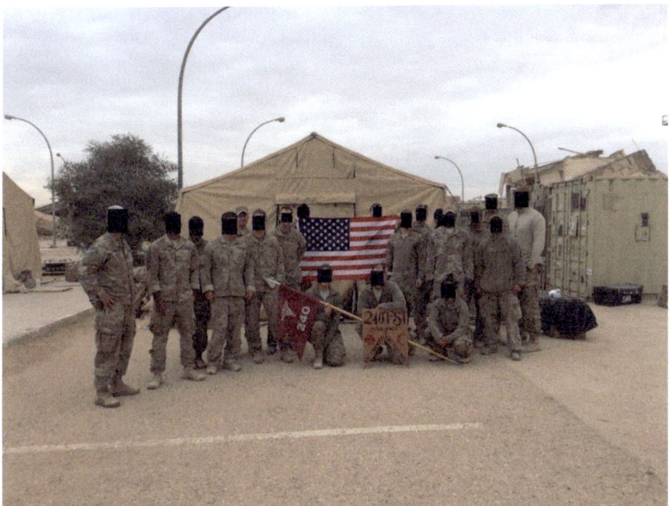

Fig. 9.1 As an Army surgeon, you will be able to deploy forward and provide trauma care to casualties in austere environments, an exceedingly rare event for your civilian counterparts. Author and the 240th Forward Surgical Team deployed in support of Operation Inherent Resolve

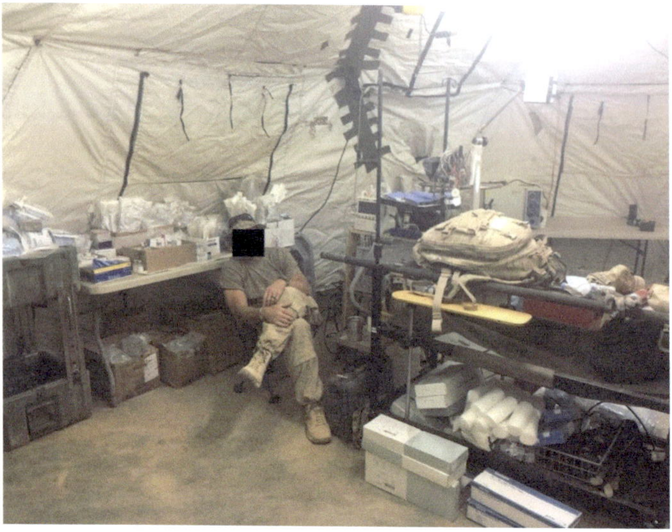

Fig. 9.2 Being prepared for surgery in a tent adds a level of complexity to surgery not usually seen. Forward Surgical Team surgical tent set up and ready for patients

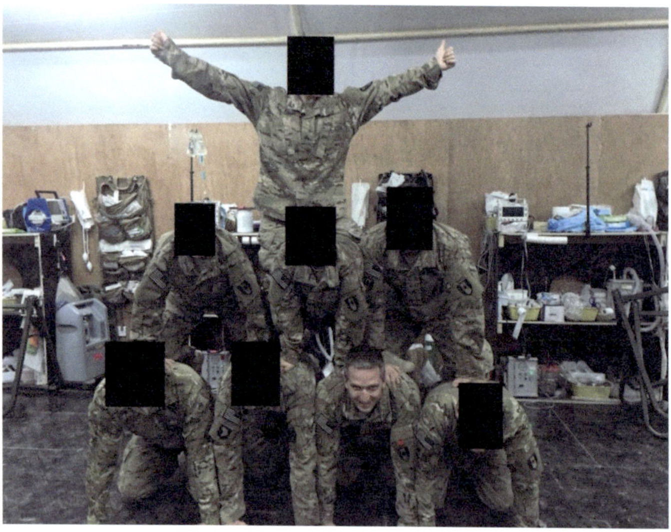

Fig. 9.3 It is not always serious. You sometimes get to practice cheerleading formations. Author deployed with 772d Forward Surgical Team in support of Global War on Terror

possible such as boards, marriage, birth of children, and illness. Deployments may result in a decrease in surgical volume particularly if over 6 months and may require a focused professional practice evaluation (FPPE) upon return stateside. Use this opportunity to have additional training and focus on maintaining surgical quality.

Depending on your specialty, maintaining surgical case volume and complexity can be challenging in addition to military requirements. The Clinical Readiness Program translates clinical operative volume into deployment-relevant "sets and reps" through the knowledge, skills, and abilities (KSA) dashboard available to everyone with a common access card (CAC) (https://jts.health.mil/index.cfm/education/jksa). The Clinical Readiness Program also includes a knowledge-based exam and hands-on surgical skills practicum through the Advanced Surgical Skills for Exposure in Trauma (ASSET) course to ensure that general surgeons maintain baseline competency in trauma and combat surgical skills. If an Army surgeon does not feel they have adequate case volume or complexity at their MTF, they should first investigate options for training agreements and memorandums of agreement/understanding through local civilian facilities for additional cases or partnering with the local VA through a VA Sharing Agreement. You can also consider augmenting your practice with off-duty employment (ODE) which allows for civilian surgical practice while on active duty to supplement your Army salary. Participating in ODE does require an Army surgeon to be in good standing, meaning up to date on all required training and any administrative requirements. Most Army surgeons will cover emergency general surgery and acute care surgical calls during ODE as it does not require responding to phone calls during non-ODE times. These jobs can be found by using a locum tenens recruiting agency, and you must be careful to not care for Tricare beneficiaries when performing ODE due to the conflict of interest as well as adhering to ODE rules set forth by the local command team.

Physical and Mental Fitness

During all the phases of an Army surgical career, you must consider and develop exercise and nutritional habits to maintain physical and mental fitness. Physical and mental fitness contribute to improved resilience in all the situations that you will be faced with during your career. As of 2024, the Army tests physical fitness with the Army Combat Fitness Test (ACFT) which requires soldiers to complete several strength and endurance exercises, including deadlifts, sprinting, pushups, and dragging and carrying weights. While physical fitness is required in the Army and tested biannually with the ACFT, it is rare for an Army surgeon to have scheduled physical fitness time, especially if you are assigned to a hospital. Because of this, it is important to remember to schedule your own physical fitness time to pass the ACFT and to be ready to deploy. Understand that failing the ACFT to include height/weight results in a flag that means that the surgeon cannot have any favorable actions to include PCS, awards, and promotion and will result in a negative officer evaluation report.

Mental readiness is a common concept for surgeons. The Army defines it as an "individual's ability to think, feel, and act in a manner that optimizes performance in a demanding environment" [10]. It is a mixture of cognitive, emotional, and interpersonal capabilities. Mental readiness is necessary for any surgeon, especially those who provide trauma and acute care surgery. Unexpected injuries, significant bleeding, and patients with strange physiology all require optimal performance in the operating room, and mental readiness helps. Training for mental readiness is complex and varies from person to person. Preparation for mental readiness will help with surgery, deployment, and your Army career.

Leadership Opportunities: FORSCOM, DHA, and Civilian Medicine

All surgeons, either civilian or military, are leaders. Army surgeons have access to leadership opportunities sooner in their careers than their civilian counterparts. These leadership opportunities can occur in academics, clinical administration, or operational units.

Army surgeons will have academic responsibilities after graduation from residency, especially in preparation for and on deployment. Medics, nurses, and technicians on the deployment teams will need education from their surgeons to be ready for forward trauma care. Some of this education is in organized settings, such as the Army Trauma Training Center (ATTC) in Miami, FL. Other times, the training will be more informal, such as training in between clinic patient encounters and surgeries. Army surgeons also have the opportunity for leadership in academic medicine. Almost every Army MTF has medical student rotations for education and training, mainly from the Uniformed Services University (USU). Army surgeons are able to apply to become assistant professors through the Department of Surgery at USU. Because of the time-in-grade requirements of 6 years for promotion to associate and full professor, it is advantageous to obtain an academic appointment at USU as soon as possible as faculty. For surgeons at GME facilities, participation in GME academic leadership, including serving as associate program director (APD), program director (PD), or other faculty leadership roles. These roles could involve leading simulation, creation of curriculum, medical student clerkship, coaching, or other academic needs. USU provides both in-person and virtual options for faculty credit to include certificates in teaching, research, academic leadership, simulation, and technology (https://fac-dev.usuhs.edu/). Army surgeons will need to participate in teaching and faculty development, and institutional service, as well as scholarly activity for academic promotion.

Army surgeons can participate in research in both military and civilian institutions. All MTFs have the facilities for some research, including institutional review boards (IRBs) and departments of clinical investigation (DCI). Some MTFs have specific research facilities such as the Institute of Surgical Research (ISR) at SAAMC and the USU research centers (https://www.usuhs.edu/research/centers) such as the Murtha Cancer Center that provides care at WRNMMC. It is not necessary to be stationed at these institutions to participate in research with them.

The DHA MTFs also have opportunities for hospital executive and clinical administrative leadership roles for surgeons. Army surgeons may start as officers-in-charge (OIC) of general surgery clinics, services, and departments to include chiefs, directors, and deputy commanders of surgical services which will generally also include oversight of the operating room and perioperative services. Leadership roles that are not specialty-specific include deputy commander roles such as the deputy commander for clinical services (DCCS), which is the equivalent of a chief medical officer (CMO). Surgeons can lead as the surgical quality officer, responsible for the implementation of the DoD-wide National Surgical Quality Improvement Program (NSQIP). Surgeons can also serve on hospital-wide committees, such as the Medical Material Standardization Board or the Risk Management Committee.

DHA MTFs are organized into Defense Health Networks (DHNs) that are led by a General Officer, usually a Brigadier (one-star) General. These DHNs will sometimes ask for assistance from subject matter experts (SMEs) which allows for surgical input at the regional level. DHA clinical communities establish the clinical practice guidelines and standardization across DHA. The Surgical Services Clinical Community (S2C2) has a chair and service leads for surgeons that represent an additional leadership opportunity to impact surgical practice at the enterprise level.

Surgeons can also opt in for consideration of command positions. Commanders of DHA MTFs and higher and in FORCES Command (FORSCOM) are chosen through a centralized selection board. FORSCOM oversees and commands all the medical units that deploy to provide forward trauma care, such as FRSDs and field hospitals (FHs). The selection board uses officer evaluations to create an order of merit list to be designated for the centralized select list (CSL) for command. To be considered, Army surgeons need to opt in for consideration and compete in the Medical Command Assessment Program (CAP) which evaluates fitness for command through a combination of mental, behavioral, physical, and peer assessments with guides available through HRC for preparation. Army surgeons should anticipate a reduction of clinical practice if selected for command. Physicians can continue to practice in a CSL position in a reduced capacity and have continued to do so to acquire first-line knowledge of challenges facing physicians within the MTFs.

While on active duty, Army surgeons can also participate in leadership roles and committees on civilian regional and national surgical societies. Participation on these committees allows Army surgeons to have influence far beyond their MTF and the Army. The mentors and peers that you meet in these societies will be with you throughout your surgical career and can help during your transition from active duty to civilian surgery. Participation in surgical societies depends on your specialty; however, many military chapters offer opportunities for leadership and engagement at a national level. SAGES provides a cost-free symposium through the Society of Military Surgeons. Excelsior Surgical Society is the military chapter of the American College of Surgeons that provides an annual surgical symposium in conjunction with the Clinical Congress to promote thought exchange for improving military surgery.

Conclusion

Navigating a successful Army surgery career is supported by the small, cohesive community of other military surgeons. You should be proactive in setting career goals and seek mentors and coaches to obtain those goals. Military medicine must constantly adapt to changing readiness requirements and prepare yourself to meaningfully contribute to change efforts that include surgical considerations. Participate in local, regional, and national surgical societies to broaden your understanding of both military and civilian surgical challenges to not only improve the delivery of care within the military but also create networks for practice following military service. Army surgeons are trained to innovate and adapt in a variety of environments with limited resources and to make the best of even the worst situations. When their Army career ends, Army surgeons bring those unique leadership skills to the civilian sector, providing diverse and innovative approaches to solving problems and fostering change.

Acknowledgements Thank you to MAJ Steve Rairdon, Career Manager for General Surgeons at the Human Resources Command (HRC) in Fort Knox, KY for his advice and guidance for Army surgeons in PME.

References

1. Plato (360 BCE) Cratylus. Translated by Jowett B. https://classics.mit.edu/Plato/cratylus.html. Accessed 15 Jan 2024.
2. Ramani S, Kusurkar RA, Lyon-Maris J, Pyörälä E, Rogers GD, Samarasekera DD, Taylor DCM, Ten Cate O. Mentorship in health professions education—an AMEE guide for mentors and mentees: AMEE Guide No. 167. Med Teach. 2024;46(8):999–1011.
3. Badawy SM. Career planning and mentorship: a few key considerations for trainees. Int J Gen Med. 2017;10:357–9.
4. Defense Health Agency Joint Medical Executive Skills Institute. Aug 1 2024. https://health.mil/Military-Health-Topics/Education-and-Training/LEADS/JMESI.
5. Pitre C, Ladd L, Welch J. Negotiating work-life integration. MedEdPortal. 2017;13:10623.
6. National Park Service. August 1, 2024. https://www.nps.gov/planyourvisit/veterans-and-gold-star-families-free-access.htm.
7. Army Family and Morale, Welfare, Recreation. Army MWR. 2020. https://www.armymwr.com. Accessed 15 Mar 2024.
8. Cureton, G new program teams army medicine with civilian hospitals. 31 January 2019 https://www.army.mil/article/216704/new_program_teams_army_medicine_with_civilian_hospitals.
9. U.S. Department of the Army. Army training and leader development: army regulation 350–1. 2017. https://armypubs.army.mil/epubs/dr_pubs/dr_a/pdf/web/arn18487_r350_1_admin_final.pdf.
10. U.S. Department of the Army. Army training and leader development: field manual 7–22. 2020. https://media.defense.gov/2023/Mar/20/2003182283/-1/-1/1/FM_7-22%20OCT2020.PDF.

10 Navigating an Air Force Career

Katherine Cameron and Christopher Mahoney

Introduction

Welcome to the General Surgery family in the United States Air Force. Navigating a career as a surgeon in the Air Force is a unique and exciting journey that blends the rigor and precision of medical practice with the patriotism of military service. This chapter aims to provide aspiring and current Air Force surgeons with a guide to thrive in this challenging and rewarding field. The path to becoming a surgeon in the Air Force demands a combination of medical expertise, leadership skills, and the ability to adapt to diverse and demanding environments. From medical education to the complex realities of surgical practice in military settings, this career is characterized by continuous learning, resilience, and honor in serving both the country and patients.

This chapter will first outline the expectations during your residency training as a member of the Air Force. Following that, it will detail the steps involved in obtaining your initial assignment and the relocation process to your first duty station. It will also address what deployments will entail for you, career development

K. Cameron (✉)
RAF Lakenheath, Brandon, England, UK

C. Mahoney
Eglin AFB, Valparaiso, FL, USA

A. T. Schlussel et al. (eds.), *The SAGES Manual for Navigating a Successful Military Surgical Career*,
https://doi.org/10.1007/978-3-031-88490-0_10

paths within the Air Force and as a surgeon, along with other crucial aspects such as your pay and benefits. By understanding the distinctive aspects of a career as an Air Force surgeon, you can navigate your career with confidence and purpose. Whether you are at the beginning of your journey or seeking to advance your career, this chapter will provide valuable insights and practical advice to help you achieve your professional goals and facilitate a positive career experience.

Residency

You have finally finished medical school and have started your journey to becoming a surgeon. Whether you are in a civilian residency program or a military residency program, you will face challenges but will be rewarded with the skills to become a competent surgeon who can take great care of your patients even in the most challenging situations and locations. You may now be wondering, "As a military surgery resident, which things should I focus on during residency?" Simply put, the most important thing to focus on is learning everything you need to become a well-rounded, competent, and capable surgeon. Following that, there are additional responsibilities that you'll assume as a resident in the military; while they may seem minor, these are critical for one's Air Force career.

There are three categories of residencies that you may be in. The first is being on active duty in a military residency program. There are five military residency programs for General Surgery in the Air Force. These programs are Travis AFB (California), Nellis AFB (Nevada), Wright Patterson AFB (Ohio), Brooke Army Medical Center (Texas), and Keesler AFB (Mississippi). At these programs, you are on active duty status and will be stationed at the associated bases and working at the hospitals on those bases. The second category is civilian-sponsored. This means you are on active duty status but working at a civilian residency program. The civilian-sponsored category does double the active duty commitment time compared to being in a military program or being civilian deferred. For a 5-year general surgery residency, a civilian-sponsored resident would owe 8 years rather than 4 years. For both of these categories, you will receive all the benefits of being on active duty, including officer pay according to rank and time in service Tricare (health and dental coverage) and time toward retirement. You will also have additional requirements due to your active duty status.

One of these additional requirements is your fitness assessment or PT test. Yes, you still have to complete this every 6 months–1 year. The components of the PT test include a version of sit-ups, push-ups, and running. There are now several options for each of these categories to choose from to complete the PT test successfully. The scoring of the PT test is dependent on age, gender, and the scoring charts, as well as passing scores and can be found here: https://www.afpc.af.mil/Career-Management/Fitness-Program/. While it may seem like an unimportant task compared to the requirements of a surgery residency program, do ensure you take the time to prepare and pass your test. The Air Force will factor your PT scores into all career decisions, including promotions, medals and decorations, and even fellowship selection. Thus, failing your PT test could have serious consequences.

Another thing you will need is training reports. These take the place of your officer performance briefs (OPB, formerly Officer Performance report, or OPR), which you will have to do after you complete residency. These are also reviewed when applying to various positions in the Air Force. If you are in a military program, chances are your institution will take care of these without you needing to do anything. If you are in a civilian-sponsored residency program, you must ensure these documents are uploaded into your personnel record every year. The Air Force Institute of Technology (AFIT) can provide assistance to ensure this is completed (Table 10.1).

If you are civilian-sponsored, make sure to buy a Common Access Card (CAC) reader for your computer, as you will need it to access Air Force websites. The Air Force Institute of Technology (https://cip.afit.edu/CIP/) will be your main point of contact for all the military requirements during residency (Table 10.1).

The last category of residency is civilian-deferred. For this category, you are a resident at a civilian program but are inactive

Table 10.1 Important air force websites

Air Force Portal	https://www.my.af.mil/	All Air Force links can be found here
My Force Support Squadron	https://myfss.us.af.mil/	Website used for fitness as well as deployment information
Air Force OKTA Dashboard	https://af.okta.mil/	Website used for all personnel information. Can access the Virtual Military Personnel Flight system through this link
Air Force Institute of Technology	https://cip.afit.edu/CIP/ Physician Phone Line: (937) 255–6565	Air Force Institute of Technology, website used to maintain personnel record

reserve status. This means you do not receive any of the active duty benefits during residency. You will receive the standard pay and insurance through your residency program, and you will not earn any time toward retirement. However, due to being inactive reserve status, you are not required to do the additional duties that your active duty counterparts are responsible for.

Fellowship

If you are interested in doing a fellowship right after residency, you will need to apply to the military fellowship match using the MODS website: https://education.mods.army.mil/MEDED/UserLogon/UserLogon.asp, which is the same application process as residency (Table 10.1). Unlike in residency and the civilian sector, not every surgical subspecialty will have an available fellowship spot available each year. Every summer, the Air Force announces which fellowships have openings and how many positions there will be. This is called the Health Professions Education Requirement Board (HPERB) and can be found through the My Force Support Squadron (MyFSS) website (https://myfss.us.af.mil/) (Table 10.1). You will have to apply through the military match to be approved to apply for and attend a fellowship program.

You will do this during the summer/fall, 2 years before you want to start fellowship. For example, if you are going to start a fellowship in 2026, you would apply to the military match in the summer/fall of 2024. The application requirements and deadlines for submission of materials will be listed on the Air Force Physician Education Branch website.

Similar to residency, there are three categories of fellowship. The first is to be on active duty in a military program. There are very few active-duty fellowship programs currently, making this one less likely for most people. The second category is civilian-sponsored. This means that you are on active duty but completing your training at a civilian program. You will also add time to your Active Duty Service Commitment (ADSC, time you have to "payback" to the Air Force), but it also means that you will receive full military pay and benefits during your fellowship training, and therefore your salary will be much higher than your non-military counterparts. The time that is added for civilian-sponsored fellowship is 1 for 1. This means you will add 1 year of commitment for every year of training. So, if you complete a 2-year fellowship, you will add an extra 2 years to your ADSC. Most fellowship slots fall into this category.

The final category is civilian deferred. This means that you are on inactive reserve status during your fellowship time. Just like for the civilian deferred residency spots, this means that you do not receive active duty pay, Tricare, or time toward retirement. If you are civilian sponsored or in a military residency program and are selected for a civilian deferred fellowship spot, you will have to separate from active duty and be assigned to the reserves for that period of time. However, due to being in a deferred status and not receiving active duty benefits, you will incur no added time to your active duty service commitment.

Preparing for Your First Attending Assignments

You have finally made it to the chief year of residency or finishing fellowship and can see the light at the end of the tunnel, but what will life look like after graduating? Where will you be headed, and what will you be doing? The first step in this is finding out where your first assignment will be. For the Air Force, assignments for new graduates and current attendings who are up for Permanent Change of Station (PCS, a military move) are decided by your Specialty Consultant. This is an individual who represents the specialty of the Air Force Surgeon General. This consultant will typically reach out in December before you graduate to give more information on possible open slots and to get your preferred list of assignment choices. Not all openings are definitively known in December, so understand that the list of openings is not final. Some Military Treatment Facilities (MTFs or military clinics/hospitals) will have an open billet, and others may not, and that may change as the spring progresses. Remember, while the consultant will try to accommodate your preference list, the needs of the Air Force have priority, so it is always possible to be stationed anywhere even if you have not ranked that base. Assignments will usually be announced in the spring of your chief year, allowing you to start planning your PCS in the last few months of training. If you are in a civilian program and you have not had any contact from anyone concerning your assignment by the end of January, you should reach out to the physician education office or AFIT (Table 10.1).

So, what are the possible locations for assignments and for how long? There are two different categories of assignments: Continental United States (CONUS) and Outside the Continental United States (OCONUS or overseas assignments to include Alaska and Hawaii). CONUS assignments usually last several years (4–5), while OCONUS positions have a defined tour length, which is typically 2–3 years. There are pros and cons to each type of assignment. OCONUS tours obviously have the advantage of getting to live in another country or a remote part of the United States, with the ability to travel in that portion of the world more easily. However, this also comes with potentially being far from home and having limited ability to participate in locum tenens opportunities.

Being stationed at a CONUS base typically allows for more flexibility in staying in one place for a longer period. Another advantage of being at a CONUS base is that some of these have Training Affiliation Agreements (TAAs) in place, which are agreements that allow military physicians to work for periods of time at a civilian hospital with the goal of maintaining surgical currency. This means that part of your duty time is spent at a civilian hospital rather than at the MTF. There are also more accessible options available for locum tenens work compared to overseas bases. While there are pros and cons to both, ultimately, every assignment has unique opportunities for you to explore (Figs. 10.1 and 10.2).

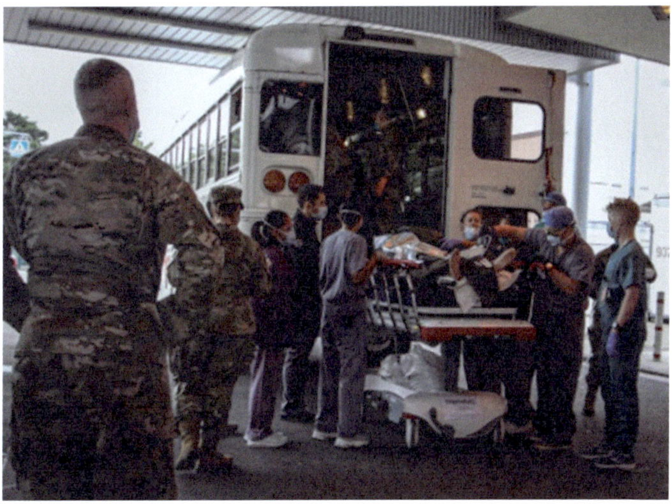

Fig. 10.1 Mass casualty event at MTF. Triage being performed on patients as they exit ambubus

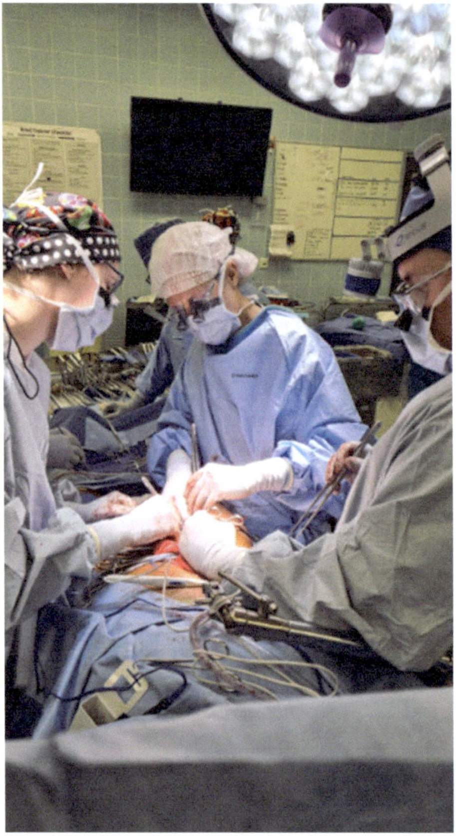

Fig. 10.2 Surgeons operating at a Military Treatment Facility

Permanent Change of Station (PCS)

You have now received your orders for your first duty assignment as a General Surgeon, so what now? After you have received your orders, if you are on active duty status, you will have an out-processing checklist uploaded to the Virtual Military Personnel

Flight (vMPF) site (Table 10.1). If you do not receive this, reach out to your Commander Support Staff (CSS), if you are in a military program, or AFIT to get this uploaded. This will be the list (including the contact information) of all the things you need to do to check out of your current duty station and move on to the next successfully. It will include things such as how to schedule your household goods shipment (packing and moving your personal belongings) and the requirements needed for your next duty station. Do not ignore this list, or your move will be delayed! If you are moving to OCONUS, there are some extra things you will need to do for the move, such as obtaining passports for your dependents, scheduling flights, and potentially additional training. These extra training items will also be noted on the second page of your orders under remarks and Personnel Processing Codes (PPC), which are specific to each assignment. You can find a glossary of PPC codes on the myFSS website (Table 10.1).

On your orders, you will also find your allotted travel days as well as your report no later than the date (RNLTD). This is the date that is the absolute latest you can check in to your new duty station. Sometimes, these will be dates that are not feasible (such as the day of written boards). If this is the case, you can submit a request for it to be changed via the vMPF website although it will need to be approved by both your losing and gaining commanders. However, most commanders understand that you need to take boards and are willing to work with you to allow you time for testing and your move.

Be aware that PCS can be expensive, and while you will be reimbursed for most of the costs you incur, you may have many expenses you will have to cover upfront. This is more common for an OCONUS PCS as you will have to pay for sometimes 4–6 weeks staying in a hotel, rental car, and sometimes flights. Due to this, consider saving some money prior to your PCS. There are options for interest-free cash advances as well, if you need them, which can be requested and coordinated through your base finance office.

Deployments

As a general surgeon in the Air Force, you will be assigned to a deployment-style surgical team. The make-up of these teams tends to change periodically, but typically, they are smaller teams than what you are used to at a large academic trauma center. Currently, the Air Force is using the Ground Surgical Team or GST, which consists of six members: a surgeon, surgical tech, anesthesia provider, nurse, ER physician, and administration person. These teams are meant to be mobile and perform damage control surgeries with limited lab and imaging capabilities (ultrasound and basic labs) and limited ability to hold patients after they have been treated (Fig. 10.3). The GST teams can be combined with other teams and specialties to make up a more substantial field hospital that has more capabilities, such as imaging, lab capabilities, ICU, and ward, as well as other surgical subspecialties. Currently, these field hospitals are known as Expeditionary Medical Support (EMEDS). All non-fellowship-trained general surgeons are assigned to these teams. You are typically required to complete specific pre-deployment training for these teams, which requires renewal every couple of years. These are the two standard ways non-fellowship-trained surgeons deploy (Figs. 10.4 and 10.5).

Deployments are typically 6 months long. There is a new deployment schedule called Air Force Force Generation (AFFORGEN), in which you will be assigned to a band that will rotate every 6 months. This means that you can typically expect a 6-month deployment followed by 18 months at home before being expected to deploy again. Most of the time, you will have several months' heads up prior to deploying, but in some instances, there is a last-minute requirement that can shorten your notice time. Outside of the time you spend preparing for deployment and the deployment itself, you will not have any significant requirements for these teams and will be able to focus on your typical day-to-day clinical duties.

Residency prepares you adequately for the medical knowledge and technical skills needed on deployment; however, it may not teach you the operational side of deployments, especially if you

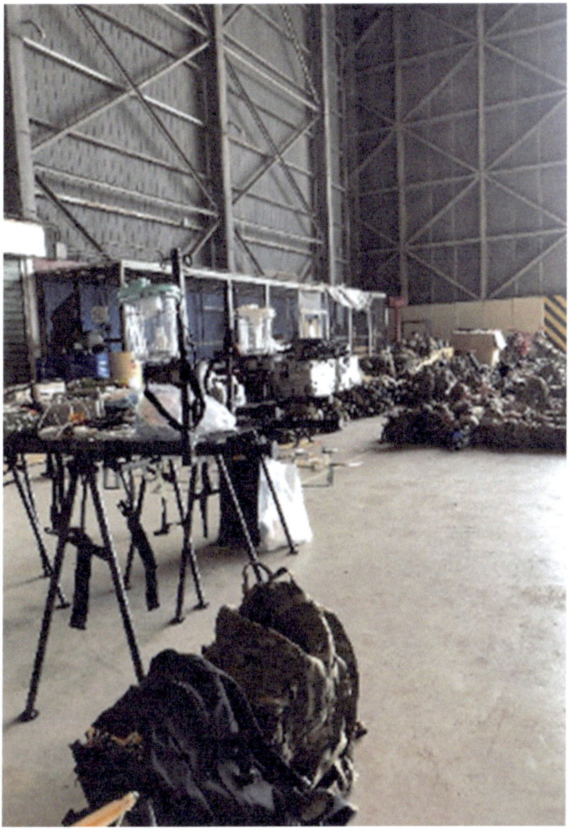

Fig. 10.3 Ground surgical team set up on a mission to receive casualties

are trained in a civilian residency program. Your first deployment can have a steep learning curve concerning all the non-medical aspects and can be quite challenging to navigate initially. Be sure to take advantage of the knowledge of those who have deployed before you and ask lots of questions regarding how to properly prepare for the operational side. It is likely they have already encountered the same problems and issues that you will face and can help make your deployment preparation and deployment itself easier.

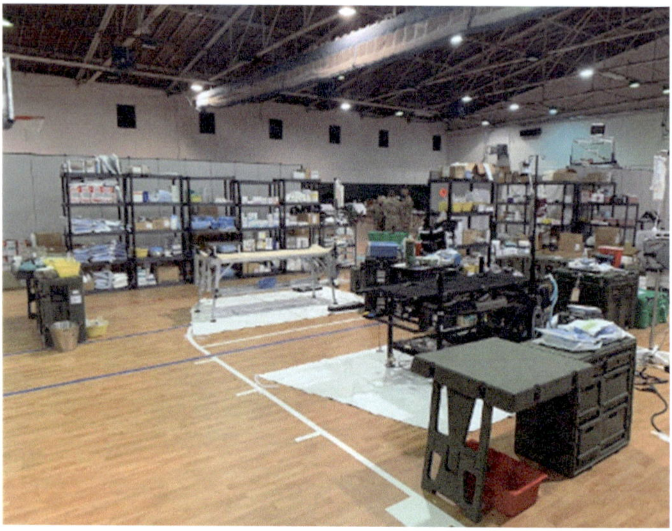

Fig. 10.4 Expeditionary medical support system set up to receive casualties

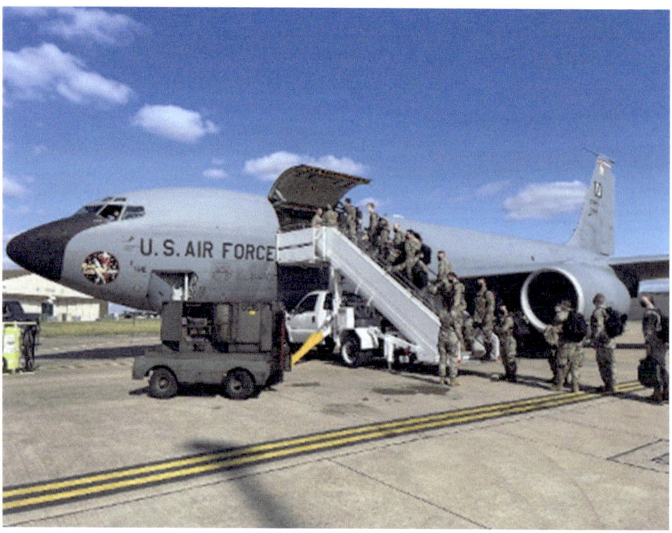

Fig. 10.5 Expeditionary medical support system deploying from home

Pay

Once you have graduated residency, you can apply for your special pay, which is an annual bonus for being a general surgeon, not in training. Single and multi-year bonuses are available, and the Medical Special Pay Plan (available on the myFSS website) outlines the amount of the bonuses for each specialty and the eligibility criteria. Also, there is an extra bonus for being board-certified, so once you have achieved board certification, be sure to apply for that bonus as well. Both of these special pay bonuses start when you submit your contract request for it, so submit it as soon as possible when you are eligible, so you do not miss out on the extra money. You can find the contracts and submit them through the myFSS website (Table 10.1).

The Air Force will reimburse you for the cost of your written and oral board exams but only for one attempt each. While not official policy, some bases will only cover the cost of your board exams if you have passed, so be aware that this may be a requirement. The exact method of having your boards reimbursed is different from base to base, so contact your flight leadership, Medical Staff office, and/or Education and Training Office for guidance at your specific base. Consider contributing to your Thrift Savings Plan (TSP), which is the military version of a 401 K and functions as it would on the civilian side. One big difference between TSP and a standard 401 K is that the maximum annual amount you can contribute increases when you are deployed to a designated combat zone, so make sure your local finance office is aware of your deployment so that this option is available for you. This increased contribution is only active while you are deployed and cannot be retroactively made after you return home, so if your finance office does not designate that you are deployed, you will lose this benefit.

Career Development

There are two portions to your career development: the military side and the surgical side. For the military side, find a mentor to help you reach your career goals. There are a few different pathways that you can take, and a senior surgeon or physician is the best person to help you figure out which one is best for you. Most MTF squadron commanders and SGHs (Chief Medical Officers) are O-6-ranked physicians who are happy to help guide you in your military career. They are a good place to start.

There are specific career development courses (Professional Military Education, PME) that you will have to take along the way for promotions. Typically, these courses are timed for promotion to the next rank. There is a Squadron Officer School (SOS) for Captains looking to be promoted to Major. However, due to residency requirements, most surgeons do not take this course as it does not affect the promotion rate for surgical trainees. The next course is Air Command and Staff College (ACSC) for Majors looking to be promoted to Lieutenant Colonel. The last one is the Air War College for Lieutenant Colonels looking for promotion to Colonel. The last two schools (ACSC and Air War College) are highly encouraged for people who are looking to achieve the rank of Colonel. There are two ways to attend these schools: online, in person, or residence. You have to apply to do these courses in person, and those spots are highly competitive, so talk to your command early if you are interested in accomplishing these courses in person so that you can put together a competitive application. How long each of these courses takes depends on whether you pursue it online or in person. The in-person will have a defined period to accomplish it, while online varies depending on how many classes you decide to take and how often.

Yearly Officer Performance Reports are another important factor for the progression of your career. Take the time to ensure as many of your accomplishments are included in these as possible. Your last three reports are included in any application that you submit.

For the surgery side of things, there are several committees and groups you can become involved with if those things interest you. The annual military surgical symposium is held in conjunction with the Society of American Gastrointestinal and Endoscopic Surgeons (SAGES). There is also the military society within the American College of Surgeons known as the Excelsior Surgical Society that you can become a member of (in fact, you do not have to wait until you graduate to join Excelsior as resident membership is encouraged). There are also military committees associated with other surgical societies, such as the Eastern Association for the Surgery of Trauma (EAST), that you can join. These have great opportunities to get involved at a national level and to get some leadership experience early in your career. These opportunities also allow you to meet both military and civilian surgeons outside your institution as well as surgeons in the other branches of military service. All of these people have the opportunity to help you in your military or surgical career, and the larger your network, the more they can help.

Conclusion

Transitioning from medical school to residency, possibly to fellowship, and finally to Active Duty as a military surgeon is an exciting journey; however, each phase demands a commitment to rigorous clinical training and fulfilling distinctive military responsibilities. Understanding all the options for medical and surgical training the Air Force offers is essential to building the foundation of one's career. Not only does the Air Force provide opportunities to work in civilian hospitals but it also offers unique and highly desirable duty stations around the globe. Identifying a strong network of peers and mentors will provide a framework for understanding your career development. A career in Air Force surgery positions military surgeons to excel both clinically and as leaders within the Air Force healthcare system.

Navigating a Navy Career

11

Miguel Cubano and Pamela Choi

Introduction

> The two most important days of your life are the day you are born and the day you find out why.
> —Mark Twain

Congratulations to you, who have earned the right to care for the men and women who risk their lives every day in defense of the Freedom and Democracy we all cherish!

Navy medicine has undergone a significant transformation over the last decade. The prolonged peacetime, the Defense Health Agency (DHA) takeover, and the conversion to GENESIS Electronic Medical Record, have all resulted in changes in Military Treatment Facilities (MTF) and subsequent changes to the Navy surgeon experience. There has also been an increasing

M. Cubano
Department of Surgery, Uniformed Services University of Health Sciences, Bethesda, MD, USA
e-mail: miguel.a.cubano2.mil@health.mil

P. Choi (✉)
Department of Surgery, Uniformed Services University of Health Sciences, Bethesda, MD, USA

Naval Medical Center San Diego, San Diego, CA, USA
e-mail: pamela.m.choi.mil@health.mil

A. T. Schlussel et al. (eds.), *The SAGES Manual for Navigating a Successful Military Surgical Career*,
https://doi.org/10.1007/978-3-031-88490-0_11

emphasis on the Expeditionary Medical Force. Despite these changes, the expectations remain the same that we will provide high-quality care in austere environments and remote locations.

As we begin, allow us a few words of advice that may prove useful in your career and life as a Navy surgeon. The key to a joyful, successful, and fulfilling life as a military surgeon is to maintain a healthy work-life **BALANCE**. That work-life balance will be different for everyone and will also be different at different points of one's life/career. Demanding schedules, frequent deployments, and educational requirements will be in constant competition with your health, both physical and mental. It is important to set boundaries and switch off to prevent burnout.

The foundation of what we do every day is to treat our patients with dignity, compassion, empathy, and **RESPECT**. The patient is the most important reason for our existence as military surgeons. Additionally, a positive atmosphere in the workplace built on mutual respect will open the door to better communication among the team members.

INTEGRITY is a fundamental core value in the life of a military surgeon. We are not only bound by the Hippocratic Oath but we have also sworn to defend the Constitution against all enemies, foreign and domestic. We operate in a high-stress environment where decisions are made based on limited resources and operational requirements, and this may test our ethics. No matter the challenging circumstances or the external pressures, adhering to the codes of conduct and judgment based on data, experience, and colleagues' input will be essential.

As an officer and surgeon, our **RESPONSIBILITIES** are demanding and diverse. The various operational settings and platforms with unique characteristics require you to be knowledgeable on equipment, mission, capabilities, and expectations. A common theme of a successful life as a military surgeon is to take care of others before yourself.

All surgeons are expected to be **LEADERS**, and this is even more true in the military as an officer. True leadership is based on combining core values with consistent actions that inspire others to a common goal. Leadership qualities include decisiveness, communication skills, integrity with a proper ethical compass, vision of the goal, and the capacity to motivate others toward a shared objective. Leadership is dynamic and complex; it is NOT proportional to the number of courses, titles, or diplomas you have on the wall.

You will without a doubt operate in high-risk environments throughout your career. **COURAGE** goes beyond physical bravery; it involves mental strength, resilience, and the capacity to lead in a high-risk situation while upholding the highest medical standards and ethics.

And finally, there is a common saying in the Marine Corps—"Semper Gumby." Situations and circumstances are always changing. The ability to adapt, improvise, and function is critical for Navy surgeons. There are many things we cannot change. We are only able to control how we react and conduct ourselves.

Fresh Out of Training (LT/LCDR)

Overnight, chief residents become staff surgeons. All surgeons are assigned to operational platforms that are embedded out of Military Treatment Facilities (MTFs). In our present high operational tempo, there is virtually a 100% likelihood that you will be deployed within the first 2–3 years of graduation.

Choosing a Billet

As a junior staff surgeon, the most important priority is to be as clinically busy as possible. The vast majority of surgeries you will be doing will be at the MTF and not through your operational platform. Thus, being attached to a smaller MTF is advantageous. Smaller MTFs do not have residents and have fewer staff surgeons to compete with for cases or calls.

When choosing a billet, it is important to talk to both your Specialty Leader and your Detailer. These are two different people who have two different but overlapping functions. The Specialty Leader is a Senior Staff Surgeon who serves as a liaison between the individual surgeon, the specialty, the detailer, and Navy

Medicine. The Specialty Leader can give important advice as he/she understands the specific needs of different commands. However, the Specialty Leader cannot write orders. Your Detailer is a senior medical corps officer but is usually a non-surgeon. Only the Detailer can write your orders. The Detailer works for PERS (Navy Personnel Command), and the Specialty Leader works for BUMED (Bureau of Medicine and Surgery). They will work together to fill all the manning needs of the Navy. It is important to have discussions with both the Specialty Leader and Detailer as early as 6–9 months before your Projected Rotation Date (PRD).

Aircraft Carrier (CVN)

CVN surgeon billets are usually only for 1 year. These are common platforms for those who are looking for a short operational tour between residency and fellowship (Fig. 11.1).

Aircraft Carriers have a fairly predictable 2–3 year cycle. Carriers spend some time "in the yards" (i.e., shipyard), where they undergo significant renovations. During this time, the ship does not go out to sea. Following this, Carriers undergo a "work-up" phase for 6–9 months, leading up to a deployment. During this time, the ship as well as the Air Wing must train and receive certifications to prepare for deployment. The ship typically does not travel far from the coastline. The "underways" may last anywhere from a few days to 6 weeks. And finally, deployments typically last anywhere from 6 to 9 months.

Each Aircraft Carrier carries a single surgeon, CRNA, and 1–2 surgery techs. The OR has the capacity for laparoscopy and endoscopy (Fig. 11.2). The surgeon will work along with their surgical techs to ensure all the surgical equipment is functional and in good order. The surgeon will also be the trauma expert for the entire ship and will often run any medical emergencies that are the result of trauma.

An Aircraft Carrier is not a casualty receiving ship. The role of the surgeon is generally there for emergencies/consultations for the ship's company and air wing as well as the entire carrier strike group. As such, the operative volume is typically low. The majority of cases are procedures that can be done under local anesthetic (lipomas, cyst excisions, and vasectomies). Common urgent pro-

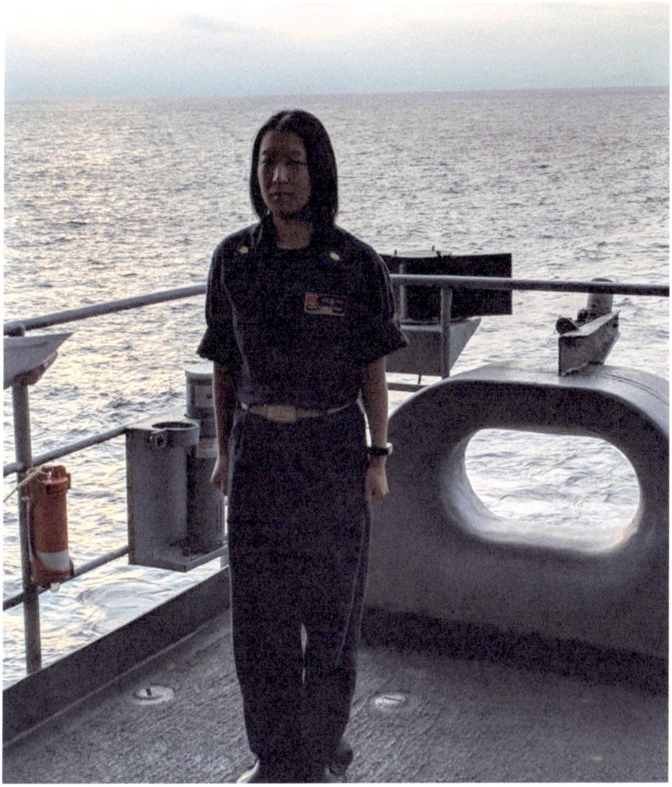

Fig. 11.1 Pam Choi, 2018, USS HARRY S TRUMAN (CVN 75)

cedures are I&D of abscesses, appendectomies, EGDs for food impactions, and complex laceration repairs.

It is important to seek your Surface Warfare Medical Department Officer (SWMDO) qualification during your tour onboard the aircraft carrier or any other shipboard duty that offers the qualification. There is a required in-person class (SWMDOIC) offered every 6 months alternating between the East Coast and West Coast, so advanced planning is needed. It usually takes at least a year to fulfill all the requirements ranging from damage control (shipboard not surgical) to the capabilities and function of the reactor, and the different weapon systems onboard the platform.

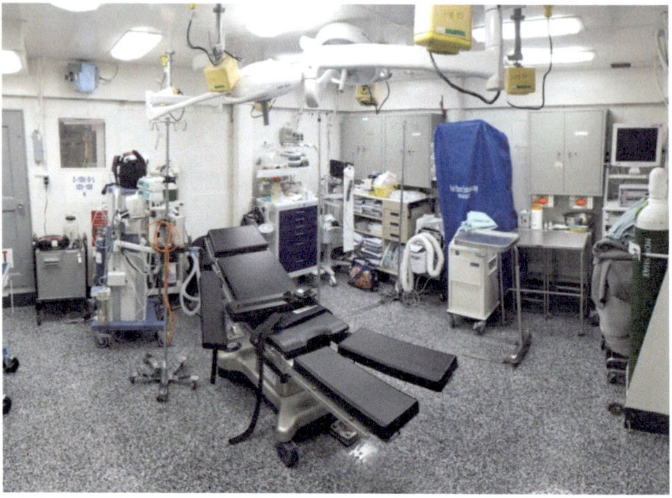

Fig. 11.2 Aircraft carrier operating room. (Source: Picture courtesy of Matthew D. Nealeigh, DO, MHPE, FACS, Commander, Medical Corps, US Navy)

Fleet Surgical Teams (FSTs)

FSTs are usually a 16 to 21-person medical support team that provides Echelon II care to the Amphibious Ready Groups (ARG). The resuscitative and damage control capabilities are vital to the readiness and support of maritime deployed forces during contingency operations.

Unlike a CVN surgeon, the members of the FST are not part of the ship's company but rather have a separate chain of command. Like many platforms, the FSTs' deployments are usually 6 months onboard the amphibious assault ship. During peacetime deployments, the volume of cases is low, but during contingency operations, there is an increased likelihood of receiving severely injured Navy sailors and Marines.

Marines ("Green Side")

Surgeons who go "Green Side" and join the Medical Battalion will experience a different culture than that of the "Blue Side." While Med Battalion surgeons are embedded out of an MTF, they are protected from "taskers" (i.e., they cannot be utilized for any "Blue Side" open assignments). However, the Med Battalion has its own schedule of field exercises (which can range from camping in the desert or going on long ruck hikes) and deployments.

Marines value and protect their "Doc" during deployments or training exercises. The relationship between the Marines and their "Docs" is built on respect, trust, and the understanding of the vital role you play in readiness. If you are fortunate enough to be assigned to a United States Marine Corps unit, make sure to work on your Fleet Marine Force qualification badge. It is a demanding qualification that you can wear with pride solidifying the bond between you and the Marines.

Expeditionary Resuscitative Surgical Systems (ERSS)

ERSS and EMF have very different expeditionary capabilities. The ERSS is only capable of damage control surgery. ERSS has no holding capabilities and depends on a medevac system to move patients immediately. The ERSS has a small footprint that can be utilized at land and sea platforms. There is typically only a single surgeon assigned to an ERSS. Deployments can be up to 6–8 months, but there may also be shorter underways (1–3 months) in which the ERSS is expected to participate.

Expeditionary Medical Facility (EMF)

The EMF is a Role 3 or Echelon III capability with expandable capabilities of up to 150 beds. EMF requires some acreage to set up and has advanced diagnostic capabilities such as a CT scanner. The EMF usually has two general surgeons as well as other surgical specialties (orthopedic surgeon and neurosurgeon).

The EMF is typically more established and has more resources available, and deployments can be anywhere from 9 to 12 months.

USNS Comfort/USNS Mercy

The USNS Comfort and USNS Mercy generally deploy with a significant complement of medical providers and staff. Thus, these deployments generally offer the most surgical volume out of any deployment, presently. However, the type of operation is dependent on the mission of the ship. As humanitarian missions, most are generally geared toward high-volume/low-risk procedures, such as hernia repairs and/or cholecystectomies.

Taking Your Boards

The American Board of Surgery (ABS) requires that surgeons must pass both the Qualifying and Certifying Examinations within 7 years of graduation. However, the Navy strongly recommends that surgeons become board-certified at the earliest opportunity. Surgeons must pass their examinations in order to start receiving additional Board certification pay. Board certification is critical for promotion and also allows for additional pay. Repeated failures may harm career progression. As such, do not be afraid to ask your fellow surgeons for help in either preparing for the examination or giving you adequate time off for studying and the examination itself.

The Navy will also reimburse you for your board examination fees (for the first time only). This generally requires starting the process months before the date of your actual examination.

The ABS also has a Military Activation Policy—those who receive orders that would preclude them from taking the examination after scheduling it will be excused from such examinations without penalty and with a full refund of any examination fees paid. It is also possible to take the examinations overseas (both the QE and CE, especially since the CE is now virtual)—the individual should contact the ABS to ensure that appropriate arrangements can be made.

Additional Qualification Designators (AQDs)

The Navy recognizes additional specialty skills/knowledge that one may have obtained throughout his/her career. Certain billets require specific AQDs. While the Navy literally has hundreds of pages of AQDs, the ones related to medicine generally refer to specific operational, leadership, clinical, research, or educational specialties.

AQDs can aid in promotion, so it is important to make sure your officer record is up to date with your AQDs. Unfortunately, like many things in the Navy, this is usually not automatic and requires some individual work. Officers may request the addition of an AQD by submitting a letter with supporting documentation to the Navy Personnel Command.

More information is available here: https://mccareer.org/2016/04/10/what-are-aqds-and-how-do-you-get-them/

A list of AQDs is available here: mccareer.org/useful-documents/

Collaterals Duties

The Navy expects that you will do other volunteer jobs in addition to your primary clinical duties. However, this is true of the civilian world as well. Civilian surgeons often play key roles on hospital committees.

There are many different possible collateral duties. These may be at the department level (i.e., making the call schedule, Morbidity and Mortality Coordinator, etc.) or command level (joining the Physician Wellness Committee, Quality and Healthcare Outcomes Committee, etc.). Operational units will also have their own collaterals (i.e., the Ship Surgeon may be the “Walking Blood Bank Officer” or on the “Medical Training Committee”).

There may be times when you will be “volunteered” to take on certain collaterals. If you do have the option, try to take on collateral duties that you are genuinely interested in. This will result in you making a positive impact in this role, which can be advantageous for promotion. Collateral duties offer an opportunity to get a better understanding of the larger healthcare/operational ecosystem as well as contribute to your department and command.

Off-Duty Employment (ODE)

ODE is a great way to supplement your clinical volume as well as earn additional money. There are many different ways to pursue

ODE. You may pursue ODE through a third party (Weatherby, Hayes Locum) or as an individual. Talk to the surgeons at your command to see what they have done for ODE.

Each command has its own rules/regulations about ODE. Typically, surgeons must be in good standing with their command prior to applying for ODE. Surgeons cannot be on duty simultaneously for your MTF and for another hospital for pay (that's why it's called OFF DUTY EMPLOYMENT). Different commands have different rules about taking leave for ODE depending on the location of the hospital.

Most importantly, ODE cannot interfere with your Navy duties. Your first and foremost responsibility is to the Navy. There may be certain situations where you may have to cancel your ODE shifts on short notice due to the needs of the Navy.

Career Progression

The most important document in an officer's career is the Fitness Report (FITREP). FITREPs are submitted at least once a year (O3-January and O4-October), but they are generally due to your reporting senior months before this (so generally O3-October/November, O4-July/August). FITREPs are also written whenever there is a change of command and detachment (i.e., whenever the individual is leaving the command).

Take time to do it correctly. Block 41 is the most important component of the FITREP. It is important to include all of the most important accomplishments within this text. If you do not have much experience writing your own FITREP, make sure your mentor or a senior officer looks at the wording and structure. You get promoted based on what that FITREP conveys to the board. It is no longer an automatic promotion if you are a surgeon.

While the nuances of the FITREP are beyond the scope of this chapter, this website provides an excellent description: https://mccareer.org/joel-schofers-fitrep-prep/

Making sure your officer record is correct and accurate is also important. The Officer Summary Record/Performance Summary Report (OSR/PSR) should accurately reflect all your education,

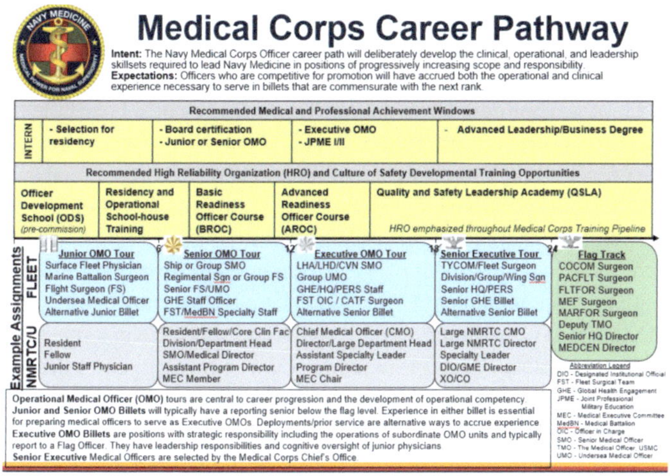

Fig. 11.3 Medical Corps career pathway

training, and certifications. Make sure that your PSR has all the Additional Qualification Designators (AQDs) that you are eligible for.

For junior officers, the most important components of promotion are gaining operational experience and passing your boards. As one advances in rank, there is a greater emphasis on the impact of collateral duties and leadership (https://mccareer.org/wp-content/uploads/2020/08/mc-career-pathway-v21.pdf) (Fig. 11.3).

Seasoned Warrior (CDR/CAPT)

At this point, officers now have a greater understanding of the Navy. Most Commanders are at least 5–7 years out from residency training. Providing excellent patient care is not enough to be promoted. Commanders and Captains are now expected to take on larger leadership roles such as Department Head, Chair of large hospital committees, or Director of Surgical Services. Once you get promoted to O5, it is time to get directorate-level positions. You will not be promoted to O6 without administrative collaterals at the level of Directorate or Department Head in a large MTF. Ask your detailer to submit your name to be a board member or recorder of a promotion board; it will help you understand the process. It is also prudent to alternate between operational and clinical duty stations to increase your chances for promotion. Advanced Readiness Officer Course (AROC) is designed to prepare medical department officers for increased responsibilities as leaders who understand the "practice and business" of Navy Medicine in operational settings and may be taken via temporary additional duty (TAD). Taking Joint Professional Military Education (JPME) is also advantageous although this is typically done in addition to one's clinical duties.

Leadership

All military surgeons are expected to be leaders 24/7. Leadership requires emotional intelligence, compassion, interpersonal skills, and empathy. Your reputation as a good leader will be tested early and often. Leadership is earned; it is constant, relentless, and sometimes exhausting. You cannot rest on your laurels. You need to prove you deserve the title and the responsibility to lead every single day. A fundamental trait in great leaders is humility. A capable leader will accept his or her mistakes, learn from them, and apologize to those affected. Strategic thinking combined with a genuine sense of care for those under your lead will foment trust, loyalty, and hope amongst your team.

The Navy does offer Intermediate and Senior Leadership Courses, which can be taken through funded TAD.

Executive Medicine

The usual progression of your career will guide you to positions of leadership within the hospital or unit. Once you get promoted to O5 and certainly O6, those responsibilities will lead you to think about Executive Medicine.

While it is an honor to be selected to be part of the command triad within Navy Medicine, your chances of remaining clinical will be diminished. Executive Medicine is not for everyone but if you decide to do it, you will need to get your MBA or an advanced degree. You don't have to have an MBA to be selected for Executive Medicine but will significantly increase your chances of selection. Attending the Naval War College can also increase your chances of being selected for Executive Medicine.

Executive Medicine is required to even have a chance to be promoted to Flag Officer. The number of Flag positions has reduced significantly. Making Flag is 25% timing, 25% luck, 25% who you know, and finally, 25% having a stellar career during your Executive Medicine tour in a large MTF (most of the time). You do need to do one or two post-command tours as a Fleet Surgeon and a tour in DC, BUMED, or DHA to be competitive. Executive Medicine and the membership at American College of Healthcare Executives (ACHE) are also good stepping stones to a career as an administrator once you retire or leave the service.

Academic Path, Research, and Graduate Medical Education

An investment in knowledge pays the best interest.
—Benjamin Franklin

Engaging in academic medicine, presenting at conferences, publishing scholarly articles, conducting or participating in research, and teaching at a training program are important activities a military surgeon should pursue during his or her career. Lifelong learning and academic growth are vital in an evolving and dynamic surgical career.

Pursue an academic position (Assistant Professor of Surgery) as soon as possible at Uniformed Service University (USU). One does not need to be attached to one of the general surgery residency programs (Portsmouth, San Diego, and Walter Reed) to achieve this. You are eligible to apply as soon as you graduate from a residency program. After 5 years as an Assistant Professor, you are eligible to apply to become an Associate Professor. If you are interested in an academic career after leaving the Navy, your new institution will have to match your prior academic title. There are also AQDs for these academic pathways.

Joining the American College of Surgeons (ACS) and other surgical societies will provide innumerable benefits to your military and surgical career. Excelsior Surgical Society (ESS) is the military chapter of the ACS created to maximize military-civilian collaboration. ESS is an important link to the past and the link of the ACS entrusted to anticipate the surgical challenges of future conflicts. ESS is a forum to assist line commanders with battlefield utilization of medical assets and to guide the next generations of military surgeons. SAGES has long supported military surgeons with a substantial discount for membership and registration for the annual meeting in addition to sponsoring the Society of Military Surgeons Symposium, which meets concurrently with SAGES.

Being involved in surgical societies will also provide another outlet for academia. All societies will have committees that you can join. This could result in publications, organizing the annual national meetings, presentations, or moderating presentations. It also provides incredible networking opportunities with other prominent members of the field.

For the few and the brave, the research track is a viable option. Research is one of the most important activities military medicine performs but comes with its own challenges (funding, additional administrative barriers, etc.).

Graduate Medical Education (GME) is another topic that is vital in the formation of the new generation of physicians. It is rewarding and time-consuming to be part of a training program. If you are committed to teaching, it is a wonderful option. This would require being at San Diego, Portsmouth, or Walter Reed.

Nearing the End

Time flies when you're having fun

Should I Stay or Should I Go?

There are many reasons why people stay in the Navy and many reasons why people leave the Navy. They are all legitimate. Each individual has different circumstances. What is right for one individual may not be the same for another. Involve your family in your decision-making. The most important thing is that you make the right decision for YOU.

If you envision a career beyond your initial Active Duty Service Obligation (ADSO), consider a Retention Bonus. While this will significantly augment your salary, it will extend your ADSO, so you will not be able to separate from the Navy until your new ADSO is completed.

Be aware that the separation process requires a 9-month notice.

Separation/Retirement

If you are leaving before retirement, the current DHA flexibility to work at civilian institutions or moonlight in different locations is the perfect scenario to get yourself a position for a smooth transition to the civilian world as a surgeon.

If you are retiring and still want to work, the flexibility provided by the new paradigm will serve you well. Attend the Transition Assistance Program (TAP) classes 1–2 years before your retirement/separation date. It is a great class with a lot of information. I would suggest you do the regular TAP and the executive TAP. It can be overwhelming; do not wait until 90 days before your departure.

You will be evaluated by the VA ideally 180 days from your retirement/separation date. Document all injuries or encounters with colleagues for back pain, fractures, infections, etc. The future care that you will need in the future will be dictated by the documentation in the medical record. This is part of taking care of yourself and your family!

Conclusion

> I am a United States Sailor.
> I will support and defend the Constitution of the United States of America and I will obey the orders of those appointed over me.
> I represent the fighting spirit of the Navy and those who have gone before me to defend freedom and democracy around the world.
> I proudly serve my country's Navy combat team with Honor, Courage, and Commitment.
> I am committed to excellence and the fair treatment of all.
> —US Navy, Sailor's Creed

Healthcare services to a defined population with a centralized government-funded structure make military medicine very similar to some socialized healthcare models. That similarity for years has been identified as one of the issues preventing efficiency.

The US Congress created the DHA to standardize and integrate healthcare across the Navy, Army, and Air Force medical departments. The goal was to centralize and streamline functions previously managed by each service. The idea is to cut costs and improve the healthcare delivery to active duty, families, and retirees. On paper, the initiative makes sense, but the reality with the current political uncertainty regarding budgets, resource allocation, and recruiting and retention issues the transition has been very challenging.

You will be frustrated by manning issues, equipment shortages, and increased deployments. Another source of frustration is that the new GENESIS electronic medical record was not designed with efficiency in mind. Credentialing takes almost a month every time you go to a new duty station. The endless number of required training in JKO and DMHRSi are just some of the reasons retention and job satisfaction are low. No other healthcare system wastes the amount of time we waste doing online courses.

This does not mean you cannot have a satisfying career.

There is no greater calling than the one we have chosen—to care for those who are willing to defend our nation. There will never be an equal for the quality of people you will meet, those who share your sense of duty and commitment. Whatever you do, put forward your best effort.

Get involved, push back against inefficiencies, and bring solutions.

The current situation is not perfect, but it is still an incredible journey, full of emotions, responsibilities, and the indescribable satisfaction of caring for our sailors/marines/retirees and their families.

12 Navigating a Career in the Army Reserve

Scott B. Armen

Introduction

Service in the United States Army Reserve (USAR) may be among the most impactful and rewarding components of a professional career in surgery. The friendships, opportunities, and experiences that result are invaluable and life-changing. However, balancing a military career with a civilian career can without question at times be challenging. To thrive and succeed in both, one must be proactive, responsive, and responsible. Key areas of focus include engagement, training, professional military education, leadership development, personal development, and operational experience.

Accession

The majority of USAR surgeons are either direct accessions who apply for and receive a commission in the Army Reserve or those who transition from the active component (Compo 1) to the Reserve Component (Compo 3). A minority are those with a

S. B. Armen (✉)
Division of Trauma, Acute Care, and Critical Care Surgery, Department of Surgery, Penn State University College of Medicine, Hershey, PA, USA
e-mail: sarmen@pennstatehealth.psu.edu

A. T. Schlussel et al. (eds.), *The SAGES Manual for Navigating a Successful Military Surgical Career*,
https://doi.org/10.1007/978-3-031-88490-0_12

break in service, who possess past experience on active duty, either enlisted or as commissioned officers, in any branch of the US military. Of note, although there are surgeons serving in medical officer and leadership roles within the US Army National Guard (ARNG, Compo 2), the ARNG possesses no clinical general surgery billets. Newly commissioned Army Reserve surgeons must complete the Direct Commission Course (DCC) followed by the AMEDD Basic Officer Leader Course (BOLC) which provides a foundation in leadership, physical fitness, mental toughness, and tactical and technical proficiency skills required of all Army medical Officers.

USAR medical officers who commission during a surgical residency or fellowship participate in the Specialized Assistance Training Program (STRAP) and are assigned to and managed by the Army Medical Department (AMEDD) Professional Management Command (APMC). Participants receive a monthly stipend of over $2300 and incur a 1-year obligation in the Army Reserve for every 6 months or portion thereof of financial assistance. Upon completion of training, STRAP participants are assigned to a Troop Program Unit (TPU), an Individual Mobilization Augmentee (IMA) position, or remain attached to the APMC. During residency and fellowship, the officer is not mandated to complete an annual Army Combat Fitness Test (ACFT), Annual Training (AT), or regularly scheduled Battle Assemblies (BAs) or "drill weekends." The service member may accumulate inactive duty for training retirement points during this time but remains protected from mobilization. After completion of training, the officer must complete DCC and BOLC within 42 months, after which they are deployable [1].

Unit Assignment and Engagement

Although there exists a variety of USAR billets for general surgeons, those medical personnel with Area of Concentration (AOC) 61J, the majority fall under Troop Program Unit (TPU) positions. A TPU is a drilling unit that typically holds one duty weekend or BA per month as well as 2 weeks of AT per year with a focus on maintaining operational readiness. Common TPU surgeon assignments include both Role 3 Field Hospitals and Hospital Centers as well as Role 2 Forward Resuscitative Surgical Detachments (FRSDs). Other assignments may include training, backfill, and support units. Unit BA dates are typically proposed, presented, approved, and scheduled months in advance of the new fiscal year. When conflicts arise, training may be rescheduled at the discretion of the Unit Commander.

Typically, a new USAR 61J will be assigned to an available TPU position located within 50 miles or a 90-min commute from their home of record. If no such available position exists, the officer may choose to apply for a vacant 61J billet or will be assigned to the APMC. Any open positions, including leadership positions such as Chief of Surgery billets, may be selected and applied for as permissible by rank. Limited funding is available to facilitate travel if there are no units located within commuting distance. Current open positions may be searched using a self-service vacancy map tool on the US Army Human Resources Command (HRC) website [2].

Assignment to the APMC is an excellent option not only for those who reside beyond commuting distance from a TPU but also for those who desire more flexibility in scheduling training requirements. The APMC's mission is to provide command structure and support to attached USAR medical officers and to conduct centralized credentialing for all USAR-privileged medical providers. The intent is to ensure individually ready, trained, and credentialed providers meet USAR training, operational, and contingency mission requirements while also focusing on recruiting and retention. Through the APMC, Memorandums of Understanding (MOUs) and Clinical Training Agreements (CTAs) may be drafted and approved to facilitate completion of inactive duty for training (IDT) or annual active duty for training (ADT) at either Veterans Affairs Medical Centers, Military Treatment Facilities, or civilian hospitals [3].

Aside from assignment to a TPU or the APMC, an additional but rare opportunity exists through the Individual Mobilization Augmentee (IMA) program. IMA billets are designed to facilitate the rapid expansion of the Active Army wartime structure to meet military manning requirements in the event of contingency, pre-mobilization, mobilization, sustainment, and/or demobilization operations. Officers assigned to the IMA have special planning and support requirements and often help to fill critical coverage gaps and staffing needs for Active Units. Similar to selecting vacant TPU positions, open IMA positions may also be reviewed and considered through the IMA website which also includes a link to an IMA Handbook. This resource helps the service member meet their administrative training requirements for both IDT and ADT/AT [4].

Despite the inherent flexibility of the APMC and IMA programs, the benefits of active participation in TPUs cannot be overstated. As subject matter experts, engaged surgeons have the ability to teach, train, mentor, and develop all unit members, markedly expanding their clinical skill sets and rendering them force multipliers. Surgeon engagement also helps strengthen unit cohesion, collaboration, and teamwork with bidirectional growth and development for every soldier. Active participation builds trust and cultivates meaningful relationships among team members. This significantly contributes to a camaraderie and esprit de corps that is rarely paralleled in civilian practice. In addition, by being actively involved, surgeons with limited military experience have the opportunity to learn military customs, courtesies, culture, and standards from team members in various roles who may possess a wealth of prior active or reserve component experience. The impact of participation on unit cohesion is clear and undeniable, resulting in highly functioning and effective teams in the operational environment.

Some Army Reserve units spend a considerable amount of time training in the field, especially FRSDs. For those with a strong interest in austere and operational medicine, field exercises may be particularly gratifying. Larger units may spend less time in the field, which may better align with the interests of others. Regardless of unit size or type, there are often periods of downtime during BA. When these idle periods occur, it is important to be proactive and seize the opportunity to train. Surgeons can be highly impactful by utilizing downtime to educate and cross-train all team members. As with most life experiences and challenges, the more time and energy an individual invests, the greater the dividends earned. The importance of finding the best unit to meet the needs and interests of the individual, even if this requires travel, is paramount.

Training

The responsibility for maintaining personal readiness to support the contingency and operational needs of the Active Army rests with the individual. Regardless of being assigned to a TPU, the APMC, or the IMA, USAR surgeons are expected to perform up to 2 weeks of AT, formally referred to ADT, and 48 4-hour blocks of IDT. Typical 2-day BA weekends with a TPU will account for four 4-hour blocks, which are known as Unit Training Assemblies (UTAs). Without predetermined scheduled BAs, APMC and IMA soldiers have the flexibility to utilize a variety of options to perform 4-hour UTAs. Examples include Continuing Medical Education (CME) Conferences, in-house unpaid clinical shifts under MOUs/CTAs, professional education courses such as BLS, ACLS, ATLS, and ASSET, performance of an ACFT or weapons qualification, and attendance at other Department of Defense educational courses, committees, and symposiums. Each UTA, irrespective of the type of training activity performed, results in one retirement point.

Similarly, TPU soldiers unable to attend a specific scheduled BA may with Command pre-approval perform rescheduled training. Rescheduled training for IDT may utilize any of the previously mentioned options to make up a drill weekend. There do exist some relatively new administrative rules regarding IDT. Overall, only two UTAs are authorized per training day, a maximum of nine UTAs are authorized per month, and a maximum of 16 UTAs are authorized per 3-month period. Ninety-day periods without a UTA must be avoided to maintain active Reserve status. Regardless, 48 paid UTAs are authorized per year, and additional UTAs beyond the 48 may be credited for retirement points (1 per UTA) without pay. To ensure a good year for retirement, soldiers must earn at least 50 points. With an additional 15 retirement points accrued for maintaining active Reserve TPU, APMC, or IMA status, achieving a good retirement year is not difficult, especially with the addition of 14 days of AT. ADT/AT or Active Duty for mobilizations result in one retirement point per day. AT may be performed with a unit, in attendance of professional military educational courses, schools, or with clinical service in accordance with MOUs/CTAs. If an individual command is not initially supportive of utilizing CME as IDT, stressing the importance of maintaining clinical competency, clinical readiness, and maintenance of certification/credentials should be helpful to facilitate command approval.

USAR surgeons may also apply for ADT to attend one CME course per year. The approval authority is HRC, with the exception of APMC for STRAP participants. Importantly, the request must be made at least 120 days in advance of the start date. The course or conference must be 3–5 days in length and include at least 6 hours of education per day. One travel day is authorized, and travel costs are covered with the exception of a rental car. Registration is reimbursed up to a variable amount depending on the program from $250 to $1500. Additional specific details may be obtained through the utilization of the HRC website [5].

Professional Military Education (PME)

During the Global War on Terrorism, the operational tempo frequently prevented surgeons from completing successive PME courses in a timely fashion. With a decreased operational tempo following the US withdrawal from Afghanistan, PME has become increasingly important, especially for promotion. Following the mandatory BOLC, the successive levels of instruction are not mandatory. Although advanced courses are optional, their completion is strongly encouraged. The next course available for enrollment, the Captains' Career Course (CCC), is presently conducted in two phases, with an online phase followed by a 14-day resident phase. For field grade officers, the Command and General Staff Officer Course (CGSOC) is a graduate-level curriculum that is commonly referred to as Intermediate Level Education (ILE). ILE may be completed in either a resident or distance learning pathway, and unlike in the past, it is becoming nearly essential for promotion to the rank of Colonel. The distance learning option, although it lasts 13–18 months, is the most common pathway utilized by USAR surgeons due to its innate flexibility to better accommodate clinical schedules and practices. This still requires up to four 2-week periods of resident phases. However, resident slots may be applied for and pursued if the individual is able to accommodate a sustained break in clinical practice of up to 10 months.

After completion of ILE, reserve surgeons possess the opportunity to compete for and enroll in the Army War College. Again, distance learning and resident course options are available. AT can be utilized to complete successive PME courses, and developing a goal-directed career map is pivotal to staying on track and remaining competitive for promotion. With less frequent interruptions for deployments, the time requisite for PME course completion is much more feasible for the majority of surgeons. Nonetheless, it is certainly possible to enroll and complete online course components while deployed. With increasing global volatility, the operational tempo and intensity of resultant missions may certainly change at any time, so personal attention to and a focus on PME must be maintained.

Leadership Development

One of the most valuable aspects of Army Reserve service is leadership development. As an Army officer, opportunities to serve in successive positions of increased responsibility are expansive. Additional duties offer broadening experiences that may be tailored to individual interests and talents. Whether the additional duty involves training, logistics, security, communications, or operations, much can be gained from voluntarily embracing these opportunities as they become available. Within each unit exist sections often led by a team that includes both a commissioned and non-commissioned officer. Examples include the OR or professional sections of an FRSD and the surgical section of a Hospital

Center. Team building and mentorship are instrumental as section leaders or officers-in-charge (OICs) assume graded responsibility for the oversight and training of additional service members. These internal leadership positions help prepare officers for command positions with increasing administrative responsibility.

Although the duties inherent to command positions require a significant time commitment, the experience and leadership skills that result are incredibly rewarding and translate extremely well to civilian career development. Command and command staff positions exist at the company, battalion, brigade, and division levels. With each subsequent level of command, a structured leadership development course is required to prepare the selected individual for the increased responsibilities of the position as well as to facilitate their effectiveness and success. While leadership is an expectation for all Army Reserve officers, realistically command may not be feasible for all surgeons, given the variability in scope and size of civilian practice. However, for those who may be interested, the command experience can be both personally and professionally rewarding. Broadening experiences also exist in command staff surgeon positions for non-medical units. These medical planning, logistics, and operations billets range from training units to non-medical commands such as civil affairs. Regardless, identifying a current commander as a mentor can greatly enhance command preparation and yield worthwhile future opportunities.

Personal Development

Aside from leadership development, there exist extensive opportunities for personal development in the Army Reserve. The Army Learning Management System and Joint Knowledge Online resources offer hundreds of courses on a diverse array of topics. Individuals may enroll and proceed online at their own pace in courses that align with personal interests. Traditional Army schools are also available to reservists, ranging from airborne basic to flight surgeon courses. Although available time may often be the rate-limiting step, the ability to pursue unique interests is a tremendous and possibly underappreciated benefit of reserve service. While some may not possess keen interests in land navigation or marksmanship, others find opportunities to develop soldier skills especially rewarding and a welcome release from the daily routines of clinical surgical practice.

Operational Experience

Mobilizations for operational deployments are predominantly managed by the US Army Reserve Command Surgeon through the 90-Day Boots on Ground (BOG) program. It is important to understand that deployments may be voluntary or involuntary. The BOG program maintains a mobilization roster, which can be reviewed by the individual surgeon. This permits the coordination of deployments around important life events as well as alignment with personal preferences regarding role 2 or role 3 missions. Attempts are made to align mobilizations with the unit of the mobilizing surgeon although sometimes this is unfortunately not possible based on operational tempo and manning requirements. The key to personal satisfaction regarding the timing of deployments is being proactive. By working with the BOG program team to understand the time frame during which they are due for deployment, surgeons may voluntarily select a mission that meets their goals and objectives. This also improves the ability of the surgeon to appropriately plan for their absence from civilian practice. In this regard, few situations are identical, as the scope of surgical practice and the size of the civilian group are highly variable. In some situations, as new urgent or emergent missions and contingencies arise, or if a surgeon is less proactive, a deployment may be assigned involuntarily. Individual responsibility improves the ability of the Army Reserve surgeon to prepare effectively and is key to both mission success and personal satisfaction regarding necessary transitions in civilian practice and personal life.

Deployments are usually restricted to "90 days boots-on-ground." Depending on manning and mission requirements, Army Reserve surgeons may voluntarily extend the duration of deployments. Although involuntary extensions are rare, they may occur based on unpredictable events and conditions in a particular theater or battlespace. In general, when planning for a deployment, it is prudent to plan for a 4-month absence from clinical practice to include in-processing (pre-deployment), out-processing (re-deployment), and approximately 1 week of leave. The pre-mobilization process begins with approximately 10 days of in-processing. Occasionally, delays in the pre-deployment process can lengthen the duration of a deployment.

The primary two preventable issues contributing to delays include privileging and medical readiness. Credentialing is managed centrally by the APMC, regardless of primary APMC, TPU, or IMA assignment, for all USAR providers on a continuous cycle. Prior to mobilization, surgeons will be contacted by email to complete any impending documentation and credentialing delinquencies and to initiate the privileging process. Failure to comply with the submission of requisite credentialing documents and failure to initiate the privileging process as directed online are the most common avoidable problems that result in at least a week-long delay in the pre-deployment process. All USAR surgeons have the ability to review their current credentials through the APMC credentialing branch website [3]. To prevent medically related delays, it is imperative to individually monitor and maintain personal medical readiness as well as optimal physical fitness. This can be accomplished by monitoring personal readiness through the MEDPROS portal and by scheduling required services through the Defense Health Agency's Reserve Health Readiness Program with QTC Medical [6, 7].

Career Management

Responsibility for managing a career in the Army Reserve predominantly rests with the individual. However, excellent resources exist to provide counseling and guidance, in order to facilitate professional growth and career development. Perhaps, the best resource is the Army Reserve Careers Group located at Fort Knox,

Kentucky. Career counselors from the Careers Group team provide personalized guidance and assist with the identification of specific assignments and broadening experiences that augment administrative and leadership capabilities. Additionally, structured Officer Development programs at the local unit level and throughout the chain of command are often extremely valuable in fostering mentorship and facilitating career management. Opportunities to serve in roles beyond the comfort zone of the individual yield significant knowledge and skills that improve performance as both an Army officer and an effective collaborative clinician [8].

Finance and Retirement

Two topics frequently resulting in questions and confusion regarding USAR 61J service include special pay and retirement. In addition to basic officer pay, there are a number of additional compensation components available to general surgeons. These include specialty, board certification, and incentive pay. To qualify, the individual must maintain a current credentialing file with the APMC. Retention bonuses are available to critical wartime specialties, which is applicable for general surgeons. Bonuses require additional service commitment contracts of variable length, which lock in the annual bonus amount for the duration of the commitment. Renegotiation is a work in progress, but currently, a longer commitment ensures the contracted amount persists in the event the annual bonus, which is adjusted annually based on manning and projected operational demands, decreases in subsequent years. Specific details are available through the education and incentives tab of the USAR G1 Self-Service website [9].

After 20 good years of Reserve or combined Active and Reserve service, a soldier is eligible for retirement. Again, to qualify for a good retirement year, a Reservist must accrue at least 50 retirement points during a 1-year period that starts not with the fiscal or calendar year but with the Retirement Year Ending (RYE) date of the individual. The RYE date is the calendar day and month 1 year after the calendar day and month they entered Army service. This may be re-adjusted if a break in service occurs but remains constant with continuous service. Attention must be paid to ensure 50 points are accrued for the year preceding the RYE date. The determination of retirement pay for Reservists is not simple. Retirement pay is calculated by totaling all points accrued throughout a career, dividing by 360, and then multiplying by 2.5%. This multiplier is then applied to the basic pay rate of the soldier for the highest 36-month average at the time retirement is requested. Given the added complexity of significant combined Active and Reserve service, the US Army Reserve Retirement Services website offers a number of key resources and support services to provide guidance and address any additional specific questions [10]. A review of the many available retirement benefits for Reservists can also be obtained online through the My Army Benefits website [11].

Summary

The most important caveats to ensure a rewarding experience as an Army Reserve surgeon are personal responsibility and responsiveness. Undoubtedly, there will exist times when navigating bureaucracy will be challenging. However, when challenges occur, patience, positivity, and perseverance will almost always prove fruitful. Although the opportunities for personal and professional growth are vast, the initiative to utilize available resources, programs, courses, and opportunities must come from the individual. Proactivity, engagement, active participation, and connection with unit members are the keys to fulfilling and impactful service. With dedication, thoughtful planning, and discipline, Army Reserve surgeons will thrive in both their civilian practice and military careers.

Additional Resources

https://www.usar.army.mil (U.S. Army Reserve)

https://ipps-a.army.mil (Integrated Personnel and Pay System - Army)

https://akoffline.us (Army Knowledge Offline)
https://jkodirect.jten.mil/ (Joint Knowledge Online)

References

1. U.S. Army Recruiting Command. Overview for army physicians. [cited 2024 Nov 21]. Available from: https://recruiting.army.mil/MRB_Physicians/
2. U.S. Army Human Resources Command. Position map – vacancy search. [cited 2024 Nov 21]. Available from: https://www.hrcapps.army.mil/portal/?page_id=12973
3. AMEDD Professional Management Command. Credentialing branch. U.S. Army Reserve. [cited 2024 Nov 21]. Available from: https://apmc2.usar.army.mil
4. Army Reserve IMA Website. U.S. Army Reserve. [cited 2024 Nov 21]. Available from: https://www.usar.army.mil/IMA/
5. U.S. Army Human Resources Command. U.S. Army. [cited 2024 Nov 21]. Available from: https://www.hrc.army.mil/
6. Defense Health Agency's reserve health readiness program. QTC Medical. [cited 2024 Nov 21]. Available from: https://smp.qtcm.com
7. MEDPROS portal. U.S. Army. [cited 2024 Nov 21]. Available from: https://medpros.mods.army.mil/portal/#/
8. Army Reserve Careers Group. U.S. Army Reserve. [cited 2024 Nov 21]. Available from: https://www.usar.army.mil/ARCG/
9. U.S. Army Reserve G1 Self-Service. Education and incentives. U.S. Army Reserve. [cited 2024 Nov 21]. Available from: https://selfservice.rcms.usar.army.mil
10. U.S. Army Reserve retirement services. U.S. Army Reserve. [cited 2024 Nov 21]. Available from: https://www.usar.army.mil/Retirement/
11. My army benefits. U.S. Army. [cited 2024 Nov 21]. Available from: https://myarmybenefits.us.army.mil

13 Navigating a Career in the Air Force Reserve

David A. Gerber

After three decades of service as a reservist in the Air Force Medical Corps, it would be easy to forget what initially piqued my interest in pursuing a career in the military. In 1990, I was beginning my second year of residency at Emory University and the Department of Defense had just launched Desert Shield in the Persian Gulf due to the escalating conflict in Iraq and the surrounding region. That military exercise quickly transformed into Desert Storm and the United States' first large-scale military deployment in nearly two decades. With the escalation of activity in the Gulf region, the branches of the armed forces were actively recruiting individuals who were interested in military service. The United States Air Force (USASF) Medical Corps had revitalized their recruiting teams after they identified a deficit in the overall number of reservists; a gap that was especially concerning in select critical skills specialties (e.g., surgeons, intensivists, critical care nurses, etc.). While rotating on the trauma service at Grady Memorial Hospital, a level 1 trauma center and part of Emory University's Department of Surgery residency, the regional USAF health services recruiter met with the surgical residents to talk about professional opportunities in the medical corps. Between

D. A. Gerber (✉)
Department of Surgery, University of Cincinnati, Cincinnati, OH, USA
e-mail: gerberdd@ucmail.uc.edu

A. T. Schlussel et al. (eds.), *The SAGES Manual for Navigating a Successful Military Surgical Career*,
https://doi.org/10.1007/978-3-031-88490-0_13

the previously mentioned escalating tensions and military activity in the Persian Gulf and my observations of the clinical training that I was receiving, I felt a calling to be a contributor to the armed services.

The US Air Force recruiter assigned to Georgia was personable and informative as he explained the Air Force's need for board-certified general surgeons with real-world civilian experience in trauma and critical care. He also laid out the responsibilities associated with commissioning as a reservist. I wouldn't be eligible to meet the Air Force's needs at that time since I was still in residency but the training that I was receiving at Emory and the various clinical sites, including Grady Memorial Hospital, made me an attractive candidate as a future reservist in the USAF Medical Corps. In essence, they were committing to the future "me" versus the current iteration. The recruiter also explained that during my surgical residency, the Air Force would allow me to be commissioned as an officer which would provide a stipend, and in turn, I would be assigned to the Inactive Ready Reserves (IRR). In this model, I would owe two "good" years of reserve payback for each year that I received the stipend. Knowing that residency would be approximately 7 years (5 clinical years in the general surgery residency +/– research years), I would be committing to a minimum of 10 active reserve years, after completing my surgical training. Getting to this point of commitment, I would encourage anyone considering this career to do the math and evaluate why they want to pursue this path. As a trainee, you are committing to a career choice that could potentially impact a third or more of your future years as a practicing surgeon.

I shared with the recruiter that my professional goals included a clinical interest in transplantation and a career in academic surgery. He was extremely knowledgeable of the various service opportunities and discussed the different ways that I could participate as a reservist that would complement my academic/civilian career. There would be support for military-based professional development and continuing medical education activities, opportunities to be assigned to various bases and units throughout the country for my reserve duty while also participating in programs such as the aerospace medicine training program, and becoming a flight surgeon if I wanted to pursue that option. He also explained the different ways I could drill with my assigned unit either in the role of a traditional reservist, what some refer to as the "weekend warrior" or in an alternative path called the Individual Mobilization Augmentee (IMA) program. In the traditional reservist role, I would be assigned to a reserve unit where I would drill one weekend per month, and I would also have 2 weeks of active duty during the year to attain a minimum of 50 points for a good year toward retirement. As an alternative, he felt that the IMA program may be a better match for someone with my academic career plan as I would have critical surgical skills that would be operationally ready, an immediate benefit for the military while simultaneously being less disruptive to my academic career because the active-duty training commitment was only 12 days per year. Another point of emphasis was that the Air Force wouldn't interfere with my decision to pursue a fellowship and would be supportive of me pursuing a career as a transplant surgeon even though the Air Force didn't have an independent transplant program. Lastly, the recruiter brought up the opportunity for professional development and growth in the military. He pointed out how a former faculty member in Emory University's Department of Surgery had become the commander of the local reserve unit while continuing his academic surgical career. This individualized approach that the Air Force brought to my recruitment allowed me to be comfortable that my commitment could be done in parallel with developing an academic surgical career while simultaneously launching the beginning of my three decades of military service.

Consistent with what the recruiter said during my recruitment, I was commissioned in the IRR, and the Air Force allowed me to complete my civilian surgical residency, including 2 years of research, without disruption. When I moved to my transplant surgery fellowship, the Air Force helped with my assignment to the 911th Airlift Wing, a reserve unit in Pittsburgh, PA, which was geographically collocated with where I was completing my fellowship. They connected me with the unit's leadership, a colonel who was a general surgeon at one of the community hospitals and the second in command who was a general surgeon at an area Veterans Affairs Medical Center (VAMC). The engagement and understanding of the unit's leadership team was incredibly important for me as the time commitment in my fellowship was 7 days/week, 51 weeks out of the year. Their approach and investment in my career development set me on a path of success in the USAF Medical Corps that lasted long after this initial assignment. While I was somewhat atypical in my background compared to the other surgeons in the unit, they were all general surgeons in the community and, on average, a decade and a half my senior. However, they embraced me and provided mentorship throughout the 2 years I was assigned to this unit. Knowing the demands of the transplant fellowship, I trained as a traditional reservist. Rather than drilling with the rest of the unit for the 2 weeks of active duty; the unit leadership suggested that I participate in the first segment of the Aerospace Medicine program in San Antonio. Part of their rationale related to the fact that the Air Force was initiating the Critical Care Air Transport (CCAT) program, and my critical skill set would align with the needs of the Air Force. CCAT was a new endeavor focused on transporting the critically ill from the battlefield while providing critical care throughout the journey to a higher level of definitive health care. The unit's leadership continued to brainstorm on ways that I could engage as a reservist after I completed my transplant fellowship, and transitioned to my first faculty position at the University of North Carolina (UNC) at Chapel Hill. They helped connect me with the 4th Medical Group at Seymour Johnson AFP in North Carolina. This marked two critical transitions as a professional. First, I would begin my career as an academic surgeon-scientist, and I would shift my role in the USAF from a traditional reservist to an IMA.

The transition to an IMA was another important decision for me and one that a future reservist should make only after they have weighed multiple factors, including how this could impact their role in the military. From the first time I heard about the IMA program, individuals in the military would remark that it stands for "I aM Alone" because your assignment is to the IMA and you, the reservist, must figure out where you will do your training and get yourself assigned to a specific unit. Thus, the individualized IMA experience can leave you without the same sense of team belonging. It works for the individual who is comfortable with some level of ambiguity in their role but would not be a good fit for everyone. To achieve a successful year toward retirement, a drilling reservist must earn a minimum of 50 points annually through a combination of activities such as active duty training, equivalent duties (continuing medical education), and compliance requirements. These points contribute to both the retirement credit for that specific year and the cumulative service time in the military. There are nuances in accomplishing satisfactory training requirements. You are accountable for identifying a training period that overlaps with both your retention/retirement (R/R) date and the fiscal year (October 1–September 30) while also meeting the needs of the unit with whom you are drilling/training. As you are building out your schedule each year, you learn that no one is looking at that calendar other than you, and if you aren't attentive to details, you could satisfy the fiscal year requirement and not get credit toward retirement, which requires a minimum of 20 years as an active reservist. This is one clear example of how being successful in the IMA program requires you to be well-organized and disciplined with respect to compliance with military requirements, including annual training and fitness testing, while also being a proactive communicator. This can be a challenge for some individuals, and when I first started on this journey, communication mainly occurred by phone and fax as email and internet-based systems were not fully developed. By the time I retired from the Air Force, the process had gone through a dramatic evolution, but the same principles of organization still applied. Even with this individual responsibility, the IMA program provides more flexibility in your scheduling than drilling as a traditional reservist.

The challenge of being in the IMA occurred within 2 years of starting my assignment at Seymour Johnson Air Force Base (AFB). The Department of Defense had just done a base reduction assessment, and it was determined that the surgical unit at this site would be permanently closed and I would need to identify another unit where I could drill. Pope AFB in Fayetteville, NC is located on Fort Bragg but it only had a primary care clinic. Fortunately for me the commanding officer of the 43rd Medical Squadron at Pope

AFB identified that Womack Army Medical Center (AMC) located on Fort Bragg was staffed by surgeons who were assigned to the 82nd Airborne Division. I was able to connect with the surgeon in charge of the unit, and they were willing to have me drill with them as an affiliate relationship. This was great, but it did lead to more paperwork on my part because I would have to keep everyone in the loop with respect to when I was going to be at Womack AMC while also remaining compliant with the Air Force's drilling requirements. Fortunately, the bureaucracy component was navigable on my end, and it was clearly outweighed by the beneficial role that I played for the surgical team at Womack AMC. My time assigned to Womack AMC covered 2002–2006 and represented a cadence of high-frequency deployments for the active-duty surgeons who were part of the 82nd Airborne Division. While the Air Force had a quicker ramp-up and ramp-down of needs for surgeons, I was able to provide support to the surgical unit at Womack while I was performing my active-duty training. Even when I was in my civilian role at UNC, I provided support for the surgical team as the entities were <2 h away from each other. This flexibility balanced with the fact that I was focusing on my academic career, and in my civilian role, I was part of a small team of transplant surgeons at UNC, so there would be a direct impact on clinical care at UNC if I were to be deployed for an extended period of time. I would describe this part of my reserve career as the learning and exploration phase. I became a facilitator and clinical consultant for the army surgeons at Womack AMC while becoming more educated on the role(s) of the reservist. Being employed in academic surgery at a public university, I had the full support of my institution as well as the support of my clinical department. I participated in some military professional development at the local level but wasn't fully engaged as I was living in this hybrid space between the Air Force and an Army Medical Center. Completing the aerospace medicine program didn't fit with my academic career, but for the interested reservist, this program provides additional opportunities to be assigned to a squadron and develop a closer relationship with a core group of active duty and reserve personnel, and the CCAT program is another good opportunity for a surgeon with critical care skills.

After several years in this role, I began my next transition to the IMA program. The military had one joint forces transplant program coordinated at the Walter Reed Medical Center in Washington, DC, and through my transplant network, I met the surgeon who was running the program. He was eager to have me transfer my assignment to their location because I was directing a civilian transplant program and would be a subject matter expert who could support the military transplant program. The benefit of being in the IMA program was that I could readily move my assignment to Walter Reed and the Uniformed Services University (USU), the military medical school, formerly known as USUHS. The medical school was going through a leadership transition, and the new chair of the department of surgery was someone with whom I developed a close multi-year relationship that transcended both my military and civilian roles and has continued beyond my retirement from the military. This period of my career in the reserves was incredibly fulfilling. I worked with the head of the transplant program on several nationwide projects to support organ donation in the DoD while also engaging USU's Department of Surgery as an adjunct faculty member. I feel that these examples show the two-way benefit of the reservist where your civilian skillset serves as a benefit to the military while the military is supporting your professional development in a manner that complements your academic growth. The chair of the Department of Surgery was an active-duty Navy surgeon, and the director of the transplant program was an active-duty Army surgeon. The Air Force remained very supportive and flexible as they valued my role on this tri-service clinical team. In addition to working on specific programs in the Department of Surgery, the Air Force provided several opportunities for me to continue with my professional military development, including several leadership programs, Air War College (AWC), and the Combined Services Senior Leadership Course. While AWC is a multifaceted educational program, it has components that focus on professional leadership that were translatable to my civilian career.

At this point in the development of my academic career, both my civilian mentors and military partners encouraged me to look for academic chair opportunities. The Air Force and the

Department of Defense's leadership programs provided an opportunity to learn how the military approaches leadership skill development and succession planning which I could compare with the development of these same skills in the academic civilian sector. In retrospect, I began the military leadership programs not fully understanding my own strengths and blind spots, but over the course of these curricula, I learned more about myself and how I could be a more effective leader. The extra benefit is that these skills along with a focus on emotional intelligence improved my performance in my civilian roles and when there was a leadership need in my academic department/health system, I was able to effectively function in new roles which included planning and navigating healthcare delivery during the pandemic. I also want to add that while interviewing for departmental chair positions, my military experience and leadership development was always a point of discussion as professional development in civilian academia does not typically focus on leadership skill acquisition the same way that it is accomplished in the military. Managing personnel and developing operational plans are a point of emphasis in military leadership along with emphasizing skills in negotiating and bias training, whereas in academics, we typically focus on individual academic accomplishments and progressively move people into positions of more complex decision-making based on institutional circumstances and the department's structure. Ultimately, I feel that my acquired skillset and experiences were critical to me being offered and accepting the next opportunity in my academic career as Chair of the Department of Surgery at the University of Cincinnati.

Integrating into my new department and new role, I have been fortunate to have a continuing relationship with the military. This unique opportunity is based on the existence of a Center for Sustainment of Trauma and Readiness Skills (CSTARS) program at the University of Cincinnati College of Medicine and UC Health. Our Department of Surgery has a long-term relationship with the team at the United States Air Force School of Aerospace Medicine (USAFSAM), the 711th Human Performance Wing and the Air Force Research Laboratory at Wright Patterson AFB. In addition to these active partnerships, the Department of Surgery and the University of Cincinnati College of Medicine established an Institute of Military Medicine to focus on translatable research activities to support the military. This framework has allowed our department to be a leader in the military-civilian medical partnership model with several active duty surgeons who operate as clinicians in our department while they run the CSTARS program and maintain skill readiness for the military. This opportunity for me as a retired reservist resonates as a way to continue my commitment and support the careers of others who are affiliated with the military and the overall mission.

In summary, I've laid out an example of one person's career as a reservist in the USAF Medical Corps, and my point of emphasis is that this is but one path. I can't emphasize enough that the components of being a reservist are the same for everyone, but there is definite variability in experiences based on an individual's assignment, branch of service, and areas of interest. Reflecting on the impact of my 30 years of service, there is no doubt that my time as a reservist was incredibly fulfilling. I didn't accomplish everything that I thought I would do but I also got involved with projects that I wouldn't have anticipated. I expanded my leadership skillset in a differentiated way that helped me at multiple junctures of my academic career, including developing strategies for navigating the pandemic, creating and launching operational plans, and ultimately expanding my foundational base as a leader.

14 Navigating a Career in the Navy Reserves

Margaret M. Morgan

I have been in the Navy now for over 24 years and the majority of that time has been as a Reservist. I'll tell my story and then try to relate that back to cover the broader topic of how to have a successful career as a Navy Reserve surgeon.

The Navy sends physicians in the Health Professions Scholarship Program (HPSP) to Officer Development School the summer before the first or second year of medical school. The only other exposure to the Navy during medical school for an HPSP student is during two, 30-day clerkship rotations at the Military Treatment Facilities. After medical school, I was commissioned as a Lieutenant on active duty and went to San Diego for my Transitional year internship at Naval Medical Center San Diego. Following internship, I "stashed" in the Emergency Department as a General Medical Officer before going to Pensacola to become a Naval Flight Surgeon. I then spent the next 5 years serving on active duty as a Flight Surgeon; first with a Marine Corps CH-46 squadron in Okinawa and then with a Special Projects P-3 squadron in Brunswick, Maine. Both tours

M. M. Morgan (✉)
Division of Trauma and Acute Care Surgery, University of Colorado Health, Memorial, Colorado Springs, CO, USA
e-mail: margaret.morgan@uchealth.org

A. T. Schlussel et al. (eds.), *The SAGES Manual for Navigating a Successful Military Surgical Career*,
https://doi.org/10.1007/978-3-031-88490-0_14

involved several trips to the Middle East which ultimately led me to pursue a career in Trauma Surgery.

It then became time to go back to residency. I wanted to train in a high acuity and high volume program. I also knew at that point that I wanted to do a Trauma Surgery fellowship immediately after residency. Many active-duty surgeons are required to do a few years as a General Surgeon on an aircraft carrier or other operational tour before they can pursue fellowship training. I therefore resigned my commission and joined the Reserves. The Reserve Component offers a program for critical wartime specialties called Training in Medical Specialties. This allows the time in service clock to keep ticking while doing a civilian residency. I completed a General Surgery residency in my hometown at Lehigh Valley Health Network followed by a Trauma Surgery fellowship at Louisiana State University in New Orleans. I stayed on as faculty in New Orleans for another 5 years before relocating to Colorado in 2020.

I have been a drilling reservist, or Selected Reservist (SELRES), since 2016. During my residency, fellowship, and first year of clinical practice, I was a member of the Inactive Ready Reserve (IRR). The IRR allowed me that necessary flexibility while I completed training and got my feet under me as a new attending. After that, I returned to a SELRES drilling status.

My first tip for success as a Navy Reservist comes down to two words: TIME and DESIRE. Many people join after their time on Active Duty without the full picture. The transition off Active Duty is difficult regardless of the occupation. There is often confusion on the time commitment, differences in Active Duty versus Reserve, or differences in military and civilian medicine. Recruiters advertise it as an easy and quick way to qualify for retirement. The Navy is currently reviewing the retirement credit policy for HPSP members. It was previously advertised as a way to get credit for those 4 years in medical school toward retirement. This credit was removed in the last few years and has been cited as a top reason physicians are now leaving the Reserves. We have recently learned that the credit is likely to be reinstated but at the time of this writing, that has yet to happen and we are not certain if it will be awarded to other HPSP recipients going forward.

The time commitment just for drill is real and to be successful, you need to acknowledge that. It's more than just *1 week a month, 2 weeks a year*. Travel to drill is often required, which if you have a busy surgical practice, requires one to take into account the travel time and therefore the time off work or not available for call. Many civilian practices are forgiving with military service, but your civilian requirements often don't change; you are just required to squeeze in your obligated number of shifts or calls, cases or clinics into the time you are available, which can put a strain on you and on your family.

The second tip for success is FAMILY SUPPORT and BUY IN. You WILL be gone essentially every month and obligated to serve 2 weeks of active duty each year. Your family has to accept the time off and the fact that when you are home and working in your civilian practice, it will be at a higher pace than the rest of your partners because of less availability due to your military service.

When I first started dating my husband, I had recently completed a fellowship and was eager to be the Trauma Surgeon I envisioned in 2007 at the Role II in Iraq. Deployments and mobilizations are advertised via a list serve for which one can sign up via a portal, or these notifications come directly from the Reserve Specialty Leader or Medical Corp Reserve Affairs officer. I was volunteering for absolutely every deployment/mobilization that came available because I had this burning desire to do what I wasn't yet trained to do 10 years prior. I said yes to a Joint Task Force Surgeon position without discussing it with him first and almost lost my relationship. He and I now have an agreement that comes to deployments: if the mission is to cut, I can volunteer (after we discuss it), and if not, I will go if specifically tagged to do so.

The next level of success in the Navy Reserve is to KNOW YOUR WHY. Why are you in the Navy Reserve? Is it to get to retirement? Do you want to deploy? Do you just want to be a part of a bigger community, serve your country, share your expertise? I have heard all of these reasons conducting Career Development Boards over the years. The Navy Reserve offers so many different options so knowing why you are serving and what you want to get out of your career and experience really helps guide your path. You have to hit certain wickets to get promoted or to select for command but if you don't have a desire to do that, then those wickets are not ones you need to pursue.

Many Reserve Medical Corps Officers would like to stay in long enough to achieve a Navy retirement. Some leave active duty with several years of service already accrued toward retirement and therefore opt to continue to serve in the Reserves with the goal of accruing 20 years. Others join the Reserves with no prior service and still would like to obtain a Navy retirement. To do so requires a total of 20 "good" years which are defined as obtaining at least 50 points during your anniversary year. An anniversary year is individualized for each Sailor and generally is based on the commissioning date. Obtaining 50 points is done by ensuring you complete at least 40 of the required 48 drill periods, or doing at least 2 days per month of drill for 10 months. The other requirement to achieve a good year is to complete 12–14 days per anniversary year of active duty or annual training. This is generally done either with your assigned reserve command or at a military treatment facility.

Even if your only objective is to get to retirement, you do have to remain engaged. Your Fitness Report (evaluation) depends on that. On Active Duty, you meet with a Detailer, often with the input of your specialty leader, and assignments are allocated more on an individual basis. Assignments in the Reserves are done through a board process and though you can seek assistance and advice from your assigned Specialty Leader and the Medical Corps Reserve Affairs Officer, in most cases, these individuals are not directly able to place you into your assignment or billet. The Navy Reserve uses a system called Junior Officer APPLY (JO APPLY) and Senior APPLY to select billets or assignments. Senior APPLY is a board run very similarly to a promotion board. Officers are required to use the Senior APPLY system for all medical corps officer billets with the exception of some flight surgery billets. Senior officer, non-command billets are generally 3-year orders, and officers are selected based on performance, letters of recommendation, fit, willingness to travel, and location. Over the last 5 years, willingness to travel for billets and the need to travel for billets have increased. Very often, travel is unfunded and typically comes out of pocket. Officers are then ranked, and the process essentially works like a manual match similar to residency. The highest ranked officer gets their highest ranked billet, the next highest ranked officer gets their highest billet if it's still available, and so on until all the officers and billets are filled. Those that are not selected can then apply in a post-APPLY process that involves phone calls and interviews. Fitness Reports and performance are absolutely critical in getting a billet that is conducive to your interests, career goals, and lifestyle. Remaining engaged and involved in your command is key to getting a good evaluation.

Can you just float in the Navy Reserve? Of course you can. Probably the best way to do that is in the Voluntary Training Unit (VTU) which is a non-pay drill status but generally keeps you local and doesn't require the 2 weeks per year. It is certainly possible to serve in that capacity until retirement and help out your local reserve center with things like Periodic Health Assessments, etc. Being in the VTU also protects you from being involuntarily mobilized which brings me to my next topic.

Navigating Deployments or Mobilizations Understand where you are in life. Are you at a point in your career and your family life where a mobilization would not be detrimental? Are you excited about the possibility of being a part of a forward surgical team and potentially providing life-saving surgery close to or on the front lines? I am and that is my WHY but not everyone is in that position and that's ok! The Navy still deploys or mobilizes surgeons for 7 months and there is often a 3–4-month work-up plus another month on the back end for redeployment. In total, you can be away from your practice and your family for a year. That's a hard thing to do. Both you and your family (and your practice!) need to be prepared for that. Involuntary mobilizations for Navy Reserve surgeons have almost entirely gone away, but if you know you are not in the position to be tagged for such a mobilization, then there are billets you can take that would put you farther down on the list (serving with the Marines, taking a leadership billet, serving as a flight surgeon, to name a few). On the opposite end, the Navy also now has a Reserve Expeditionary

Resuscitative Surgical System (ERSS) that would put you closer to the top of the list should a need arise. There are many different options within the Navy Reserve that allow for all different opportunities and experiences. It is impossible to list all of them which is why I now bring up a couple more keys to success.

Get a Mentor A mentor is critical. A mentor can help you navigate the wide array of options and decide what exactly you want to do with your Navy Reserve career. My mentor is now a 2-star Admiral and someone with whom I served both during my intern year and while deployed to Iraq. We talk a couple of times a year, and she has always provided me with sage and frank advice as I navigated the different time periods in my life, my changing goals, and my Navy career.

Go to the Symposiums The Navy Reserve has an annual Operational Medicine Symposium which is a great way to network with other surgeons and to learn of any upcoming operational needs. You are also afforded the chance to speak with one of the Admirals in attendance and get some career advice. There are other leadership symposiums but this one is the most well-attended and geared most specifically to the operational side of the Navy Reserve. Announcements and notifications regarding officer development symposiums, the aviation medicine conference, and others will come out from either the respective specialty leaders or the Reserve Affairs Officer.

Sign up for the ListServ The ListServ, or Gov delivery, provides you with current Navy announcements letting you know immediately of openings for various schools and scholarships and upcoming mobilization needs. It is the fastest, most direct way to learn about opportunities in the Navy that otherwise may take a long time to trickle down through your chain of command.

Then There Are the Basics These are the little things that will keep you in favorable conditions with the Reserve Center and your command: Keep your email address current, maintain your access to all the various Navy-specific websites, complete your annual General Military Training, be aware of deadlines, ensure your records are in order, etc. These are the details that if you can keep in compliance, will simply make your life easier.

I have immensely enjoyed my 24 years in the Navy and have had the opportunity to truly see the world. Knowing my WHY and having my family's support have been the absolute key to my success.

Stationed Abroad in the Military

15

Tiffany C. Cox and Eric P. Ahnfeldt

Introduction: The What and Why of the Overseas Surgeon

One of the allures and uniqueness of the military surgeon career is an overseas assignment. In fact, it ranks the second most common reason behind financial incentives for the reason why Navy physicians join in the first place [1]. To be stationed in Italy, Spain, Japan, Germany, and the United Kingdom, to name a few, holds both personal and professional benefits compared to a civilian practice. Yet, prioritizing how to remain clinically relevant, academically minded, and remain CONUS engaged with pertinent societies can be challenging. Balancing the needs of the military which requires these strategic locations to remain active with the retention of a surgeon's own professional discipline will be discussed herein to convey considerations for a successful overseas practice.

Why does the Department of Defense (DOD) have overseas assignments for active duty (AD) surgeons? While there are many strategic reasons beyond the mission as a medically ready force during wartime that are outside the scope of this chapter, funda-

T. C. Cox (✉) · E. P. Ahnfeldt
Department of Surgery, Uniformed Services University of Health Sciences, Bethesda, MD, USA
e-mail: tiffany.cox@usuhs.edu

A. T. Schlussel et al. (eds.), *The SAGES Manual for Navigating a Successful Military Surgical Career*,
https://doi.org/10.1007/978-3-031-88490-0_15

mentally where there are high concentrations of AD personnel, there are typically accompanying medical supporting services. Not only do the AD members themselves take comfort in being stationed overseas where they know they will receive medical care by surgeons who practice to United States (US) national standards, allowing dependents to have the confidence of being cared for while co-located. As well, many contractors, government service civilians, and even North Atlantic Treaty Organization (NATO) allies are treated by the US surgeon within these environments. While there are still times to refer to local national networks for certain low acuity subspecialty needs, there is often the collaboration between facilities across services that allows for the true feel of the military network to do our best for patients when they are at their worst.

Integration and learning from our local national counterparts are opportunities for professional development that few experience unless in societies with colleagues worldwide. Opportunities such as collaborating with the local Italian Trauma System and providing podium presentations to global surgical leaders allow for a shared conceptual model and best practices to form. Current world events provide occasions for shared practices with Ukrainian plastic surgeons and the development of a curriculum for trauma management strategies and reconstructive options. The overseas assigned military surgeon has these types of real-time, globally collaborative, opportunities which few in the medical field would otherwise have. This concept extends to other allied partners wherein there are developing systems to respond to large-scale near-peer combat situations including Europe (EU), Africa, South-East Asia, and South America. Even our own US deployed ready forces can receive continued training efforts as is done for underway Marine squadrons serving as Role 2 light maneuvering teams. These efforts can be supported in the same time zone by surgeon educators overseas providing maintenance of skills developed by Navy Medicine Readiness and Training Command (NMRTC) Naples, Italy Society for Simulation in Healthcare™ (SSH) accredited Simulation Healthcare Advanced Practice Environment (SHAPE) Center. The continued mission of this hospital to be a training platform throughout the EU merges the need for maintenance of skills for those deployed [2, 3] while maintaining professional and academic engagement for the Outside Continental United States (OCONUS) surgeon.

Unique Environment

Serving in an overseas assignment can be incredibly rewarding as well as frustrating. Each surgeon's experience depends on a multitude of both internal and external factors. It is the impact of the external factors on the internal characteristics of each surgeon that ultimately defines how rewarding or frustrating is the experience of serving as an OCONUS surgeon.

External Factors

There is a litany of unique external factors that exist at OCONUS duty stations. The most prominent external factors concern hospital staff, supplies, and the relationship of the Military Treatment Facility (MTF) with the local national health system. Each of these factors affects the individual surgeon to varying degrees depending on the temperament and circumstances of the surgeon.

Hospital staff, including colleagues, live and work in a unique cultural bubble. Most of the staff undergo a permanent change of station (PCS) move every 2–3 years. This cultural bubble forces the hospital community to live in a closed work environment. For these short-tenure overseas assignments, individuals must work together with no other possibility for outside employment. Furthermore, the workforce is limited to the pool of people that have relocated to the OCONUS MTF. This can lead to resource constraints and unique skillset limitations. In the CONUS environment, this lack of depth or skillset limitation can be augmented by training or contracting solutions that utilize outside personnel or training platforms. Whereas in the OCONUS setting, most training solutions must be within the organization. Contracting solutions to utilize outside personnel from the US are extremely costly. Thus, the relationships with the host-nation hospital system become critically important. Additionally, with a turnover of staff every 2–3 years, it is difficult to maintain institutional memory. Maintaining legally vetted memorandums of understanding (MOUs), hospital policies, and standard operating procedures (SOPs) can help mitigate the loss of institutional memory.

Working with the host-nation medical system presents significant opportunities for international collaboration but is filled with cultural and legal challenges. Healthcare delivery outside the US can be very different from that which the US surgeon and their patients are accustomed to. Furthermore, the concept of "local practice" or "standard of care" is relative when several international borders are all within close proximity. Each country has its own medical norms and standards, licensing requirements, and maintenance of said licensing. These international requirements can be dramatically different from one country to another. The pertinent question to the military surgeon then becomes, "Who's standard of care do we use?", especially when referring a patient to the local economy for specialty services.

It is critically important for the military surgeon to establish professional relationships with their host-nation counterparts within the civilian healthcare delivery system. Avenues of opportunity to do so include attending their local national conferences as well as being a liaison with the surrounding hospitals as it is also a part of the mission of the military hospitals to regularly perform on-site visits. These relationships are personally, professionally, and strategically important and rewarding. The local national surgeons share the love of surgery and intellectual curiosity enough to facilitate the fostering of a professional relationship. Through this relationship, the military surgeon can gain situational awareness about how healthcare is delivered in their host nation. Furthermore, this relationship allows ease of patient transfer back and forth from the DOD system to the host nation. It also generates continuity and facilitates introductions with other host nation medical professionals. When a legal review is required to formalize transfer agreements, these relationships typically provide a starting point for gaining the host nation's legal confidence and concurrence. However, the military surgeon must understand that these professional relationships must be continually nurtured and protected. If these relationships become fractured or neglected, the resulting rift can have a devastating impact on access to care for beneficiaries.

There is no better example in recent history of the benefit to well-nurtured professional surgeon relationships between military and local national surgeons than the medical care rendered during the US withdrawal from Afghanistan. The relationships between the military surgeons at Landstuhl Regional Medical Center (LRMC) in Germany and their German counterparts in the surrounding region had been developed over the preceding 3 years as LRMC sought to gain American College of Surgeons (ACS) Level 2 Trauma Center status [4]. These relationships facilitated MOUs for certain subspecialties and transport capabilities not available at LRMC. Because these professional relationships had been founded in the years preceding 2021, the military and German surgeons had a solid respect for each other's clinical skills and understanding of the capabilities of the local German hospitals. This facilitated the American and German surgeons' emergency international credentialing at LRMC allowing them to operate and round together on Afghans and American Marines when LRMC was overwhelmed with casualties after the Abbey Gate Bombing on August 26, 2021, at Hamid Karzai International Airport [5]. Without these well-established relationships, many of the lives that were saved could have had worse outcomes; however, the aforementioned is a crystalline example to be immolated across the globe.

Internal Factors

Internal factors to consider when beginning an OCONUS surgeon's assignment include personality type, marital status, family dynamic, career experience, rank, and specialty. There are advantages to surgeons that can foster diverse and cross-cultural relationships. Due to that cultural bubble, the OCONUS MTF creates surgeons that do not prefer the small community in which they work will struggle to thrive.

Both single and married surgeons have their own rewarding experiences OCONUS. However, there are some significant challenges for working spouses. Teleworking is a viable option under certain status of forces agreement (SOFA) which is unique to each location and should be researched in advance of an upcoming assignment. However, even when teleworking is possible, time-zone differences can be an obstacle. Work visas can also be difficult to obtain. Government service jobs may be available, but the application and onboarding process is very lengthy and burdensome. For those spouses that temporarily leave the workforce during the OCONUS assignment, there are volunteer opportunities through the American Red Cross [6] allowing maintenance of professional acumen.

Accompanying children can significantly impact the experience. One of the major benefits of an OCONUS assignment is the ability to travel and do so as a family. The varying ages of the children can impact when and how to travel. But the enrichment by this multicultural experience as a family is priceless. They can gain a deeper appreciation for the regional history, geography, art, architecture, music, and cuisine. Navigating the local national schools is an opportunity to expose your children in an immersion style to a culture that broadens their global perspective. Similarly, many children, including those of the authors, enjoy the DOD schools as a unique student body experience. The students at the DOD school attend for 2–3 years due to billing assignments and can be admixed with other NATO international students. This short tenure at the schools creates an atmosphere where all students are relatively new to the school. The students at the DOD schools have the unique and shared experience of being an expatriate. In addition, the faculty caters to the unique needs of expatriate students. Many families have their kids enrolled in community and school sports programs. This furthers the enriching experience and coincides with stateside opportunities. However, in the OCONUS environment, "away" games typically, even in the DoD system, necessitate international travel to compete with other EU or DOD teams.

The stage in a surgeon's career, along with their rank, plays a significant role in the experience of the OCONUS surgeon. These two elements usually increase simultaneously as a career progresses. The higher the rank, the further the surgeon is in their career. However, there are occasions where the rank lags the stage in a career. These instances usually include either delays in promotion or joining the military after civilian training and corresponding employment. Both situations in the OCONUS environment should be a consideration of accepting the billet at the right time advancing a surgeon's career from leadership positions in ways they might otherwise not have an opportunity to do so in the larger stateside facilities.

For the clinically active surgeon with years of service, overseas assignments can provide deployment opportunities and the chance to see how different MTFs and their medical command structures function. Prior clinical and administrative experience allows the military surgeon to navigate the complexities of the OCONUS environment with its corresponding resource constraints. Recent surgical residency graduates do not have this depth of experience or confidence and may struggle when presented with clinical or administrative challenges. Therefore, if recent graduates are going to be placed in OCONUS assignments, it is critical that more experienced clinically active surgeons be co-located.

Lastly, type of specialty plays a critical role in the experience of the OCONUS surgeon. For example, a surgical oncologist would find that many of the resources available to treat their patients are not present in the OCONUS environment. Thus, they would be highly dependent on the local national health system to reach their expected standards. This, in turn, would limit the practice of the surgical oncologist, and their skills could potentially atrophy. However, a highly motivated surgical oncologist could turn this dependency on the host nation into an advantage for their professional career. The resourceful OCONUS surgeon will use this opportunity to develop relationships with host-nation surgeons and develop professional and academic associations. With this comes invitations to attend international conferences and meetings. This networking can give the OCONUS military surgeon face-to-face access to internationally renowned surgeons with varying breadth and depth of experience to learn and enrich one's own practice. This is an opportunity that CONUS DOD surgeons will never have had exposure to.

Strategic Utility for Deployments Abroad

The DOD needs surgeons to provide surgical services to areas that have military personnel. Prior to World War I (WWI), the United States maintained an international policy of isolationism. The lessons learned in the early and mid-twentieth century, however, resulted in an increased US military presence globally. After the Korean conflict, Germany became the major platform in the EU for medical care and evacuation. Likewise, Okinawa Japan became the major platform for surgical care in the Asia-Pacific region with evacuation routes to Tripler Army Medical Center in Hawaii. Meanwhile, there continue to be mobile surgical assets in the form of hospitals or small surgical teams (Army, Navy, and Air Force) as well as hospital ships (Navy) and on-ship surgical suites (Navy) following shifting troop populations and geopolitical conflict areas.

Many of these platforms and configurations were developed in the mid-twentieth century and have been adapted to meet the needs of the current theater of operations. The major hubs of military evacuation post-WWII have also become the major locations for OCONUS surgical assignments. The twenty-first century has seen the most rapid advances in the application of technology in both warfare and healthcare delivery. While these hubs of surgical care were developed in response to conventional symmetric type warfare, asymmetric warfare with non-conventional forces such as seen in Afghanistan has dominated their use since 2001. However, with the advent of Russian aggression in Ukraine including the crisis in Crimea in March 2014 and more recently in Donbas, Zaporizhzhia, and Kherson in February 2022, the resultant increased defensive posture of NATO strategy [7, 8] has shifted to include conventional symmetric warfare again. These hubs for medical care abroad also serve to provide quality surgical care and final quality control function before MHS beneficiaries are transported across the ocean for medical evacuation back to the United States.

The Military Health System (MHS) must work in partnership with host-national health systems. These DOD MTFs serve to allow the MHS to engage with international partners. NATO, EU, and other partners across the globe regularly perform training exercises with DOD facilities and joint resources. This prepares all the organizations for eventualities including large-scale military engagements. Such operations would quickly overwhelm military medical resources. Thus, partnerships with integrated local national established healthcare delivery systems will expand the ability to care for large numbers of military and civilian injured patients [9].

Contingency planning requires multiple international locations with surgical capabilities. At the time of this publication, the conflict zones that are most likely to escalate to multistate levels are in the Eastern European theater and the Asia-Pacific theater. In these areas, healthcare collaborative agreements need to be well-established and functioning. With the destructive power of current warheads, no single healthcare system will be able to absorb the number of casualties that would be generated during large-scale warfare. Thus, shifting patient loads internationally to offload the healthcare system in closest proximity to the conflict will be important. On a smaller scale, this was seen during the Afghanistan evacuation of over 120,000 people to safety [10] and again during the Ukraine invasion in 2022.

These strategic OCONUS locations serve the purpose of providing military medical reach into the international community. Surgeons that choose to serve in these locations play a critical role in providing this strategic surgical care. As previously stated, the role of the surgeon is much greater than just performing surgery. They are surgical ambassadors, bridging the gap between DOD and host-nation facility capabilities. If their role in this capacity goes unrecognized by the OCONUS surgeon, the mission of the MTF is degraded. Uniformed Services University of Health Sciences (USUHS) Global Health Engagement among many other online or in-person courses exist if a surgeon knows they will be going overseas and can immerse themselves ahead of time to gain perspective in global health.

Exceptional Clinical Circumstances

OCONUS Environment Preparation

Preparing for the OCONUS assignment starts prior to boots on the ground at the overseas station. Knowing you are billeted for overseas, considerations for expanding skills start months before packing. Partnering with gastroenterology, interventional radiology, gynecology, cardiothoracic, urology, plastic surgery, and neurosurgery can expose you to skillsets that may be useful in an environment where you otherwise do not have these subspecialists readily available at one's facility. Scrubbing these cases can assist in improving already attained skills to benefit from just-in-time repetition or provide exposure to cases you may have never seen and have more familiarity thereafter with the steps of the procedure. While these skills aren't standard to general surgeons' practice, there may be circumstances where you cannot refer a surgical patient out of one's facility and could otherwise have less confidence to provide surgical care necessary for the environment [11, 12]. Simulation cannot be understated as another avenue of preparation prior to an overseas assignment. Programs such as Advanced Trauma Life Support (ATLS), Advanced Surgical Skills for Exposure in Trauma (ASSET), and Advanced Trauma Operative Management (ATOM) are highly recommended. This is true not only for the possibility of needing to acutely treat a trauma patient at a small overseas facility but more importantly the intent of overseas locations as strategically embedded to remain poised for its primary mission as the Role 2 or Role 3 deployment medically ready force. These courses have shown efficacy both to improve skills through the course as well as improved bedside performance and confidence [13]. Other non-trauma subspecialty procedure-specific simulation physical models and proficiency curricula, such as urologic emergencies [14], have been developed by military educators to assist surgeons who are billeted to go to these types of environments and can be utilized to prepare the individual prior to ever leaving the US.

Access to Care

Local national network referrals can assist in access to care for our patients that need specialists outside the capabilities of the smaller overseas medical facility. However, the OCONUS environment provides additional opportunities for patients to receive US standard of care. Transfer to a nearby Military Training Facility (MTF) or even to a higher echelon CONUS are available when time allows. When time does not allow, the exposure to these cases prior to being stationed to an often solo-practice OCONUS MTF provides understanding and preparedness. There are opportunities for subspecialists to rotate at one's facility from other OCONUS locations or CONUS surgeons through either Temporary Duty Travel (TDY) or the Visiting Surgeon Program (VSP) [15]. When overseas surgeons are preparing before their assignment, they can gain the benefits to first assist cases outside of their normal practice. This will not only add to the complexity of their own case volume prior to arrival but also gain experience to then provide meaningful assistance to those traveling from afar once in the OCONUS atmosphere. Additionally, OCONUS facilities can allocate surgical specialists for TDY to provide credentials to specialists and expand surgical capabilities at that hospital as needed.

Using All the Tools in the Toolbox

Supply chains, budget constraints, and access to nuanced procedure-specific tools can be quite challenging overseas. Efforts have been focused and partnered with overseas vendors to improve access to deliverables [16], but the process is still lacking in consistency and timeliness. At the same time, working to try and keep patients in our facility and minimize transfers out for causes such as not having the tools you would at a CONUS MTF is vital. Understanding how to operate, not just how to do an operation, becomes paramount. For instance, many overseas MTFs lack gastroenterology complete with endoscopic retrograde cholangiopancreatography (ERCP) capabilities. In conjunction with this limitation, the lack of a choledochoscope may limit a surgeon's capability to perform stone retrieval for a retained stone. Ordering one takes time and money and for the frequency with which this may be seen at one's facility may be hard to justify cost and maintenance expenditure. However, at our facility, the combined need for a ureteroscope when our regional urologist would visit and its dual use as a choledochoscope for the instances it would be required was able to justify the cost and increase capability.

A novel solution set arose from issues with supply chains to obtain endoscopic tattooing ink which was no longer available. The facility still needed to maintain the ability to mark locations for concerning polyps identified on screening colonoscopies. Utilizing the endoscopic clip at the excision site (Fig. 15.1) and postoperatively obtaining an abdominal x-ray (Fig. 15.2), localization was maintained and provided an alternative to performing the procedure effectively while thinking outside of the "standard" toolbox. Even after 8 weeks, the clip localization had remained in place (Fig. 15.3). In some circumstances, this technique was used as an endoscopic marker for any larger piecemeal resected polyps to re-survey the same location, marker for more advanced endo mucosal resection or verify complete resection. While it is expected that the clip will slough, short-interval scopes can utilize this in their armamentarium of endoscopic options. More so, even in more austere environments with less access to consumables, innovative thinking can minimize referring patients out for procedures you can commonly perform when considering the supplies you do have at hand.

Maintaining Diversity and Complexity of Skills

Even as a fellowship-trained surgeon, maintaining skills for complex cases is possible through collaboration with one's surrounding DOD network. Limitations of the facility and personnel can seem to limit one's ability to practice these cases as you would normally do. For example, as a bariatric surgeon having an intensive care unit (ICU) and supporting multidisciplinary

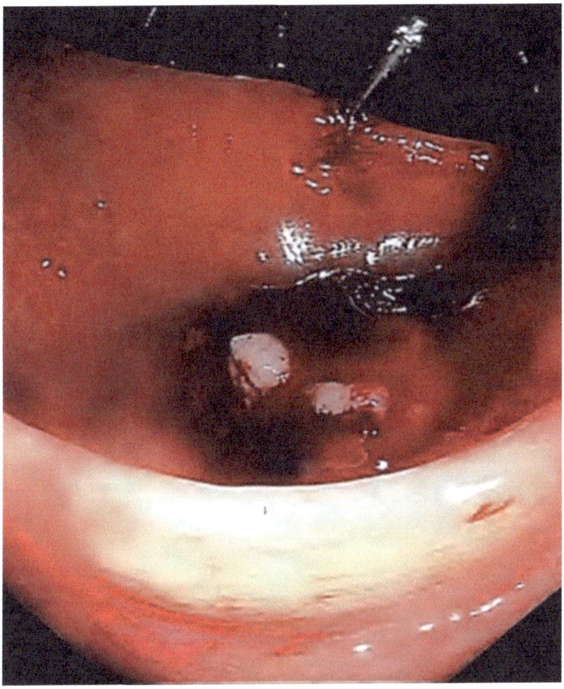

Fig. 15.1 Clip at the time of initial scope to mark piecemeal resection due to lack of inking resources

staff such as bariatric nutritionists and bariatric behavioral health specialists is necessary. In the case of bariatrics, the local facility lacked these aspects but a regional network facility that had an already established Bariatric Program at Landstuhl, Germany, collaborated with the local site. Through this, fellowship-trained surgeon skills were able to be maintained by partnering with their program, utilizing the expansion of virtual medicine to accomplish the multidisciplinary visits necessary and provide exposure to these cases to feel confident and remain privileged in these non-core cases. Additionally, platform-based approaches not available at a smaller MTF collaborate with the more expansive MTFs to create the mutual benefit of utilizing the equipment at the larger facility while maintaining the skills

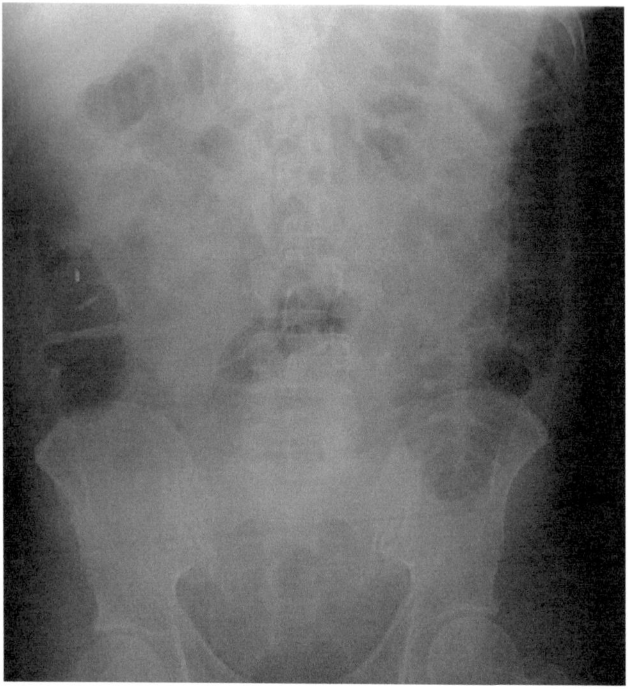

Fig. 15.2 Abdominal X-ray denoting the location of clip anatomically confirming area of right colon involved

of robotic surgery for the individual overseas surgeon at a smaller facility. Quarterly rotations are ideal to provide skill maintenance as rotations more frequently for the smaller MTF surgeon who may be coming from a practice where they are 50–100% of the duty is not feasible. As the continued Defense Health Agency (DHA) focus on improving Knowledge, Skills, and Attitude (KSA) for the military surgeon, this concept as described supports the needs of the DHA, the needs of overseas surgeons, and needs of the patient to improve their regional access to care. Traveling with one's primary facility personnel can expand team training to one's surgical technicians and anesthesia providers if they accompany the surgeon for these cases and thereby improve their own KSAs simultaneously.

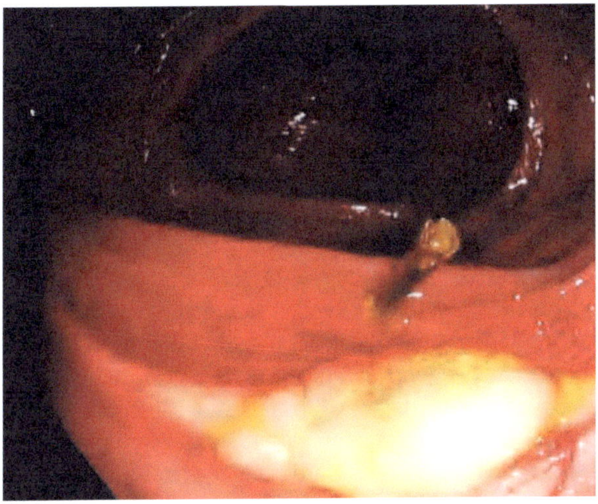

Fig. 15.3 Interval scope demonstrating residual polyp burden with the clip still in place

At the very least, most overseas MTFs have more than one surgical discipline practice at the location. With that, double scrubbing cases can afford the general surgeon experience and understanding of cases they would otherwise not gain experience with a stateside practice and diversify their case volume to strive to achieve improving KSAs. Military-civilian partnerships are commonplace stateside for residents and surgeon faculty. This concept has expanded overseas and is successful for the Air Force surgeon in the United Kingdom as well as for the Army surgeon with European civilian partners.

Sustaining Academic Engagement

For the military surgeon, CONUS or OCONUS, the USUHS remains a cornerstone of academic engagement opportunities. General surgeons from across the globe can apply as an assistant professor through USUHS. USUHS students rotate during medical school both stateside and OCONUS. This affords the student the opportunity for exposure to overseas challenges as well as improving their knowledge and attitudes making them more confident to serve overseas through these early experiences [17]. Residents have similar exposure through humanitarian missions and proven to gain acquaintance with diverse cultures and worldly perspectives while performing cases that are required through the Accreditation Council for Graduate Medical Education (ACGME) guidelines [18].

US Society engagement is highly encouraged and attainable. Many societies today have virtual platform committee meetings and online virtual conference sessions to attain CME, and overseas commands support continued research efforts through their Research Integrity Officer affiliated with an Institutional Review Board (IRB) stateside for approval of any research proposals. The military supports accredited continuing medical education (CME) both globally and at one's own facility when events are registered [19] and can allow you to receive ongoing CME credits. USUHS is also partnered with Naval Postgraduate School (NPS) and provides further prospects for degrees and certificates; a highly recommended asynchronous course allowing certification in Healthcare in Simulation [20] is an ideal certification for the overseas academically minded surgeon.

Future Directions

The OCONUS surgeon will always be a necessity for the military. With the changing global political landscape and the rise of the Defense Health Agency (DHA), who determines how that surgeon is utilized is also shifting. LMRC, the military's only OCONUS trauma center, became a DHA facility in 2022. With that transition, all civilian positions historically being Army positions have now also become DHA positions. The same is true as the rest of the OCONUS facilities make the DHA transition. These two entities, the MHS and the DHA, have different and overlapping missions. For example, the mission of the DHA is to provide a medically ready force and ready medical force to Combatant Commands in both peacetime and wartime. For the Army, the

Medical Corps's mission is to conserve the Army's fighting strength by providing the highest quality healthcare to soldiers, families, retirees, and other eligible beneficiaries. With each additional entity that controls the forces or the facilities comes competing interests, requirements, and metrics with which to measure the performance of the facility and clinicians. However, the mission of the military, according to the 2022 National Defense Strategy [21], is to safeguard and advance vital US national interests, working alongside other agencies to protect the security of the American people, expand economic prosperity and opportunity, and realize and defend the values at the heart of the American way of life. As long as there are military surgeons, there will be a need to provide surgical care overseas as the United States seeks to expand its influence throughout the world. Thus, whether in peacetime or war, the role of the military surgeon abroad will continue to be an essential key to providing access to life-saving surgical services when and where the country needs it most.

Disclosure The views and opinions expressed herein are those of the authors and do not represent the opinions of the United States Army, United States Navy, the Uniformed Services University of the Health Sciences, or that of the DOD.

References

1. Goodrich E. Joining the navy to become a physician: the typical experience. Mil Med. 2022;187(9–10):e1209–15. https://doi.org/10.1093/milmed/usac117.
2. Hall A, Qureshi I, Vasquez M, et al. Military deployment's impact on the surgeon's practice. J Trauma Acute Care Surg. 2021;91(2S Suppl 2):S261–6. https://doi.org/10.1097/ta.0000000000003279.
3. Cant MR, Naumann DN, König TC, Bowley DM. How do deployed general surgeons acquire relevant skill sets and competencies and mitigate skill fade? BMJ Mil Health. 2021;167(3):209–13. https://doi.org/10.1136/bmjmilitary-2020-001641.
4. Knudson MM, Rasmussen TE. The Senior Visiting Surgeons program: a model for sustained military-civilian collaboration in times of war and peace. J Trauma Acute Care Surg. 2012;73(6 Suppl 5):S536–42. https://doi.org/10.1097/TA.0b013e31827548c9.

5. Bozzay JD, Murphy TP, Baird MD, et al. The last days: the medical response of United States and allied military teams during the Afghanistan exodus. J Trauma Acute Care Surg. 2023;95(2S Suppl 1):S13–8. https://doi.org/10.1097/ta.0000000000004062.
6. American Red Cross International Services. [cited 2023 Dec 5]. Available from: https://www.redcross.org/about-us/our-work/international-services.html
7. Wolff AT. The future of NATO enlargement after the Ukraine crisis. Int Aff. 2015;91(5):1103–21.
8. Chesnut M. US/NATO-Russian strategic stability and the war in Ukraine. CNA; 2023.
9. Lebeda FJ, Scheerer JB, Dembek ZF. A systems perspective of DoD global health engagement. Mil Med. 2020;185(7–8):e1024–31. https://doi.org/10.1093/milmed/usz461.
10. US Transportation Command Afghanistan evacuation support [Online]. Ustranscom.mil; 2021 [cited 2023 Dec 5]. Available from: https://www.ustranscom.mil/cmd/neo.cfm
11. Nealeigh MD, Kucera WB, Bradley MJ, et al. Surgery at sea: exploring the training gap for isolated military surgeons. J Surg Educ. 2019;76(4):1139–45. https://doi.org/10.1016/j.jsurg.2018.12.008.
12. Nealeigh MD, Kucera WB, Artino AR Jr, Bradley MJ, Meyer HS. The isolated surgeon: a scoping review. J Surg Res. 2021;264:562–71. https://doi.org/10.1016/j.jss.2020.12.032.
13. Mackenzie CF, Tisherman SA, Shackelford S, Sevdalis N, Elster E, Bowyer MW. Efficacy of trauma surgery technical skills training courses. J Surg Educ. 2019;76(3):832–43. https://doi.org/10.1016/j.jsurg.2018.10.004.
14. Hafer AS, Sweeney WB, Battista AL, Meyer HS, Franklin BR. Development and implementation of Urologic Care Army/Air Force/Navy provider education, a urologic emergency simulation curriculum. Mil Med. 2023;188(3–4):817–23. https://doi.org/10.1093/milmed/usac003.
15. Fox JP, Latham KP. The Air Force Visiting Surgeon program: development, outcomes, and future application. Mil Med. 2021; https://doi.org/10.1093/milmed/usab507.
16. Koerner SD, Anaya MA. The implementation of Prime Vendor Europe and its successful impact on an overseas naval medical treatment facility. Mil Med. 1996;161(10):607–13.
17. Mancuso JD, Garges EC, Hickey PW, et al. Outcomes from U.S. military-supported overseas training rotations in tropical medicine and global health, 2006–2015. Mil Med. 2017;182(9):e1796–801. https://doi.org/10.7205/milmed-d-16-00408.
18. Jensen S, Tadlock MD, Douglas T, Provencher M, Ignacio RC Jr. Integration of surgical residency training with US military humanitarian missions. J Surg Educ. 2015;72(5):898–903. https://doi.org/10.1016/j.jsurg.2014.12.004.

19. MODS. 2023 [cited 2023 Nov 18]. Available from: https://education.mods.army.mil/NavyCME/Default.aspx
20. School NP. 2023 [cited 2023 Nov 18]. Available from: https://movesinstitute.nps.edu/healthcare-certificate
21. Austin LJ III. 2022 National defense strategy of the United States Including the 2022 nuclear posture review and the 2022 missile defense review. U.S. Department of Defense; 2022.

Part III

Developing Your Career as a Military Surgeon

Success in Your First Job: How to Maximize Time and Overcome Low Surgical Volume

16

Walter B. Kucera
and Romeo C. Ignacio Jr.

Introduction

In the early years of a surgical career, transitioning from training to practice can be both exhilarating and daunting. Junior military attendings, who have recently graduated from residency or fellowship training and are stationed at their first duty station, are faced with challenges that are unique and much different from civilian-trained surgeons. These difficulties include managing low surgical volume, adapting to a new environment, and thriving

W. B. Kucera
Department of Surgery, Naval Medical Center San Diego,
San Diego, CA, USA

Department of Surgery, Uniformed Services University of Health Sciences, Bethesda, MD, USA

R. C. Ignacio Jr. (✉)
Department of Trauma, Rady Children's Hospital San Diego,
San Diego, CA, USA

Division of Pediatric Surgery, Rady Children's Hospital San Diego,
San Diego, CA, USA
e-mail: r1ignacio@health.ucsd.edu

A. T. Schlussel et al. (eds.), *The SAGES Manual for Navigating a Successful Military Surgical Career*,
https://doi.org/10.1007/978-3-031-88490-0_16

amidst the complexities of military life. This chapter aims to provide guidance on how to navigate these obstacles effectively.

Constant Dilemma of the Deployed Surgeon

For many military surgeons, the reality of working in both deployed and garrison environments can pose significant challenges. A critical issue is the decline in surgical skills that occurs when operative volume is low. Studies have shown that surgeons with periods of reduced operative experience often face deterioration in their technical skills. A review of the literature reveals that the frequency of procedures is directly correlated with the maintenance of technical proficiency, which can affect patient outcomes [1]. For instance, research by Dalton and colleagues has demonstrated that surgical skills can decline significantly with extended periods of low operative volume [1], highlighting the challenges in maintaining medical readiness [2]. Therefore, it is important to identify ways to counteract these effects when assigned to such billets.

A study by Hall et al. (2021) illustrates that surgeons deployed in selective overseas assignments often face fewer routine surgical cases, which can impede the maintenance of technical skills [3]. The lack of regular practice means that even experienced surgeons can see a decline in their abilities. This issue is compounded by the diverse and often high-complexity cases that military surgeons may encounter, requiring a level of proficiency that might be difficult to maintain with infrequent practice. Additionally, many smaller military treatment facilities (MTF) have fewer resources when it comes to available consultants and equipment than most training institutions.

Lastly, the transition from a training environment to a new military treatment facility can be challenging. Junior surgeons who have recently completed their training may find the low case volume at their new duty station disheartening, especially when compared to the high-volume environments they experienced during training. The first years after graduation are critical for the development of young surgeons, so it is important for the surgeon to recognize this and work hard to develop professionally.

Key Takeaway
The transition from a training program to either a deployed setting or an MTF can be associated with decreased resources and case volume that can negatively impact readiness.

Operative Skills Training

To address the issues related to low surgical volume, junior military surgeons must *proactively* seek ways to enhance and maintain their operative skills. Here are several strategies to consider.

Simulation

Simulation training has become an invaluable tool for surgeons aiming to maintain and improve their skills [4]. Modern simulation technologies provide realistic scenarios that replicate various surgical procedures and challenges [5]. These simulations allow surgeons to practice techniques, refine their skills, and build confidence in a controlled environment. According to Atesok et al. (2017), simulation training can help bridge the gap between infrequent operative cases and the need for continuous skill development [6].

Utilizing simulation platforms available at military treatment facilities or through specialized training programs can provide significant benefits. Engaging with these tools regularly can help you stay sharp and prepare for a wide range of surgical scenarios.

Assisting in Non-General Surgery Cases

Another effective method for maintaining surgical skills is to assist in cases outside the general surgery realm. Collaborating with subspecialty surgeons in fields such as orthopedics, urology, or vascular surgery can offer valuable exposure to different surgical techniques and procedures. This cross-training helps broaden your skill set and provides insights into various surgical approaches, which can be beneficial in both routine and emergency situations.

Some emergency procedures performed by these subspecialists can aid in uncommon traumatic injuries that a general surgeon may face in the combat theater, such as compartment syndrome of the lower extremity, renal or bladder injuries, and penetrating vascular trauma. As elucidated by Nealeigh et al. (2019), even on non-combat shipboard deployments, orthopedic, urologic, and gynecologic emergencies represent some of the most required procedures to be performed by general surgeons [7].

Nadaud et al. (2024) emphasize that exposure to diverse surgical specialties enhances overall surgical competence [8]. By participating in non-general surgery cases, you can gain experience with different types of procedures and improve your adaptability in the operating room.

Trauma Skills Courses

Participating in trauma skills courses is another excellent way to enhance surgical skills. Courses such as Advanced Trauma Life Support (ATLS) and Advanced Surgical Skills for Exposure in Trauma (ASSET) focus on trauma management and advanced surgical techniques. These courses are specifically designed to improve decision-making, procedural skills, and trauma care, which are critical in both deployed and non-deployed settings. Additionally, as will be discussed later, these courses can be ideal for team building as other members of the team, such as scrub techs, can often participate. This is also an opportune time to consider becoming an instructor for these courses. This affords the junior surgeon additional training and professional growth in learning how to educate their peers.

Surgical societies, such as the American College of Surgeons (ACS) and the Society of American Gastrointestinal and Endoscopic Surgeons (SAGES), also offer advanced courses that provide hands-on training in various surgical techniques. Engaging in these courses not only sharpens your technical skills but also helps you stay updated with the latest advancements in surgical practice.

Video Review and Quality Improvement (QI)

Young surgeons should also look for ways to improve their skills and decision-making by performing an intense review of 100% of their cases. Long-term outcomes and quality assessments of patient care should also be done routinely and reviewed either weekly or at least, monthly. Surgeons should also record 100% of their laparoscopic cases and review them, especially if they had an intraoperative misadventure. Recorded cases can be shared with other providers, too, so they can offer constructive criticism. This will not overcome fully low volume and acuity, but it may help prevent the surgeon from making the same mistake twice or prevent them from getting into intraoperative trouble.

Off-Duty Employment (ODE)

Surgeons should also consider doing off-duty employment while in garrison or in port in the US. Adding 1–2 days of work per month in addition to their military duties can help to maintain operative and decision-making skills. Even doing this less frequently will help. Of course, this must be balanced against further time commitments and time away from family. Additionally, it requires command permission, and sadly, some local commanders do not recognize the need for surgical skill maintenance, and they may not allow their doctors to do locums work. In those instances, reaching out to the surgeon's consultant or specialty leader may be helpful to help convince the commander.

Key Takeaways
The use of simulation, hands-on courses, ODE, and QI initiatives can mitigate some of the effects of low volume and acuity while at the MTF or deployed environments. These options are available from many different organizations both within and outside of the military.

Enhancing Nontechnical Skills

While technical skills are crucial, nontechnical skills play an equally important role in a successful surgical career. These skills can enhance your effectiveness as a leader and team member, improve patient care, and contribute to overall career growth.

Leadership

Leadership is a key component of success in any military role. For junior military surgeons, developing strong leadership skills is essential for managing surgical teams, making strategic decisions, and guiding others. Leadership in the military context involves understanding and motivating your team, managing resources efficiently, and making decisions under pressure.

Engaging in leadership training programs, both in and out of the military, and seeking mentorship from experienced leaders can help you develop these skills. Volunteering for leadership roles within your facility or participating in military leadership exercises can also provide valuable experience. Specific leadership development opportunities in the military are discussed later in the Specialized Training section, but you should seek out mentors for help in military-specific areas such as award and evaluation writing.

Communication

Effective communication is critical in both clinical and military settings. Surgeons must be able to convey information clearly and concisely to their teams, patients, and other healthcare professionals. This includes delivering briefings, providing feedback, and facilitating discussions.

Developing strong communication skills involves practicing active listening, presenting information clearly, and engaging in constructive dialogue. Regularly seeking feedback and participating in communication training workshops, such as those offered by the Faculty Development Program with USUHS, can help you improve these skills. Additionally, taking the time to attend Commander's Update Briefs and other organization-wide meetings can demonstrate how best to communicate with stakeholders in the combat arms community who may or may not have medical familiarity.

Team Building Skills

Collaboration and teamwork are fundamental aspects of surgical practice. In a military setting, you often work as part of a multidisciplinary team, which may include other medical professionals, support staff, and military personnel. Building effective teamworking skills involves learning how to work collaboratively, respect diverse perspectives, and contribute to a cohesive team dynamic.

Participating in team-based activities, such as joint training exercises or collaborative projects, can enhance your ability to work effectively with others. Developing these skills not only improves patient outcomes but also fosters a positive work environment. One of the best ways to develop your team is to operate together. If you are assigned to an operational unit, such as a Fleet Surgical Team or Forward Surgical Team, work with your local MTF to secure a time when your team can fully staff a day of cases. If you are assigned to an MTF, work with your OR leadership to schedule days to work with nurses, techs, and anesthesia providers with whom you will deploy.

Decision-Making

Decision-making skills are crucial for surgeons, especially in high-pressure situations. In a military environment, decision-making can be further complicated by factors such as limited resources, time constraints, and competing priorities.

Developing strong decision-making abilities involves practicing critical thinking, assessing risks and benefits, and making informed choices under pressure. Engaging in simulation exercises and participating in scenario-based training can help you improve your decision-making skills.

Situational Awareness

Situational awareness refers to the ability to perceive, understand, and anticipate the dynamics of a given situation. For military surgeons, this means being aware of the broader context in which you operate, including the operational environment, patient needs, and team dynamics.

Enhancing situational awareness involves staying informed about the operational context, understanding the needs of your patients, and being mindful of the dynamics within your team. Regularly reviewing relevant information and participating in scenario-based training can help you improve your situational awareness.

Key Takeaways
Working with teams from your assigned unit or deployment group prior to deployment is crucial for later success in the field. Utilize your educational and simulation resources to maximize your non-technical skills.

Development of Military/Promotion

Career advancement within the military framework involves more than just clinical proficiency. It requires strategic planning and active engagement in various professional and educational opportunities.

Volunteer for Leadership Opportunities

Taking on leadership roles within the military can significantly impact your career development. Not surprisingly, the convening orders for the promotion selection boards routinely mention that "officers fully qualified for promotion should show a readiness for leading and solving problems at larger and larger scales." [9] Junior surgeons should actively seek out opportunities to lead projects, participate in command roles, or contribute to strategic planning. Volunteering for these roles demonstrates initiative and a willingness to take on additional responsibilities.

Importantly, leadership roles are present across a wide spectrum. One does not necessarily need to be a director of surgical services or department head in order to effect change. Active membership of a hospital-wide committee can build important long-term relationships with others in the command in addition to making an impact on operations. Such relationships often can be the difference in securing more senior positions later in one's career.

Advancement of Educational Opportunities and Specialized Training

Pursuing further education and specialized training can open doors to new opportunities and enhance career prospects. Junior surgeons should explore options for additional certifications, advanced degrees, or specialized training programs. One of the top priorities when getting out of training is obtaining board certification in your specialty. Board certification will not only result in a larger paycheck each month through Board Certification Pay, but it is also an important consideration for promotion boards [9].

While numerous opportunities for in-person and distance education exist for advanced degrees, such as an MPH or MHPE, there are also opportunities for increasing the breadth of medical knowledge into other areas. One such example is the Military Tropical Medicine (MTM) course offered by the Uniformed Services University of the Health Sciences (USUHS) [10]. With an option in an asynchronous virtual format, the MTM course allows deployed surgeons to increase their familiarity with uncommon diseases that may be present in their Area of Operations, which can increase their operational efficacy in addition to their medical proficiency.

In addition to medical courses offered both in person and online, participation in military-specific training is another key factor for selection boards. Of note, Navy or Joint Professional Military Education (PME) programs are a particular point of emphasis for promotion [8]. The PME programs through the services' War Colleges not only provide valuable insight into the higher level workings of the military but also afford a useful Additional Qualification Designation (AQD) (JS7) for naval officers. Available as an asynchronous 7–10-month program, these courses can be accomplished during a deployment even with limited internet connectivity. This course can be combined with online programs from the Joint Medical Executive Skills (JMES) Institute, notably the JMSE-Intermediate course, which fulfills the requirements for the Executive Medicine AQD (67A) [11]. While the Army and Air Force do not have AQD equivalents for their officers, they do have service schools available for medical officers. It is highly recommended that junior surgeons use their early career years to discuss their goals with their assigned branch corps or service specialty advisor. This advisor is an expert in providing guidance on successfully advancing your military career and ensuring you meet all necessary requirements for ranks and desired future positions. For junior officers with the ability to travel for courses, numerous in-person courses are also available for personal advancement in healthcare administration and military education. The USUHS MedXellence course, which is offered throughout the year in numerous locations both within the US and worldwide, provides instruction on healthcare administration and insight into the workings of the Defense Health Agency [12]. Combined with the JMES-I online course, these two courses provide useful groundwork for new graduates that may find themselves in division officer or department head positions. Military leadership courses, such as Intermediate Leadership Course and Advanced Readiness Officer Course for the Navy, Captain's Career Course and Intermediate Level Education for the Army, and Squadron Officer School for the Air Force, provide service-specific instruction on the processes of the larger institution, which grows understanding of the "practice and business" of military medicine [13–15].

Continuing education not only broadens your knowledge and skills but also reflects a commitment to personal and professional growth. Engaging in educational opportunities can help you stay updated with the latest advancements in surgical practice and contribute to career progression.

Participation in Scholarly Activities

Engaging in scholarly activities such as research, teaching, and publishing can contribute to professional development and academic advancement. Junior military surgeons should consider participating in research projects, presenting at conferences, or contributing to medical journals. Another option for engaging in scholarly activity is volunteering as a peer reviewer for medical journals. While some journals require an invitation to review, others such as Military Medicine, have a self-nomination process [16]. Serving as a reviewer for one journal can open opportunities for others. If participating in an IRB-approved research project leads to a peer-reviewed publication, the Researcher AQD (6ZF) can be awarded for naval personnel [17].

For surgeons who are not immediately pursuing fellowship training, an alternative way to engage in academic medicine is by applying to join the faculty at USUHS. The Department of Surgery at USUHS requires board eligibility, engagement in scholarly activity, and evidence of institutional citizenship to be considered for an assistant professor appointment [18]. Appointment to Assistant Professor also confers the 6ZB AQD for Navy surgeons [17].

Participation in scholarly activities enhances expertise, builds a professional network, and supports career progression. It also demonstrates a commitment to advancing the field of surgery and contributing to the broader medical community.

Engagement in Local and National Surgical Organizations and Committees

Active involvement in surgical organizations and committees can provide valuable networking opportunities and access to professional resources. Junior surgeons should consider joining local or national surgical societies, participating in committee work, and attending relevant conferences. Many societies have specific Young Surgeon committees made up of and advocating for recent graduates. These committees can be important stepping stones to gaining other opportunities in those societies.

Many societies also offer reduced rates and specific military education. Registration to the annual SAGES conference, for instance, is free for surgeons on active duty or reservists deployed to the combat zone during that year. Membership to SAGES is also only $60 annually for active-duty surgeons. Because SAGES provides combat care education, attendees can develop their combat skills as well as their non-combat surgical skills at a very low personal cost. The American Society of Metabolic and Bariatric Surgeons (ASMBS), the American Association for the Surgery of Trauma (AAST), and the American College of Surgeons (ACS), each have discounts and benefits for active-duty surgeons. Engagement in these organizations helps build connections, stay informed about advancements in the field, and contribute to professional development. It also provides opportunities for collaboration and knowledge-sharing with other professionals in the field.

Attainment of Overseas and Combat Experience

Gaining overseas or combat experience can be a significant asset in a military career. The selection boards are instructed to "give favorable consideration" to officers who have deployed to combat environments, and they acknowledge that such deployments may lead to atypical career paths [8]. Such experience provides exposure to diverse medical and surgical challenges, enhances adaptability, and contributes to professional growth. Additionally, ground-based deployments with the Navy can earn the Fleet Hospital Assignment (6OU) and Trauma Team Trained Officer (6OW) AQDs [17].

In addition to combat deployments, assignment to operational platforms also provides opportunities for career advancement. For Navy surgeons assigned to Marine Corps billets, the Marine

Corps Medical Department Officer (6FA) AQD is available after 90 days of assignment is completed. For those assigned to US Naval surface warships, such as ship's surgeons for a CVN or a member of a Fleet Surgical Team, the Surface Experienced Medical Officer (6FD), Shipboard/Hospital Ship Assignment (6OB/6OC), and the Surface Warfare Medical Department Officer warfare device (LA7) [17]. For the Army, service schools, such as the Basic Airborne Course and the US Army Medical Center of Excellence, courses are available to demonstrate operational readiness [13]. Similarly, Air Force Surgeons can attend service schools such as Basic Airborne Training for additional operational experience [14].

Junior surgeons should seek opportunities for deployment or assignments that offer the chance to gain valuable field experience. This experience can enhance your skills, broaden your perspective, and support career advancement.

Key Takeaways
A low clinical volume and acuity allow for the development of other important aspects of one's military resume. Taking the time to invest in these skills early in one's career can pay outsized dividends later.

Personal Growth and Maintaining Well-Being

Maintaining personal well-being is essential for long-term success and fulfillment in a military career. Junior surgeons should focus on several key areas to support their personal growth and well-being.

Family

Balancing professional responsibilities with family life can be challenging, especially in the military. It is important for junior surgeons to prioritize family time, communicate openly with loved ones, and seek support when needed.

Building a strong support system and managing work-life balance contribute to overall well-being and job satisfaction. Ensuring that you have time for family and personal activities helps maintain a healthy and fulfilling life.

Health, Exercise, and Wellness

Maintaining physical health is crucial for managing the demands of a military career. Regular exercise, a balanced diet, and adequate rest are important for sustaining energy levels and overall health.

Junior surgeons should make time for physical activity and self-care to stay fit and resilient. Incorporating exercise into your routine helps manage stress, improve mood, and enhance overall well-being. It is important for physicians to maintain their military bearing, as well.

Young surgeons should also dedicate some time to non-surgical activities that interest them. After nearly a decade of intense education between medical school and surgical training, there was likely little to no time spent on their favorite hobbies. The surgeon could take advantage of being less clinically active by doing so, which may help them better deal with burnout or stress in their life. Adnan Alseidi, MD, is currently the Vice Chair of Education at the University of California—San Francisco and became a certified chef while at sea during one of his ship assignments in the US Navy. Not only is he a well-respected surgeon at one of the world's leading academic institutions, he is also one of its city's restauranteurs.

Mentorship

Having a mentor can provide invaluable support and guidance throughout your surgical career. Junior military surgeons should seek out mentors who can offer advice, review cases, share experiences, and provide career development support. Many national and regional surgical societies offer free mentoring programs for recent graduates.

Mentorship helps with navigating career challenges, setting goals, and achieving professional growth. Building strong relationships with mentors can contribute to long-term success and fulfillment in your career.

Key Takeaways
It is important to use the time provided in the first years out from training to regain the balance in your life that may have eroded during medical school and GME training.

Conclusion

Navigating the early years of a military surgical career can be challenging, particularly when faced with low surgical volume. By actively seeking out training opportunities, enhancing non-technical skills, engaging in career development activities, and focusing on personal well-being, junior military surgeons can overcome these challenges and achieve success in their roles.

Success in your first job as a military surgeon involves a combination of technical proficiency, leadership, communication, and personal growth. By embracing these strategies, you can maximize your time, maintain your skills, and build a fulfilling and successful career in military medicine. Furthermore, low clinical volume is not a predictor of success as a clinician, a military leader, or as a surgical leader after leaving the military. There are many examples in this book of military surgeons overcoming low-volume assignments and being successful.

References

1. Woods MS, Liberman JN, Rui P, Wiggins E, White J, Ramshaw B, Stulberg JJ. Association between surgical technical skills and clinical outcomes: a systematic literature review and meta-analysis. JSLS. 2023;27(1):e2022.00076. https://doi.org/10.4293/JSLS.2022.00076.
2. Dalton MK, Remick KN, Mathias M, et al. Analysis of surgical volume in military medical treatment facilities and clinical combat readiness of

US military surgeons. JAMA Surg. 2022;157(1):43–50. https://doi.org/10.1001/jamasurg.2021.5331.
3. Hall AB, Qureshi I, Gurney JM, Shackelford S, Taylor J, Mahoney C, Trask S, Walker A, Wilson RL. Clinical utilization of deployed military surgeons. J Trauma Acute Care Surg. 2021;91(2S):S256–60.
4. https://postgraduateeducation.hms.harvard.edu/trends-medicine/simulation-training-helps-surgeons-refine-their-skills-strengthen-leadership-potential
5. Seymour NE, Gallagher AG, Roman SA, O'Brien MK, Bansal VK, Andersen DK, Satava RM. Virtual reality training improves operating room performance: results of a randomized, double-blinded study. Ann Surg. 2002;236(4):458–63.
6. Atesok K, Satava RM, Marsh JL, Hurwitz SR. Measuring surgical skills in simulation-based training. J Am Acad Orthop Surg. 2017;25:665–72.
7. Nealeigh MD, Kucera WB, Bradley MJ, Jessie EM, Brian Sweeney W, Matthew Ritter E, Rodriguez CJ. Surgery at sea: exploring the training gap for isolated military surgeons. J Surg Ed. 2019;76(4):1139–45.
8. Nadaud JM, Heidel RE, Daley BJ. Rural surgery preparedness after graduation from a surgical residency. Am Surg. 2024;90(9):2253–7.
9. Hogue RD. Order convening the FY-25 promotion selection boards to consider staff corps officers on the active-duty list of the navy for permanent promotion to the grade of commander. Department of Defense; 2024 April 24. Available from: https://www.mynavyhr.navy.mil/Portals/55/Boards/Active%20Duty%20Officer/documents/FY25_Promotion%20Board_Materials/FY-25_AO4S_CO.pdf?ver=dNZyk02vWwLNN-0rdiNvNQ%3D%3D
10. Navy Medicine. Military tropical medicine. Available from: https://www.med.navy.mil/Naval-Medical-Leader-and-Professional-Development-Command/Officer-Training/Military-Tropical-Medicine/
11. Medical Corps, United States Navy. Executive Medicine (67A) AQD. 2023 Aug. Available from: https://safe.menlosecurity.com/doc/docview/viewer/docN5ABE3CAB759Aea644738f58adc011fd4cc2b103b2eb-fe32b3ed94519e9e3c9295ae30c2d7c37
12. Uniformed Services University. About MedXellece. Available from: https://medschool.usuhs.edu/pmb/education/medxellence
13. U.S. Army. Specialized skill training. Available from: https://myarmybenefits.us.army.mil/Benefit-Library/Federal-Benefits/Specialized-Skills-Training?serv=120
14. U.S. Air. Military specialized skills training. Available from: https://www.myairforcebenefits.us.af.mil/Benefit-Library/Federal-Benefits/Specialized-Skills-Training?serv=26
15. Navy Medicine. Advanced readiness officer course (AROC). Available from: https://www.med.navy.mil/Naval-Medical-Leader-and-Professional-Development-Command/Officer-Training/Advanced-Readiness-Officer-Course-AROC/

16. Association of Military Surgeons of the United States. Military medicine reviewer guidelines. Available from: https://academic.oup.com/milmed/pages/reviewer_guidelines
17. United States Navy. Part D. Additional qualification designator (AQD) codes. Available from: https://www.mynavyhr.navy.mil/Portals/55/Reference/NOOCS/Vol1/Manual_1_83_PTD_AQD_Apr23.pdf
18. USU Walter Reed Department of Surgery. Faculty appointment and promotion. 2024 Mar 3. Available from: https://sites.google.com/usuhs.edu/sur/faculty/faculty-promotion

Maintenance of Wartime Medical Skills

17

John Christopher Graybill,
Shaun R. Brown, Jeffrey A. Bailey,
and Brian J. Gavitt

In 2013, the medical director of the United Kingdom's Military Health Services, Commodore Alasdair Walker, described a concept known as the "Walker Dip." Beginning with the Crimean War, where British Forces received abysmal medical care, he demonstrated a cycle between conflicts, where military medical

J. C. Graybill (✉)
Joint Trauma System, Fort Sam Houston, San Antonio, TX, USA

Walter Reed National Military Medical Center, Bethesda, MD, USA

Uniformed Services University of the Health Sciences, Bethesda, MD, USA
e-mail: John.C.Graybill.mil@health.mil

S. R. Brown
Joint Trauma System, Fort Sam Houston, San Antonio, TX, USA

Uniformed Services University of the Health Sciences, Bethesda, MD, USA

Army War College, Washington, DC, USA

J. A. Bailey
Joint Trauma System, Fort Sam Houston, San Antonio, TX, USA

Uniformed Services University of the Health Sciences, Bethesda, MD, USA

Washington University, St. Louis, MO, USA

A. T. Schlussel et al. (eds.), *The SAGES Manual for Navigating a Successful Military Surgical Career*,
https://doi.org/10.1007/978-3-031-88490-0_17

departments "forgot" the lessons learned in the previous wars, resulting in much higher levels of death and disability than seen at the end of prior conflicts [1]. Recent examples of lessons lost are numerous, for example, the use of tourniquets, which were prevalent in Vietnam but fell out of favor due to concerns about limb loss. The 75th Ranger Regiment reinstituted the use of tourniquets in Operation Iraqi Freedom, showing a survival benefit that led to the DoD's broad adoption of their use in Iraq and Afghanistan on September 1, 2006 [2]. Similarly, before the invention and widespread utilization of gunpowder, soldiers wore armor. However, armor fell out of favor for centuries due to its heavy weight, lack of mobility, and minimal protection against ballistic wounds. Body armor was reintroduced by the time the US Military was involved in a conflict in Mogadishu, Somalia, on October 3 and 4, 1993. The reintroduction of body armor resulted in a reduction in fatal chest wounds (14% vs 39%) compared to Vietnam [3]. This led to the widespread reimplementation and use of body armor in the DoD for the recent conflicts in Iraq and Afghanistan. A third lesson is utilizing whole blood as the resuscitation fluid of choice. Whole blood (WB) was routinely used in World War I and II [4]. It fell out of favor and was replaced with crystalloid resuscitation, followed by unbalanced resuscitation and, subsequently, by balanced resuscitation strategies. However, recent scientific evidence has resulted in WB once again being implemented as the first-line resuscitation agent of the US Military, in the form of low titer O-whole blood.

Another contributing factor to the "Walker Dip" is the lack of provider exposure to high-acuity, complex trauma patients and experience in performing critical procedures needed to save lives and function. Two factors have led to this: medical specialization and low patient volume in MTFs. The operational (deployed) med-

B. J. Gavitt
Joint Trauma System, Fort Sam Houston, San Antonio, TX, USA

Uniformed Services University of the Health Sciences, Bethesda, MD, USA

88th Surgical Operations Squadron, Wright Patterson Air Force Base, Cincinnati, OH, USA

ical force's structure relies on generalists, specifically, people who can function as jacks-of-all-trades. The general medical officer, or GMO, is a combination internist, family practitioner, pediatrician, and psychiatrist. The ideal surgeon is a general surgeon with a heavy familiarity with trauma, vascular surgery, cardiothoracic surgery, and open general surgery with some knowledge of orthopedics and neurosurgery. However, the US medical system has steadily increased individual provider specialization due to the vast increase in specialty-specific knowledge, science, technology, personal professional preferences, and economic pressures and factors [5]. The increasing specialization of medicine has created a paradox for the Department of Defense (DoD), creating a workforce that needs increasingly specialized knowledge and skills to practice in the garrison while still requiring a broad medical foundation to perform as a physician in a deployed environment.

Care for the traumatically injured also requires quick thinking and action, sometimes using complex but infrequently performed procedures, on an often-unstable patient. To obtain the knowledge and skills needed to master the care of the traumatically injured, one needs frequent exposure to the traumatically injured and other acutely ill patients with complex surgical problems. Unfortunately, due to laws and policies regarding healthcare insurance for DoD beneficiaries' access to high acuity patients can prove challenging.

The DoD healthcare insurance is legally broken into three separate components. Active-Duty service members are insured under a program called Tricare Prime. Unless care capacity is exceeded, they receive all their care in military treatment facilities (MTFs) and clinics. Dependents (e.g., spouses, children, and retirees under 65) can receive their care under Tricare Select. Tricare Select is a managed care support contract run by third-party insurance companies. The contract is divided into the Eastern US (currently managed by Humana Military Health Services) and the Western US (currently managed by TriWest Healthcare Alliance). Those contracts run as a self-managed, preferred provider organization, in which patients can see any provider within a pre-approved network, whether primary care or specialty care. Tricare for Life is a Medicare supplement insurance for retirees and dependents over 65, which the same companies manage. Medicare is the primary payor with Tricare being the supplementary payor. Like the Tricare Select group, those beneficiaries can see any provider within their network, including any provider that accepts Medicare. Finally, many former service members receive care from the Veterans Health Administration.

Unfortunately, most patients with acute, complex medical conditions fall within the over-65 cohort, the majority of whom receive their care outside the MTFs. The active-duty population is predominantly healthy and does not require complex care outside of orthopedic sports injuries. This combination of factors has led to a decrease in the MTFs volume and acuity of patients. Historically, most military healthcare providers have worked primarily within the MTFs. The low volume and acuity of patient care has put their medical readiness at risk to care for high-acuity trauma in the deployed environment.

Within the limitations defined by law concerning Tricare and delivery of care to DoD beneficiaries, multiple attempts have been made to maintain the clinical proficiency of medical providers, especially for surgeons who have degradable skills.

Numerous attempts have been made to recapture care at MTFs. These are primarily focused on preventing something known as "leakage." Leakage occurs when a clinic, whether primary or specialty care, lacks the capacity or capability to care for patients. Under current policy, if a clinic does not have availability within 28 days, a Tricare beneficiary, regardless of category, can receive care outside the MTF and within the network. Primary care appointments that are deferred to the network that require further subspecialty referrals often stay within the network rather than return to MTF specialty clinics. Most attempts at recapturing care are through marketing and customer service efforts to Tricare Select and Tricare for Life patients. Few of these endeavors have yet succeeded. There are no special incentives for Humana or the TriWest Healthcare Alliance to utilize MTFs and military clinics for beneficiary care they manage.

Fortunately, several other efforts have had much more success. One of the significant efforts has been the Joint Knowledge,

Skills, and Activity (JKSA) program. The JKSA focuses on building and maintaining the foundations needed to deliver high-acuity trauma care in a resource-restricted environment. These foundations include knowing not only trauma care but care specific to wartime injuries, the skills necessary to access and repair those injuries, and enough clinical proficiency, as measured by a busy clinical practice, to do so expeditiously. While this may sound intuitive, many surgeons do not have exposure to trauma patients in their routine clinical practice. As such, trauma care is not part of their regular academic endeavors either. The JKSA program has worked with the Joint Trauma System (JTS) and the American College of Surgeons to develop curricula focused explicitly on wartime trauma and best practices as defined in the JTS Clinical Practice Guidelines. The Emergency War Surgery Course and the M-curricula are two such endeavors. Likewise, the JTS and JKSA programs run surgical skills courses for military providers to allow them to train on traumatic exposures, repairs, and some reconstructive procedures. They also include skills outside the normal scope of general surgery that a deployed surgeon may have to perform downrange due to the lack of specialists, including craniotomies, lateral canthotomies, external fixator placement, and control of obstetrical traumas. The two most taught courses are ASSET+ for general surgeons and surgical subspecialists and COTS+ for orthopedic surgeons. The final component focuses on measuring clinical and operative activity and educating commanders on improving provider exposure to high-acuity care. While care of the traumatic patient is the best way to prepare to care for wartime casualties, this may only be realistic for some surgical subspecialists in their stateside clinical practices. Specific high-complexity care, like open oncologic and colorectal cases, utilizes many of the same skills as trauma operations and may serve as a surrogate for traumatic care. In short, the JKSA program emphasizes that delivery of large volumes of high acuity, high complexity care results in better outcomes for combat casualties. This is true of both individual providers as well as entire hospital systems. KSA scores for surgical specialties were developed in meetings held by the Military Health System Strategic

Partnership with the American College of Surgeons. Specialty leaders, consultants, and senior surgeons with deployment experience from each military service gathered and developed a scoring system based on case complexity and relevance to combat casualty care. One's KSA score can be found at: https://info.health.mil/hco/JKSA/Pages/Clinical%20Specialty%20Rosters.aspx

Another significant effort has been the establishment of military-civilian partnerships (MCPs). The goal of the MCPs is to provide active-duty service members from critical wartime specialties the ability to practice (within their expeditionary scope of practice) in a high acuity, high volume environment not available to them in the direct care system (MTFs). MCPs generally fall within two categories: strategic (managed at the Service Level by the Army, Navy, or Air Force) and local (managed at the MTF commander level). Strategic MCPs generally involve embedding providers in active level 1 trauma centers. Those centers are almost all large academic centers, providing high volumes of other specialty care. The Air Force was the first service to adopt this model with their Center for the Sustainment of Trauma and Readiness Skills (C-STARs) Programs. The C-STARs program partners with a growing number of academic partners to include the University of Maryland Shock Trauma Center, the University of Cincinnati, and Washington University and St. Louis University in Saint Louis. Providers are embedded within their affiliated hospitals and work on the trauma teams as their primary duty assignment; they deploy on the same schedule as those located in the MTFs. The US Army more recently followed suit with the Army Military-Civilian Trauma Team Training (AMCT3) partnerships. This program includes partnerships with Harborview Medical Center in Seattle, Oregon Health and Sciences University in Portland, the University of Chicago, Vanderbilt University in Nashville, Emory University in Georgia, and Cooper University in Camden, New Jersey. The Navy has a long-standing partnership with the University of Southern California at Los Angeles County General Medical Center and has also recently partnered with the University of Pennsylvania.

Local MCPs are organized and initiated at the MTF level where providers are stationed but spend part of their time practicing at local civilian hospitals for skill sustainment. Regional Veterans Administration Medical Centers also frequently serve as local MCP locations. These partnerships are not necessarily trauma-focused but instead focused on the specialties of the participating providers. Local MCPs provide an opportunity for surgeons to increase their case volume and acuity while providing a needed sub-specialization or surgical service needed within the local community of the MTF. Various MTFs within the three services (Army, Navy, and Air Force) have agreements with local private, public, academic, and Veteran's Administration Medical Centers. These MCPs include numerous specialties to include: colorectal surgery, surgical oncology, general surgery, minimally invasive surgery, trauma, cardiothoracic, vascular, plastics, otolaryngology, urology, neurosurgery, obstetrics/gynecology, cardiology, gastroenterology, critical care, and others. The patient population at these partnerships are diverse. Most patients are civilians whose insurance identifies those facilities as in-network providers. Others are DoD beneficiaries, allowing surgeons to provide timely care when the capacity at the MTFs is exceeded. The addition of local MCPs has been shown to increase case volume and complexity among all surgeons within the specific service of the MTF, regardless of whether the surgeon participates in the MCP or not [6]. The capacity limitations of the MTFs are almost universally a result of shortages in support staff, not a lack of surgeons. Local MCPs create a diversified surgical platform for the surgeons and provide case volumes that are resilient to fluctuations in staffing and operating room availability.

Examples of agreements include but are not limited to:

(a) External Resources Sharing Agreement (ERSA): ERSAs involve a TRICARE contractor whereby the MTF sends MHS providers to a local hospital to provide healthcare services not available at the MTF, usually due to a lack of support personnel or equipment. This avoids a referral to a network provider and examples include endoscopy, robotics, critical care, and nuclear medicine.
(b) Veteran Affairs (VA) Sharing Agreement: This allows you to evaluate and treat patients at the VA with full privileges. This

partnership can significantly help foster relationships between your VA and MTF, especially if there is a shortage of surgeons at the VA facility or a shortage of operating room, endoscopy, or other clinical space at your facility. Since the MTFs are lending their personnel to VA hospitals to care for VA beneficiaries, many MTFs request compensation to the DoD for the provision of their providers.

(c) Support Agreements: Memorandum of Agreement (MOA) which involves resources and Memorandum of Understanding (MOU) which has no resources involved. MOUs and MOAs are written contracts between two or more parties that outline the terms and understanding of their collaboration, particularly in the delivery of healthcare services. MOUs and MOAs may be used to establish agreements between military medical treatment facilities and civilian medical facilities or between military treatment facilities and other government agencies. MOAs are typically more formal and legally binding than MOUs because they may be used to allocate resources, define roles and responsibilities, and establish performance standards and metrics.

The details of the local MCPs are varied. The most significant variance is in malpractice coverage. Most DoD attorneys agree that providers working in these partnerships as part of their official duties are covered under the Federal Tort Claims Act (FTCA). However, some local MCPs recommend or require supplemental insurance, which is usually, but not always, provided by the civilian facilities. Outside of the Mission Zero Act, civilian facilities do not typically receive direct funding for MCPs from the government; however, the facilities can bill for services provided by the military surgeons and thus offset the cost of malpractice coverage. One point in common with all these agreements is that DoD providers cannot receive supplemental pay at a civilian facility where they practice as a part of an MCP.

The government has several agreements with foreign hospitals outside the United States to maintain providers' medical skills. The most noteworthy is a trauma partnership with the Sheikh Shakhbout Medical City (SSMC) located in Abu Dhabi, United

Arab Emirates, where multiple tri-service medical personnel are embedded. SSMC serves as this Emirate's primary trauma and burn center for a population of 1.57 million people. Service members' tours of duty at SSMC are for 2 or 3 years, and all assignments are accompanied. Other agreements exist with hospitals in England and Korea but are rotational rather than embedded partnerships.

Another type of foreign partnership is referred to as Global Health Engagement (GHE). These partnerships are typically transitory, lasting 2–4 weeks at a time and are team focused. The Uniformed Services University of the Health Sciences partners with a university hospital in Tegucigalpa, the capital of Honduras. Providers covering a variety of services (from ENT and ophthalmology to pediatrics) rotate through the hospital for several weeks to provide care for the local population. The State Department, which has limited medical resources but is the official first liaison with any foreign government, will frequently set up a partnership with a country as part of an outreach and goodwill program. They will engage the appropriate geographic combatant command to staff the collaboration. A specific type of GHE is the Medical Readiness Training Exercises (MEDRETES). Army field hospitals routinely fill these exercises in West and Central African nations such as Ghana, Senegal, and Chad. MEDRETES are usually 4 weeks long and involve various hospital providers, from physicians and nurses to pharmacists, scrub technicians, radiology technicians, and medics. Even though many providers participate in these events, MEDRETEs are typically focused on specific care areas, such as obstetrics, otolaryngology, plastic surgery, or general surgery.

One effective method for healthcare professionals to maintain their medical skills is through Off-Duty Employment (ODE) [6]. ODE involves government employees working in civilian roles outside their official duties while receiving supplemental income from these civilian sources. While ODE is often associated with medical personnel, it is prevalent across the (DoD), with enlisted personnel working as Uber or Lyft drivers being among the most common examples.

Rules and regulations govern ODE within the DoD, including restrictions on the number of hours an employee can work per week without taking leave and the required time gap between an ODE shift and duty at a military hospital. It is essential to note that healthcare providers engaging in ODE are not covered under the Federal Tort Claims Act (FTCA) and must obtain additional malpractice insurance, either independently or through their employer. Additionally, when providing services during ODE, physicians are prohibited from charging Tricare beneficiaries for their care. Providers must report their ODE activities, even if they use leave (vacation time).

While the DoD aims to standardize ODE policies across its services and hospitals, the reality is that there is considerable variation. Specific hospital commands may impose additional requirements, such as mandatory military training and specific medical documentation standards. These requirements can vary significantly from one institution to another. Generally, providers assigned to operational units face fewer restrictions compared to those working in Military Treatment Facilities (MTFs). Enforcement of DoD policies regarding ODE also varies widely among institutions and even within institutions.

It is crucial to understand that violating ODE policies carries inherent risks. Consequences may include punitive actions under the Uniform Code of Military Justice and adverse credentialing actions. These actions can be reported to state medical and civilian credentialing boards, potentially impacting one's ability to secure civilian employment after military service. Charging Tricare beneficiaries for care outside the DoD and failing to report for duty are among the most common violations of ODE policy.

In summary, healthcare professionals in the DoD have opportunities to maintain their medical skills through ODE though the availability and regulations for ODE can vary significantly based on one's assignment. To identify the specific opportunities available to you, consider consulting with colleagues within and outside your surgical department. Their experiences can provide valuable insights into navigating ODE effectively.

References

1. Mabry RL, DeLorenzo R. Challenges to improving combat casualty survival on the battlefield. Mil Med. 2014;179(5):477–82.
2. Cordts PR, Brosch LA, Holcomb JB. Now and then: combat casualty care policies for operation Iraqi freedom and operation enduring freedom compared with those of Vietnam. JTACS. 2008;64(2):S14–20.
3. Mabry RL, Holcomb JB, Baker AM, et al. United States Army rangers in Somalia: an analysis of combat casualties on an urban battlefield. JTACS. 2000;49(3):515–29.
4. Cap A, Beckett A, Benov A, et al. Whole blood transfusion. Mil Med. 2018;183(2):44–51.
5. Detsky AS, Gauthier SR, Fuchs VR. Specialization in medicine, how much is appropriate? JAMA. 2012;307(5):463–4.
6. Sheldon RR, Bozzay JD, Brown SR. Case volume and readiness to deploy: clinical opportunities for active-duty surgeons outside of military hospitals. JAMA. 2023;347(2):221–8. https://doi.org/10.1097/XCS.0000000000000697.

Establishing and Progressing an Academic Surgical Career in Both the Military and Civilian Worlds

18

Marissa Beiling, Jenifer Edmondson,
and Kenneth S. Azarow

Introduction

A recurrent theme in this textbook is how military surgeons can progress along in their careers while still meeting the military's non-medical requirements. For those who wish to pursue an academic career, the concerns are no less prominent. The young military surgeon may wonder how they can pursue academic endeavors in a system that typically does not provide research resources, with local leaders who are not prominent in their surgical field, with the requirements of deployment or military skills, and while trying to become proficient as a surgeon. There is not one straightforward answer, but the military has a long history of surgeons who have gone on to have great academic success in the civilian world.

M. Beiling · K. S. Azarow (✉)
Department of Surgery, Oregon Health and Science University,
Portland, OR, USA
e-mail: azarow@ohsu.edu

J. Edmondson
Darnell Army Medical Center, Ft. Cavazos, TX, USA

A. T. Schlussel et al. (eds.), *The SAGES Manual for Navigating a Successful Military Surgical Career*,
https://doi.org/10.1007/978-3-031-88490-0_18

As with our civilian counterparts, the process of an academic career begins in medical school, continues during primary surgical residency training, and becomes focused during their initial practice or during subspecialty/fellowship training. The level of achievement/progression at both the junior and senior faculty levels is dependent upon one's own initiative and creating an atmosphere of inquiry as a matter of course in one's daily activities regardless of the employment environment. Opportunities do, however, become more plentiful the further one advances into their career. Learning that exists in formal military education and during deployments translates well into academic work. This chapter will examine the careers of eight individuals who effectively managed a military medical career through retirement (minimum 20 years) and then were able to translate that experience to achieve success as leaders in the civilian sector [1–8]. We will detail each of these individuals as they traveled through the five phases of their careers. The eight individuals are:

- Dr. Norman Rich, founding Chair of Surgery Uniformed Services University of the Health Sciences (USUHS) (1977–2002), started in this role as an active-duty Army officer and transitioned the role to a civilian position (Image 18.1).
- Dr. James Ficke—Chair of Orthopedic Surgery at Johns Hopkins (Image 18.2).
- Dr. David Jaques—fully retired. Vice Chair of Surgery and Program Director at Memorial Sloan Kettering Cancer Center followed by a role as Vice President for Surgical Services Barnes Jewish Hospital, Washington University, St. Louis (Image 18.3).
- Dr. Allen Morey—Past Distinguished Chair in Reconstructive Urology at the University of Texas-Southwestern (UTSW) (Image 18.4).
- Dr. Annesley W. Copeland—Clinical Professor of Surgery, Uniformed Services University of the Health Sciences and Walter Reed National Medical Center (Image 18.5).

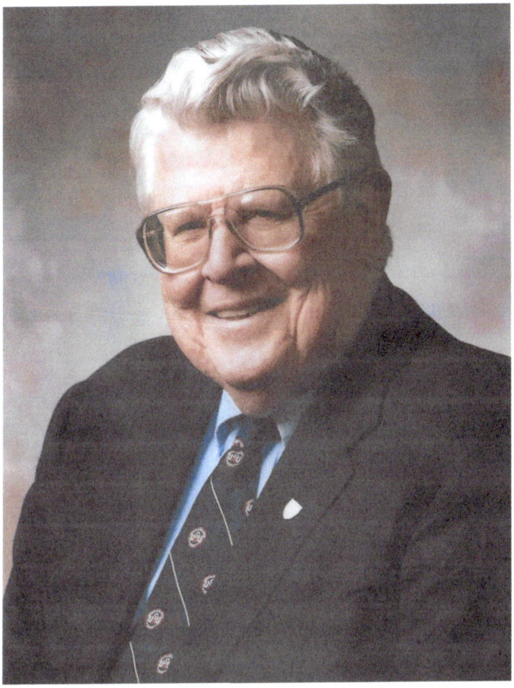

Image 18.1 Dr. Norman Rich, founding Chair of Surgery Uniformed Services University of the Health Sciences (USUHS) (1977–2002)

- Dr. Kenneth Azarow—Chair of Surgery at Oregon Health and Science University (OHSU) (Image 18.6).
- Dr. Mary Edwards—Chief of Pediatric Surgery, Surgeon-in-Chief, Bernard and Millie Duker Children's Hospital, Albany Medical College (Image 18.7).
- Dr. Eric Elster—Dean, Uniformed Services University of the Health Sciences (USUHS) (Image 18.8).

While the careers of these individuals were built upon the generations of military surgeons that preceded them, each serves as a modern-day example for the next generation of academic

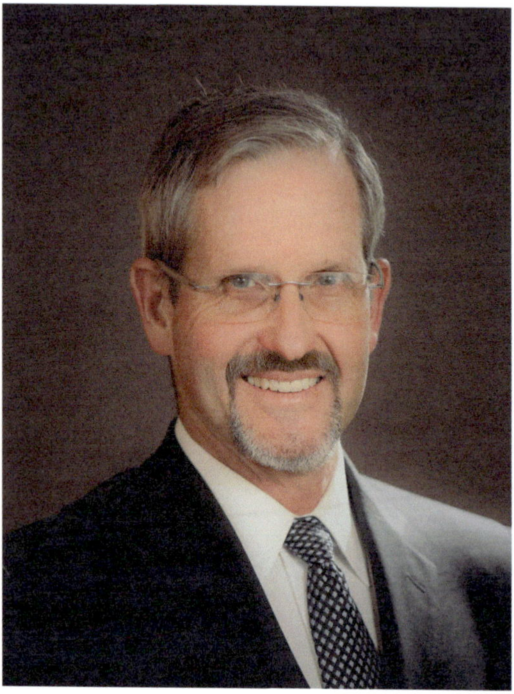

Image 18.2 Dr. James Ficke—Chair of Orthopedic Surgery at Johns Hopkins

military surgeons. Finally, one advantage of a military career is that there will be leadership positions available, whether at a small military treatment facility, on a combat surgical team, or as a department chair. Because there are fewer military surgeons than civilian ones, it is not unusual for a recent graduate to be the section or clinic chief upon arrival at their first duty station. The personnel management and clinical lessons learned from those positions give the average career military surgeon much more experience as a leader.

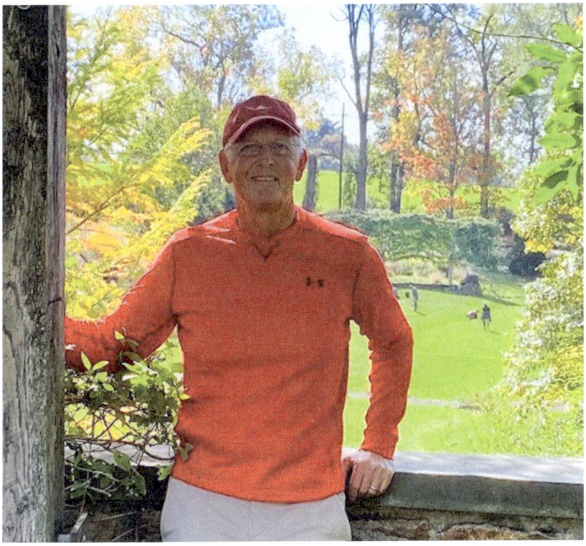

Image 18.3 Dr. David Jaques (ret)—Vice Chair of Surgery and Program Director at Memorial Sloan Kettering Cancer Center and Vice President for Surgical Services Barnes Jewish Hospital, Washington University, St. Louis

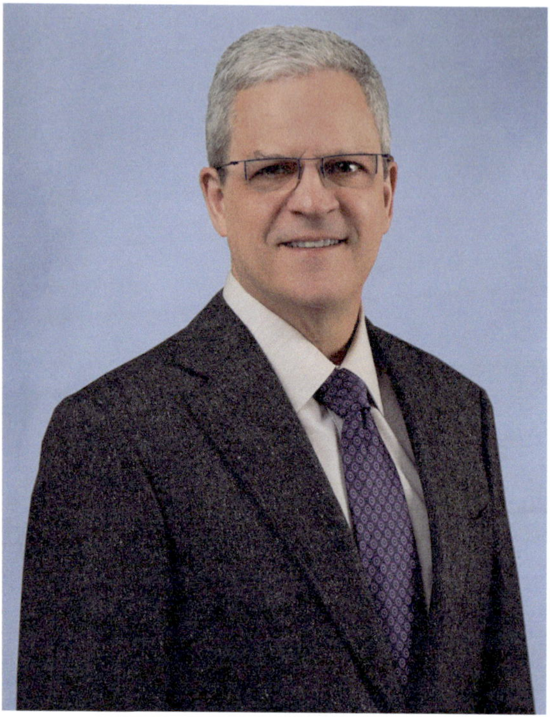

Image 18.4 Dr. Allen Morey—Past Distinguished Chair in Reconstructive Urology at the University of Texas-Southwestern (UTSW)

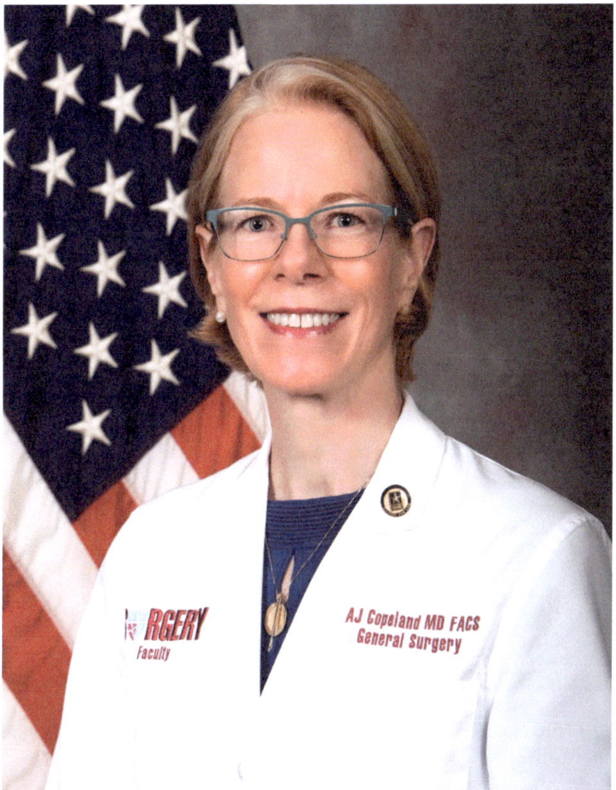

Image 18.5 Dr. Annesley W. Copeland—Clinical Professor of Surgery, Uniformed Services University of the Health Sciences and Walter Reed National Medical Center

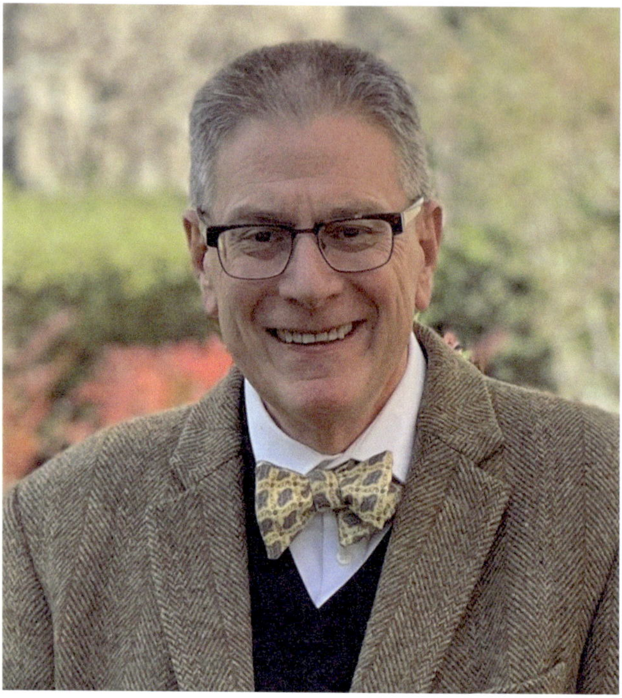

Image 18.6 Dr. Kenneth Azarow—Chair of Surgery at Oregon Health and Science University (OHSU)

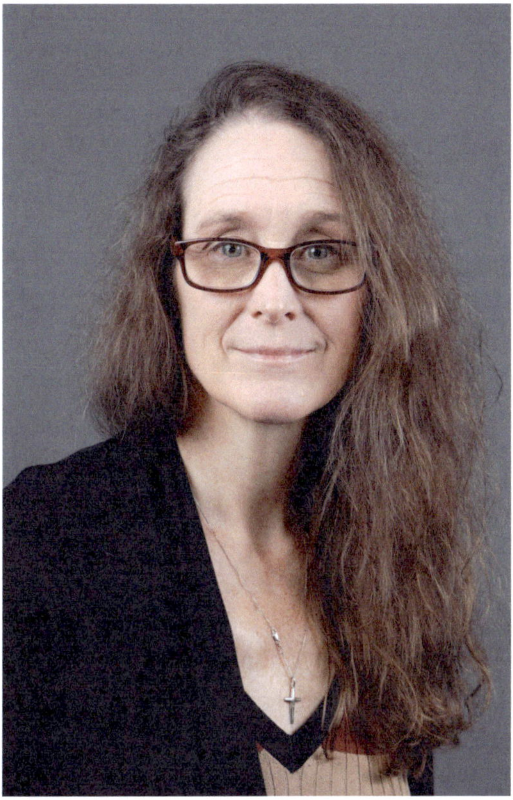

Image 18.7 Dr. Mary Edwards—Chief of Pediatric Surgery, Surgeon-in-Chief, Bernard and Millie Duker Children's Hospital, Albany Medical College

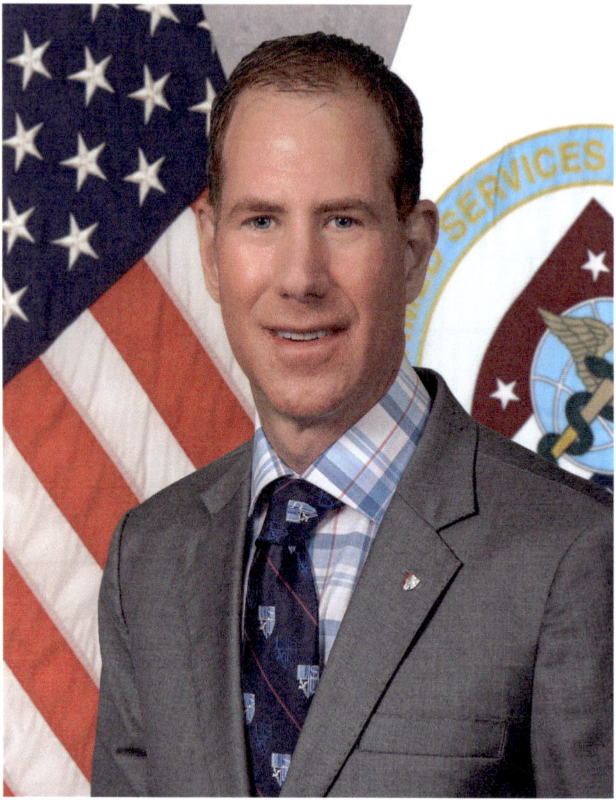

Image 18.8 Dr. Eric Elster—Dean, Uniformed Services University of the Health Sciences (USUHS)

Medical School and Residency

It is apparent from our cohort that sustained academic excellence began in medical school. In schools that had alpha omega alpha chapters at their schools, four of six individuals achieved membership [1, 2, 6, 7], and two schools did not have AOA chapters [3, 5]. One individual was valedictorian of the graduating class [2]. However, only two individuals, Jaques and Morey, had major peer-reviewed publications as students [5, 6]. All of our cohorts graduated from their respective officer basic course, a military requirement, and five of the eight completed either the expert field medical, air assault, or airborne badges, mountain warfare training, aerospace medical training, and aviation indoctrination [1–8]. Graduating from USUHS or on an HPSP scholarship from a nonfederal institution appeared to make no difference within this cohort. The transcendent theme is one of success. Put in other words, success at one's current job/position is still more vital than academic extracurricular activities. Earning high marks in coursework is more important than pursuing an optional research project during medical school.

During the summer or time off from medical school, it is extremely valuable to gain additional medical or military training. If you are in a civilian medical school, then the requirement may be to attend military training, such as the officer basic course, which is branch-specific, or a clinical rotation on active duty. If you are a student at USU, you could receive a military assignment, such as filling a temporary billet as a medical administrative officer. Medical students are not given clinical medical corps assignments due to their lack of clinical experience. However, they can rotate clinically on an elective basis, attend a variety of military training schools, and also have temporary administrative assignments consistent with medical support missions.

Military surgeons aspiring to an academic career do not need to complete a civilian residency with a strong academic reputation. All of our examples graduated from military surgery residencies [1–8]. Four of the eight joined their first professional or societal organizations as residents [1, 5, 7, 8]. Considering the significant number of leadership positions these individuals have achieved within their societies, it is difficult to determine the impact of early membership in professional organizations. What is quite evident is that residency is the point where academic excellence transitions from high grades in coursework and rotations to expansion into research, publishing in peer-reviewed journals, authoring book chapters, editorial reviews of peer-reviewed submissions, etc. Here is a list of academic achievements accomplished during residency and how many of our cohort achieved each one [1–8]:

Peer-reviewed scholarly paper(s)	5 of 8
Book chapter(s)	2 of 8
Presentation at National Meeting	6 of 8
Additional military training	4 of 8

As far as their first year after their primary surgery residency [3, 7, 8], three of the eight had medical corps assignments as general medical officers (GMO) after their first year of residency. A GMO is a military physician who, after completing their intern year, serves as a clinician in a military unit without having completed residency training. The presence or absence of an operational tour at this stage does not negatively affect the long-term trajectory of our cohort. Academic opportunities, though, clearly emerge during one's residency and need to be taken advantage of. Furthermore, performing one's residency in a military healthcare facility did not limit or influence these opportunities. Two of the three authors of this chapter are current military residents embedded in a civilian healthcare facility, and their opportunities are similar to those of their counterparts who are training in military healthcare facilities. The great importance of general surgery residency, beyond the essential surgical training, is to prepare oneself for success in either surgical subspecialty training or their first surgical job assignment, which may include a leadership position. The progression through academia is not solely determined by the structure of one's residency program; however, the individuals themselves must be willing to partake in the academic work.

Post-Graduate Years

Following residency, all individuals in our cohort completed rigorous surgical fellowships or narrowed their practice to specialize in a specific disease pattern. Over half of them first did clinical practice as general surgeons before opting to matriculate into a fellowship or narrowing their practice. It is evident that this phase marks an extension into research and education, including publishing, embarking on assistant professorships, and receiving grants [1–8].

Peer-reviewed scholarly paper(s)	5 of 8
Book chapter(s)	2 of 8
Presentation at National Meeting	7 of 8
Additional military training	4 of 8

It is readily apparent that advanced training, in addition to providing surgical aptitude, offers pivotal professional networks and habits vital to academic success. One last point to emphasize about advanced specialty training is that beyond networking and research productivity, there is no substitute for clinical excellence. This is how a surgeon will be characterized, and all other opportunities and work will assume this characteristic.

Many members of our group used the research conducted during their fellowship years as a springboard for their subsequent academic careers. It was during this period that they began to concentrate their academic efforts. COL Azarow developed a keen interest in congenital diaphragmatic hernias and their subsequent pulmonary injuries [1]. He published the article "A Tale of Two Cities" in the *Journal of Pediatric Surgery* during his time in Toronto, then participated in multiple clinical trials, and received related grants in the field. He published more than 15 additional articles on this topic and educated other surgeons from California to Switzerland, with his contributions shaping the current approach to the management of these patients [1].

Similarly, CAPT Elster's proclivity toward immunology, which began as a surgical resident and was fostered in fellowship, has defined his academic career and contribution to the medical field [3]. He began by conducting research with the Naval Medical Research Center's (NMRC) Immune Cell Biology Program and published numerous articles regarding immune cell gene expression as it relates to the subject of transplantation. CAPT Elster also adapted his work to trauma, making advancements in the understanding of the immune response to trauma and biomarkers involved in traumatic injury and wound healing. He has authored dozens of articles on these topics and has also lectured across the globe, with a more recent interest in precision medicine—how a patient's own genome should guide their medical care [3].

Dr. Morey, an internationally renowned urologic reconstruction specialist, also nurtured his academic interests during his fellowship. During his fellowship, he published several articles about buccal mucosal grafts for repairing traumatic urethral injuries and strictures, and he has contributed dozens more since. He has lectured on the topic of buccal grafts all around the US and internationally, including at the Urologic Congress of Central America and the Caribbean in Honduras [6].

Dr. Ficke completed fellowships in both orthopedic trauma and foot and ankle surgery, preparing him to become the founder of the Orthopedic Amputee Service at Brooke Army Medical Center [4]. He is considered a world expert in combat-related extremity injury. Dr. Jaques was mentored by Dr. Murray Brennan during his fellowship and published on clinical outcomes of melanoma and retroperitoneal sarcoma [5]. This rigorous analysis of outcomes led to a career of scholarly activity making improvements in clinical care in a variety of surgical situations, namely outcomes in surgical palliative care and reporting and improving upon surgical-related adverse events. While Dr. Rich, a vascular surgeon, has the most extensive bibliography of our cohort, much of his academic career started during deployment [7]. We will highlight his academic start later in the chapter.

As mentioned before, a unique aspect of a military career is the opportunity for advanced education and command experience. Drs. Azarow, Edwards, Morey, Copeland, and Ficke are graduates of the Advanced Officer Course (now the Captain's career course) and the prestigious Command and General Staff College [1, 2, 4, 6, 8]. The latter is the equivalent of Masters level training in leadership. All five of these individuals, along with Dr. Jaques, have earned the "A" proficiency designator (the equivalent of "professor rank in the civilian sector—given to only 5% of physicians) and the Order of Military Medical Merit [1, 2, 4, 5, 6, 8].

Operational Assignments

Equally important, though, is the operational work these surgeons have done. Dr. Azarow served as Deputy Commander for Clinical Service (DCCS) of the 86th Task Force in Iraq and transformed the 86th Combat Support Hospital into a functioning trauma hospital [1]. Dr. Ficke was the DCCS of the 228th Combat Support Hospital and then Theater Consultant for the 44th Medical Brigade Commander during Operation Iraqi Freedom [4]. Dr. Copeland served as DCCS for the 28th Combat Support Hospital (Forward) Tuzla, Bosnia-Herzegovina [8].

Dr. Edwards's deployment leadership is almost too extensive to list but here is a brief synopsis: Consultant for Pediatric Surgery, Task Force Strength, Afghanistan; 256th Combat Support Hospital, Al Asad Detachment, Operation New Dawn, Iraq, Chief of Surgery and Chief of Professional Services; Joint Trauma System, Combat Surgery Casualty Care Committee Planning Group and committee member/physician reviewer of the Afghanistan medical evacuation protocols, 25th Combat Aviation Brigade.

Dr. Rich was chief of the surgical service, 2nd Surgical Hospital, Ft Bragg, and the Republic of Vietnam, An Khe, during the Vietnam War. Dr. Elster, while on deployment, was director of surgical services and chief of surgery at Role 3 MMU Kandahar [7]. The theme here is that acquiring and implementing military training can lead to elevated positions of authority during deployment, which serves as an impetus for future leadership roles. The skills developed in these positions do indeed translate into civilian academic and organizational executive positions. These experiences develop and hone the skills required for leadership, and there are very few experiences in life or education that allow one to hone communication and organization skills like a leadership position during deployment. Furthermore, it is apparent that the ultimate common requirement for a successful career in academic medicine is excellence in these two skills. Everything else can be learned or taught on the job.

Junior Faculty

The next area of progressive academic development and contribution for this group occurs during deployment as junior faculty. In one's clinical work, the conscientious young surgeon should be looking for ways to improve their work and the system. A classic example of this is the individual who set the standard for the rest of this generation of surgeons, Dr. Norman Rich. During his deployments in Vietnam, he began collecting the fragments retrieved from the munitions that caused vascular injuries [7]. This meticulous documentation of the injuries, surgical procedures performed, and their outcomes led to the development of the Vietnam Vascular Registry. Scholarly contributions from this registry have led to the principles guiding the modern-day surgical management of vascular injuries. Dr. Rich has given dozens of named national and international lectures and received multiple awards for this contribution [7].

COL Jaques deployed to Saudi Arabia and Iraq in support of the 82nd Airborne Division during Operations Desert Shield and Storm and served as the senior general surgeon for this division. He established a surgery center in Saudi Arabia, developed a combat surgery course, oversaw the founding of a blood program that was used across the theater and led the first surgical capability into Iraq [5]. From infection to disability, Dr. Ficke documented extremity orthopedic injuries and best practices in our most recent conflicts in Southwest Asia [4]. COL Edwards completed multiple deployments to both Afghanistan and Iraq where she made substantial clinical contributions by documenting the physiologic impact of blast injuries in children and educating the international surgical community on this topic [2]. COL Azarow also published about his experiences with pediatric trauma at a combat support hospital in Iraq as well as improving combat readiness [1]. He also served as the senior surgeon in theater in Afghanistan in 2007 and concentrated on preparing surgeons for deployment in vastly under-resourced regions. What can begin as simple documentation of one's clinical experience can identify gaps in surgical care that lead to policy or even a fundamental change in care. In each of these cases, the surgeons looked at their deployments as a way to improve surgical care.

These clinical experiences should become publications when possible. While the science may not compare to a randomized clinical trial, the experience in combat is unique and has direct clinical applications. As such, quality academic work can be done without a robust research team behind the military surgeon. Again, the development of the Vascular Registry is a prime example [7]. The prospective data collection and organization took place during deployment; however, data analysis, follow-up programs, and multiple publications took place while a faculty member was at home. The diligent analysis of this work along with a solid performance in an operational/administrative role will likely lead to one to mature into senior leadership roles. As senior faculty, all our examples have attained senior leadership positions. This first occurred as part of their military service, then as educators training the next generation of military surgeons. This helped translate them into leaders within their professional societies and executive positions in their post-active-duty careers. We will review some very brief selected examples in our cohort.

Senior Leadership Positions

Dr. Azarow has served as program director for the general surgery residency at Madigan Army Medical Center and was the chief of surgery at that institution. After retirement, he was selected to serve as chair of the Pediatric Surgery Board, director of the American Board of Surgery, chair of the Advisory Council of the American College of Surgeons (ACS) on pediatric surgery, and on the Accreditation Council for Graduate Medical Education (ACGME) review committee for surgery. This led to his current role as chair of surgery at OHSU [1].

Dr. Edwards's senior leadership career started in education as she served as program director for the general surgery residency at Brooke Army Medical Center. From there, she rose to become the general surgery Consultant to the Surgeon General of the Army. The consultant position recognizes one as a subject matter expert and as an advisor to the Surgeon General on that specialty. Additionally, the consultant is intimately involved in the deployment and professional development of all military surgeons in that specialty. Because of her success there, she was elected to the pediatric surgery Board of the American Board of Surgery (ABS) and sits as a member of the ACGME review committee on surgery. Currently, she is the chief of pediatric surgery and the surgeon-in-chief of Bernard and Millie Duker Children's Hospital at Albany Medical College [2].

Similarly, Dr. Jaques began as an educator when he served as general surgery program director at Walter Reed Army Medical Center, where he eventually became chair of the Department of Surgery. He, too, became a consultant to the Surgeon General of the Army. After retirement, his military success led Dr. Jaques to become program director of the surgical oncology fellowship program and vice-chair of the Department of Surgery at Memorial Sloan Kettering Cancer Center. He then went on to become vice president of surgical services at Barnes Jewish Hospital in St. Louis [5].

Dr. Copeland has progressed through her academic career through the tract of teaching and education. She transitioned from the Army to civilian status but stayed within the Department of Defense. Her progression at USUHS led to the role of medical student clerkship director which she took over in 2012 and still holds as of the writing of this chapter. For over a decade, she has been a primary mentor to future surgeons who aspire to have a military career. Nationally, she has been an examiner for the American Board of Surgery, and she is most notable for her leadership within the Association of Women Surgeons (holding all executive positions including that of President) [8].

Dr. Morey's work eventually led him to become chief of urology at Brooke Army Medical Center and the urology Consultant to the Surgeon General of the Army. His success there enabled him to serve as president of the Society of Genitourinary Reconstructive Surgeons (GURS). This, in turn, led him to hold multiple national committee positions in the American Urologic Association (AUA) and serve as a member of the ACGME Review Committee in Urology. He later became the Paul C. Peters Professor and Distinguished Chair of Reconstructive Urology at UTSW in Dallas [6].

Dr. Ficke eventually became chair of orthopedics and rehabilitation at Brooke Army Medical Center and consultant to the Army Surgeon General in orthopedics. His work during the wars in Iraq and Afghanistan along with his success in military leadership enabled him to hold national positions in the ACS's Committee on

Trauma, the American Orthopedic Association, the Orthopedic Trauma Association, and the American Academy of Orthopedic Surgeons. Dr. Ficke is currently the Chair of the Department of Orthopedic Surgery at Johns Hopkins Hospital [4].

After his time in Vietnam, Dr. Rich became chief of the vascular service at Walter Reed and Director of the Vascular Fellowship. While on active duty, he became the founding chair of the USUHS Department of Surgery and transformed that position after retirement into one that could be maintained by a civilian, which he held for 22 years. Dr. Rich was a founding member of the American Trauma Society, president of the Society for Vascular Surgery, president of the International Society for Cardiovascular Surgery, as well as four other professional societies, held multiple executive positions in the ACS and held positions of influence in over 40 professional societies with honorary membership in over 25 international societies. Dr. Rich was named as an "Icon of Surgery" and received a lifetime achievement award from the ACS. Finally, Dr. Rich was a Founding Member in 1994 for the Diploma in the Medical Care of Catastrophes under the auspices of the Apothecaries of London with NGO participation [7].

Our last example, Dr. Elster, also did not progress from educational roots and was less of an operational one. His translational and clinical research led him to be a senior staff scientist at the Naval Medical Research Center. His success there allowed him to progress to Chair of the Department of Surgery at USUHS. From there, he recognized the gaps in combat care surgery training and helped found the Military Health System Strategic Partnership with the American College of Surgeons (MHSSPACS) whose main mission was to collaborate with civilian trauma surgeons to help prepare military surgeons for combat care and advance the lessons learned from combat to the civilian systems. He was the natural choice and the inaugural president of the Excelsior Surgical Society, which functions as the military state chapter of the ACS. He has held numerous executive positions and chaired committees in multiple organizations including the ACS, the American Society of Transplantation, and the Halsted Society. This has all led to his current position as Dean of USUHS [3].

Conclusion

In summary, we have taken a general/breast surgeon, transplant surgeon, orthopedic surgeon, urologist, surgical oncologist, two pediatric surgeons, and a vascular surgeon out of dozens (if not hundreds) of instances to illustrate that prominent surgical careers in American medicine can develop within full military careers. Furthermore, skills gained can translate into successful civilian careers after retirement. There are three common themes among these surgeons:

1. They all took advantage of their deployment situation by recognizing gaps in clinical care, analyzing them, and publishing their findings. Surgeons do not need to be at the busiest military base or have a research team to achieve this.
2. They all were successful in their operational roles. The crux of military work is caring for one's soldiers, organizing the work well, and having effective communication. These principles and the operational experience will help surgeons become strong leaders.
3. All of them have clinical excellence. These examples began during their fellowship. It is not essential for those who desire an academic career to be fellowship-trained, but it does allow for networking, which makes some opportunities more readily available. In lieu of fellowship training, the path toward clinical excellence may be achieved with a mentor and rigorous examination of one's outcomes. It is certainly incumbent for the current senior leadership or even those retired from the military to help develop the junior surgeons.

It is the author's sincere hope that these living examples will inspire military surgeons in the future to pursue academic surgery as a viable and fulfilling option for their careers.

References

1. Azarow KS. Curriculum vitae. 1 July 2023. Personal communication.
2. Edwards MJ. Curriculum vitae. 2 July 2023. Personal communication.
3. Elster EA. Curriculum vitae. 1 Jan 2022. Personal communication.
4. Ficke JR. Curriculum vitae. 30 Aug 2023. Personal communication.
5. Jaques DP. Curriculum vitae. 1 Mar 2020. Personal communication.
6. Morey AF. Curriculum vitae. 1 July 2023. Personal communication.
7. Rich NM. Curriculum vitae (abbreviated). 1 July 2018. Personal communication.
8. Copeland AW. Curriculum vitae. 1 July 2024. Personal communication.

19 Academics and Research

Joshua Dilday and Matthew J. Martin

Overview of Benefits of Military Academic Surgical Career

Military surgeons play a crucial role in advancing surgical knowledge and innovation. However, productively engaging in academic surgical research within the constraints of military service requires a strategic approach. This chapter aims to provide a roadmap for military surgeons to successfully navigate the multifaceted landscape of academics and surgical research, spanning the initiation of research projects, interacting with the local Institutional Review Board (IRB), conducting animal research, and securing academic appointments. Drawing on the experiences of military surgeons, this chapter seeks to empower practitioners in balancing the demands of military service with the pursuit of a meaningful and impactful research career in the field of surgery.

J. Dilday (✉)
Division of Trauma and Acute Care Surgery, Medical College of Wisconsin, Milwaukee, WI, USA

M. J. Martin
Division of Trauma and Acute Care Surgery, Keck School of Medicine, USC Medical Center, Los Angeles, CA, USA

Division of Upper GI and General Surgery, Keck School of Medicine, USC Medical Center, Los Angeles, CA, USA
e-mail: matthew.martin@med.usc.edu

A. T. Schlussel et al. (eds.), *The SAGES Manual for Navigating a Successful Military Surgical Career*,
https://doi.org/10.1007/978-3-031-88490-0_19

Early Involvement

Research Mentors

Academic surgery does not exist in a silo. In fact, trying to perform relevant research without guidance, support, and mentorship will likely lead to early burnout without a sense of accomplishment. Early career surgeons should take full advantage of the opportunities for mentorship that exist throughout the military academic landscape. Collaborating with colleagues, seeking mentorship from experienced researchers, and leveraging military research priorities can help military surgeons identify meaningful research topics. Understanding the unique demands of military service ensures that research aligns with the broader goals of the armed forces. One challenging aspect of this may be the lack of academic mentorship within one's own division or department at the military facility. In this case, it is critical to research who are the active academic surgeons in the military in a given field of interest and contact them for advice and mentorship.

Research Year During Residency

Most military surgery residencies will provide, or at least allow for a dedicated research year. While this year is variable in both timing and experience, it remains a valuable asset to beginning a career in academic surgery. This year should be used to familiarize oneself with research methodology, terminology, and protocol development. Additionally, it allows for dedicated time to perform clinical and/or laboratory research without the simultaneous equal time commitment dedicated to direct patient care. A thoughtfully planned research year can propel a young surgeon's academic trajectory. Planning consideration should include opportunities for protocol development, experiment/research methodology, data analysis/statistical methods review, manuscript writing, and possible conference abstract submission. Of note, due to the timing of abstract submission, the research performed during the research year is often presented at a conference the following year. However, the goal should be to submit at least one research project to a national conference—even if the project will not be presented until the research year is over. Hazards to avoid during the dedicated research year(s) are focusing on non-research or academic activities or taking on too many projects with the result that very few or none of them come to fruition. A good mentor is critical to helping maintain focus and an appropriate workload.

National Membership Engagement

National surgical societies and organizations can be phenomenal resources for the early academic surgeon—especially for those in the military. Surgical societies often have specific military committees that can help promote military-relevant academia and research endeavors. The American Association of the Surgery for Trauma (AAST), Eastern Association of the Surgery for Trauma (EAST), Association for Academic Surgeons (AAS), Society for Gastrointestinal and Endoscopic Surgery (SAGES), and American Society of Metabolic and Bariatric Surgery (ASMBS) all have military-specific committees and/or groups that specialize in advancing relevant military research and careers. Additionally, the Excelsior Surgical Society (ESS), a subgroup of the American College of Surgeons (ACS) is a military society dedicated to military surgeons. Early involvement in these organizations can provide opportunities to present at their respective conferences and create strong mentorship ties. Additionally, local chapters of the ACS and the Committee on Trauma (COT) may have opportunities for involvement for those interested in an academic career.

Starting a Research Project

Develop a Question

Before embarking on any research endeavor, it is essential to identify a research question that is relevant to both military and civilian healthcare. Collaborating with colleagues, seeking mentorship from experienced researchers, and leveraging military research priorities can help military surgeons identify meaningful research topics. Understanding the unique demands of military service ensures that research aligns with the broader goals of the armed forces.

However, it can be difficult to identify a research question worth pursuing. Often, the military surgeon is not stationed at a location where a robust network of academic collaboration is already developed. In such cases, research questions must be generated from the "ground up." It will behoove the researcher in this situation to look for topics that are generated from everyday experiences. Local "morbidity and mortality" conferences, process improvement meetings, quality metric reviews, and individual patient experiences can all be areas where research questions are conceived.

Although there are many ways to develop a research topic/question, the following may serve as an initial guide.

- *Identify a Gap in Knowledge*
  Begin by conducting a thorough literature review to identify existing gaps, controversies, or unanswered questions in the field. Ensure that your research question is both novel and relevant to the current state of knowledge. Remember, originality and relevance may not always be positively correlated; a research mentor can help review if an ordinal study question is relevant enough to pursue answering. Always do an in-depth literature review before embarking on a new project, as you may discover that your research question has already been addressed and may not be worth pursuing or may be worth pursuing with adjustment of the research question and goals.
- *Formulate a Clear and Specific Question*
  Craft a research question that is clear, specific, and focused. Avoid overly broad or vague inquiries. The question should be answerable through empirical investigation and contribute meaningfully to the existing body of knowledge. Without a clear question, a clear study path is impossible to plan—let

alone walk. Many studies have started as vague questions only to be terminated after many painfully lost hours.

- *Consider Feasibility*
  Evaluate the feasibility of your research question, taking into account available resources, time constraints, and local considerations. Ensure that the research can be conducted within practical boundaries afforded at one's local institution. Additionally, the feasibility of project completion should be considered. A well-intended project will falter if the resources and researcher are no longer available during its later stages. In the event a project is expected to grow beyond its local confines, incorporate a strategy early to utilize outside resources in the event that comes to fruition.

Create a Project Outline

A research endeavor started without a plan will be doomed from the start. Taking the time to develop a clear and detailed framework is essential in order to ensure success in the development and implementation of a project worth publishing. Some steps to follow are listed below.

- *Define Research Objectives*
  Before drafting a research protocol, clearly define the objectives of the study. Identify the specific research questions, hypotheses, and potential clinical applications. This should flow from the clearly defined research question and highlight why vague research questions should be avoided. Ensure that the research aligns with military healthcare priorities and contributes to advancements in surgical practice.
- *Literature Review*
  Conduct a thorough literature review to understand the existing knowledge in the field. Identify gaps, controversies, or areas where additional research is needed. This will inform the rationale for your study and help position your research within the broader context of surgical science. Involving a librarian can help with the literature search and provide an important per-

spective when obtaining previous background on the subject. A careful and deliberate literature review can pave the way for a well-written manuscript. One way to maximize the benefit of the literature review is to document the findings in an annotated bibliography. This can be done manually by the researcher or librarian. Additionally, external products can also provide this service (e.g., Endnote, RefWorks, etc.).

- *Study Design and Methods*
  Outline the study design, including the type of study (e.g., observational and experimental), data collection methods, and statistical approaches. Detail the procedures to be followed, ensuring clarity and replicability. Clearly articulate the methods for data collection, measurements, and statistical analyses. Consider ethical considerations and animal welfare (if applicable) principles in the design phase.
  Consulting with a statistician and/or research mentor is crucial during this step. Regarding research design, it is important to remember that a poorly conceived study will lead to poorly accepted outcomes. Thus, discussing plans for statistical analysis, power analysis, planning for subgroups, and tailoring the methodology to the question will avoid future headaches later in the process.
  It is also helpful to review the relevant guidelines regarding outcome reporting based on the main study designs (e.g., STROBE, SQUIRE, CONSORT, etc.). These guidelines, found at, www.equator-network.com, should be implemented early during the methodology.
- *Budget and Resources*
  Develop a realistic budget that accounts for research-related expenses, such as materials, participant compensation, and data analysis tools. Create a detailed timeline outlining key milestones and deadlines.

Analysis With/Without a Statistician

As mentioned previously, collaboration with a statistician early in the research process can avoid unnecessary headaches and errors later in the research process. Once the data has been collected, a careful analysis of the results is warranted. This should follow the previously planned methodology laid out in the research proposal. If a statistician is available, discuss the most appropriate statistical tests, potential confounding variables, and strategies for handling missing data. Collaborate closely during the interpretation of results to ensure accurate and meaningful conclusions. Remember, "garbage in equals garbage out"—a good analysis cannot overcome poorly planned or collected data.

If a statistician is not available for consultation, the onus of the analysis falls on the researcher. For this, a statistical software tool may be required (SPSS, R, SAS, etc.).

Manuscript Preparation and Submission

The manuscript is the penultimate goal of the research project. If planned appropriately, the manuscript will come together from the logical flow of the initial research proposal. However, that is often easier said than done. Early career researchers may not be as savvy regarding scientific writing. However, with mentorship and practice, writing the manuscript will become less daunting. Some simple steps to follow are below.

- *Data Analysis and Interpretation*
  Conduct rigorous data analysis using appropriate statistical methods. Interpret the results in the context of the study objectives and existing literature. Clearly articulate the implications

of your findings for both military and civilian surgical practice. Remember that a good interpretation of the results must be free from the bias brought in by the researcher. If the results do not support the initial hypothesis, that is ok and still warrants a presentation and publication. Be careful not to skew the results in order to blindly support the original hypothesis.

- *Manuscript Preparation*
  Prepare a well-organized manuscript that logically flows from the research design. Clearly outline the background, objectives, methods, results, and conclusions. Collaborate with co-authors and acknowledge the contributions of all team members, researchers, and support staff. Key points to include are a clear hypothesis and research question, a clearly articulated description of the methodology, the strengths of the findings compared to other relevant articles, and a thorough description of the recognized limitations of the study.
- *Selecting a Journal*
  Choose a reputable journal that specializes in surgical research and is likely to reach the target audience. Consider the scope, impact factor, and editorial policies. Tailor the manuscript to fit the specific requirements of the chosen journal. Each journal will have its own manuscript submission requirements and guidelines. Often, each conference will have an associated journal for encouraged and/or mandatory submission.
- *Submission and Peer Review*
  Submit the manuscript to the selected journal, adhering to their submission guidelines. Keep in mind that most journals accept <50% of submissions. Therefore, do not get discouraged if the research is rejected on the first submission. This is an opportunity to revise and strengthen the paper for submission to another journal. While there are a variety of reasons for rejection, some preventable ones include obvious grammatical errors, lack of a clearly defined research question and/or hypothesis, incomplete methodology, and failure to describe the benefit to the academic literature. Ensuring these components in the original manuscript can decrease the rate of reflexive rejections. Prepare for the peer-review process by addressing potential critiques. Respond thoughtfully to

reviewer comments to strengthen the final publication. Responding to the reviewers should not be treated as argumentative; a polite and humble response to the reviewers will go a long way.

- *Dissemination and Knowledge Translation*
  Once published, actively disseminate your research findings within the military community, academic circles, and relevant medical societies. In the current age of social media, the promotion of research and conference presentations can increase its visibility. Academic careers may be influenced by the visibility of research endeavors. However, a publication being "visible" will not change its perception if it is a poorly designed study. Careful promotion of clinically relevant research endeavors can help launch an academic career.

Navigating the Department of Clinical Investigation

In many healthcare institutions, research and clinical investigation activities are overseen by a specialized department. Military hospitals frequently utilize the nomenclature "Department of Clinical Investigation" (DCI). This department is responsible for managing all research endeavors at its institution. A good relationship with the DCI is paramount to efficiently navigating protocol development and acceptance. Often, the hospital statistician will fall under the jurisdiction of the DCI. Additionally, the Institutional Review Board (IRB) and the Institutional Animal Care and Use Committee (IACUC) will be housed within the DCI.

IRB

The IRB plays a crucial role in protecting the rights, welfare, and well-being of human research participants. Its primary function is to review and oversee research involving human subjects to ensure ethical conduct and compliance with regulatory standards. The

IRB carefully reviews research proposals and assesses the study's design, methodology, participant recruitment strategies, and procedures to ensure that ethical and regulatory standards are met. This includes ensuring that research participants provide informed consent, that their privacy is protected, and that the risks associated with the research are minimized and justified. A risk analysis is performed by the IRB, ensuring that the potential benefits outweigh the risks and that the research contributes valuable knowledge without imposing undue harm on participants. For ongoing research, the IRB conducts periodic reviews to ensure that the study is progressing efficiently, ethically, and safely. This includes assessing any changes to the study protocol and reviewing adverse events or unanticipated problems involving risks to participants. Researchers are required to promptly report any adverse events or deviations from the approved protocol.

While each local IRB may have its own proposal submission regulations, the following is an example outline of some relatively common proposal components.

- *Introduction*
  - Background:
    Begin your proposal by providing context for the surgical research project. Clearly outline the significance of the research problem, emphasizing its relevance to healthcare and the potential impact on surgical outcomes.
  - Objectives:
    Clearly state the research objectives. Define the specific aims of your study, highlighting the gaps in current knowledge that your research aims to address. Again, this should flow from the previously defined research question.
- *Literature Review*
  - Current State of Knowledge:
    Summarize relevant literature that provides the foundation for your research. Identify key studies, methodologies, and gaps in current understanding. It is important to demonstrate a comprehensive understanding of the existing body of knowledge.

- Rationale for Military Relevance:
  Articulate why your research is particularly relevant to military healthcare. Often, the relevance and/or benefit may pertain to more than just the military community. In that case, the IRB simply wants to see that military education, proficiency, or outcomes will be impacted. Discuss any unique considerations or challenges that military populations may present in the context of surgical interventions.

• *Research Design and Methods*
  - Study Design:
    Clearly specify the study design (e.g., randomized controlled trial, cohort study, etc.) and justify your choice. Discuss how the design aligns with your research objectives and the feasibility of its implementation within a military healthcare setting. This should flow easily from the research question and objectives.
  - Participants:
    Define your target population, including specific inclusion and exclusion criteria. Provide details on recruitment strategies, considering the unique characteristics of military personnel.
  - Interventions or Procedures:
    Clearly describe the surgical interventions or procedures under investigation. Include information on any innovative techniques or technologies being employed and justify their selection. This section will be tailored based on the research design. Not every research project will have interventions or procedures evaluated.
  - Data Collection:
    Outline your data collection plan, specifying the variables to be collected and the methods for capturing, recording, and storing data. Address any challenges related to obtaining data from military healthcare records and explain your approach to overcoming them. It is important to address how this data will be kept in compliance with HIPAA standards. Often, the data should be kept in one centralized location that allows for de-identification of the data to minimize the potential for subject harm.

  - Statistical Analysis:
    Provide a detailed plan for statistical analysis. Specify the statistical methods you will use to analyze the data and justify their appropriateness for addressing your research questions. If available, the local statistician can help with this section. Often, a power analysis should be employed to determine the number of patients needed to identify a statistically relevant outcome.
- *Ethical Considerations*
  - Informed Consent:
    Describe your approach to obtaining informed consent from participants. Address any challenges related to the unique circumstances of military personnel, such as deployment status or restrictions on consent processes.
  - Confidentiality:
    Detail how participant confidentiality will be maintained, particularly considering the sensitive nature of military health data. Explain any data anonymization or de-identification procedures. Keeping all patient data on a centralized, protected platform is often recommended.
- *Budget and Resources*
  - Budget Justification:
    Provide a detailed budget for your research project, including personnel, equipment, supplies, and any other relevant expenses. Justify each budget item in relation to the research objectives. Not every project will require a budget.
  - Resources:
    Outline the resources required for the successful execution of the research. This may include collaboration with military healthcare facilities, access to specialized surgical equipment, and any additional support needed.
- *Timeline*
  Present a realistic timeline for the different phases of your research project. Include milestones, data collection periods, analysis phases, and any other key events. Clearly outline how you plan to adhere to the proposed timeline. The goal project completion date should be included in the proposed timeline.

- *Conclusion*
  Summarize the key components of your research proposal and restate its importance in the context of military surgical care. Emphasize how the proposed study has the potential to advance knowledge and improve surgical outcomes for military service members.
- *Appendices*
  Include any additional documents that support your proposal, such as consent forms, data collection tools, and letters of collaboration from military healthcare facilities.

While not exhaustive, this step-by-step guide can help to prepare and present a structured research proposal tailored for submission to a military IRB. Remember to adhere to the specific local IRB guidelines and continually refine the proposal based on mentor and collaborative feedback.

IACUC

Animal, specifically large animal, research is a vital component of surgical investigation, providing a bridge between preclinical studies and human trials. For military surgeons engaged in academic research, conducting studies on large animals offers unique opportunities to simultaneously perform relevant research and refine surgical techniques. Many important military surgical advances have been conceived in an animal lab. Because the ethical and humane treatment of animals in academia is of paramount importance, the IACUC exists to safeguard the welfare of animals in research. This includes assessing the justification for the use of animals and evaluating the potential benefits of the research, ensuring that all animal-based research activities adhere to relevant laws, regulations, and guidelines and conducting regular inspections of animal facilities to ensure compliance with housing, husbandry, and veterinary care standards. A key member of the IACUC is a local veterinarian. The importance of early and frequent veterinary collaboration cannot be overstated. It behooves the researcher to consult with the veterinary team to help refine the protocol and ensure the well-being of the animals through the research process. An early collaborative approach may help streamline the protocol through to IACUC approval. These projects will almost always require dedicated research funding to pay for animals, supplies, administrative support, and other items. Look for funding opportunities internally at the medical center, from local or regional academic surgical organizations, and from external funding agencies. The general principle is to start locally and build up a body of research that can lead to larger external grant funding. It is also important to look at both DOD and civilian funding sources for opportunities.

Below are important points to consider unique to animal research.

- *Rationale and Objectives*
  Clearly articulate the scientific rationale for using animals in the study. Define specific research objectives and explain why animals are necessary to achieve these goals. Consider alternative methods that could reduce or replace animal use if feasible. If alternative methods are either not available or feasible, clearly document the reasons. The IACUC is looking for a proper and clearly defined justification for animal use in the proposed research plan.
- *Species Selection*
  Not all research endeavors require the same animal species. While some are more suited for large animals, others may be performed with smaller animals. The most common large animals used in military research are swine. However, the research must justify the choice of animal species and provide information on their biological relevance to the research question. Consideration should be given to the availability of alternatives and the ethical implications of using a particular species.
- *Experimental Procedures*
  This is often the part of the proposal that prompts the most discussion. Again, early and frequent collaboration with the veterinary team can help in this area. Be careful to detail all experimental procedures, including anesthesia, surgery, and data collection methods. Clearly outline steps taken to minimize pain, distress, and potential harm to the animals. Any

deviation from this plan must be clearly documented with updates given to the IACUC. A timeline for procedures and a plan for addressing potential adverse events is requested.

- *Animal Welfare Considerations*
  The veterinary team is paramount to writing this section. Animal research should only be performed with the utmost attention to animal safety and ethical treatment. The IACUC will require the description of measures taken to ensure the welfare of animals throughout the study. This includes housing conditions, environmental enrichment, veterinary care, and humane endpoints for animals experiencing pain or distress. The committee may also request documentation of the qualifications and training of personnel involved in the study. The veterinary team can help highlight the expertise of individuals responsible for animal care, handling, and the implementation of experimental procedures.

Large Database Research

Large databases play a pivotal role in outcomes-based research, providing a wealth of clinical data for diverse research inquiries. This section aims to guide researchers through the process of performing outcomes-based research using three prominent databases: ACS NSQIP, NTDB, and NIS. While this list is not exhaustive, they are likely the most commonly used databases for most military academic surgeons. There is a plethora of local and national databases sponsored by surgical societies, collaborative initiatives, and hospital resources that are also available. While the specific data captures may vary for each database, the premise of utilization remains similar for each product. The following describes the most commonly utilized and available databases relevant for military surgery research.

ACS NSQIP

The American College of Surgeons National Surgical Quality Improvement Program (ACS NSQIP) is a robust database capturing detailed clinical information from diverse surgical procedures.

Researchers can leverage this database for outcomes research, focusing on surgical complications, mortality, and other perioperative outcomes. The ACS NSQIP database has also expanded to capture certain "targeted" variables in subsequent data pools. Some of these "targeted" databases are specific to vascular, colorectal, and bariatric cases.

NTDB/TQIP

The National Trauma Data Bank (NTDB) is a comprehensive resource for trauma-related outcomes research. Researchers interested in trauma surgery can access a vast array of data on injury severity, patient demographics, and outcomes to investigate factors influencing trauma care and patient outcomes. Additional factors can be elicited from the Trauma Quality Improvement Program (TQIP). The TQIP database is a subset of the NTDB that has additional quality metrics extracted from TQIP-involved ACS trauma centers.

NIS

The Healthcare Cost and Utilization Project's Nationwide Inpatient Sample (NIS) is a large database encompassing a representative sample of hospital inpatient stays across the United States. Researchers can explore a wide range of clinical and demographic variables to study national trends, healthcare utilization, and outcomes.

DoDTR

The Department of Defense Trauma Registry (DoDTR) stands as a comprehensive and invaluable resource for surgical research, providing a wealth of data on military trauma cases. Established by the US Department of Defense, the DoDTR serves as a centralized repository that captures detailed information on traumatic injuries sustained by military personnel. The primary purpose of the DoDTR is to facilitate the analysis of trauma-related data to enhance the quality of care provided to military personnel. It captures information from the point of injury through the entire continuum of care, including pre-hospital interventions, surgical procedures, and post-operative outcomes. The DoDTR includes a range of demographic variables, such as age, sex, rank, and branch of service, enabling researchers to stratify and analyze data based on specific population characteristics. Detailed information on the nature and severity of injuries is recorded in the registry, including the mechanism of injury, anatomical location, injury severity scores, field resuscitation and transport times, as well as information on hospital care, including surgical procedures, transfusions, and complications.

Research Funding

In some cases, obtaining funding for research can be necessary, but funding for research can be beneficial in all cases. Studies requiring extensive staff or technological support (e.g., prolonged data collection, database servers, animal care facilities, etc.) may have their feasibility maintained by external funding. However, research funding is frequently sought after without success. By exploring diverse funding opportunities, crafting strong research proposals, and leveraging collaborations, researchers can position themselves to obtain financial support from sources such as military grants, scholarships, and private foundations. Some good starting places to consider are outlined below.

Local Institution

The first logical place to check for funding opportunities is within the local institution. There may be funding available through the offices of DCI or Graduate Medical Education (GME). If these are not directly available, the DCI and GME offices may have contacts or known local scholarship opportunities. Some of these funding sources may be allocated to certain types of research (e.g., animal, injury prevention, etc.), but a quick inquiry as to their availability is worthwhile.

DoD

The DoD offers a range of funding opportunities specifically tailored to support military health research. This includes grants from agencies such as the Defense Health Agency (DHA), the Congressionally Directed Medical Research Programs (CDMRP), and the Uniformed Services University of the Health Sciences (USUHS). These funding resources, although competitive, can provide substantial financial backing to a well-designed research proposal.

National Organizations

A lot of national organizations offer scholarships and funding opportunities. These offerings range from being focused on conference travel and scholarship to full research grants. In some cases, there are specific funds allocated to the early researcher. While not an exhaustive list, the ACS, AAST, EAST, ASMBS, AAS, and SAGES all offer some sort of funding/scholarship for early researchers. These are excellent opportunities for both funding and conference participation, as many of the national organization-linked funding resources are associated with conference presentations and exposure.

Building an Academic Career in the Military

In addition to becoming involved in academic pursuits and doing high-quality research, successfully developing an academic career should focus on obtaining an academic appointment, meeting requirements for academic promotion, developing a network of colleagues and collaborators, and becoming involved in locoregional and national organizations to develop a local and then national presence and reputation.

Academic Appointment

Any military surgeon with teaching responsibilities and/or academic aspirations should apply for an initial academic appointment with the Uniformed Services University of the Health Sciences (USUHS) as early as possible. This is typically done after completion of residency and any fellowship upon initial duty assignment as an attending surgeon. The initial appointment is typically at the Assistant Professor level and then proceeds through promotions to Associated Professor and Full Professor. It may also be possible to obtain an appointment as a resident or fellow at the Clinical Instructor level. Fellows and residents in their chief years can apply to be a Clinical Instructor and then apply to be an Assistant Professor upon graduation. The initial application for Assistant Professor is typically very straightforward and does not require significant academic accomplishments outside of the usual for a new attending surgeon. Contact and application information can usually be obtained via the administrative leadership for your assigned division or department or by directly contacting USUHS for further instructions. It may also be possible to obtain a civilian academic appointment through any local partnership programs with civilian universities or academic medical centers. This pathway is usually very well-defined with set criteria and an application packet that can be obtained similar to that listed above for USUHS. The time to then start thinking about and planning for promotion to the next level is immediately upon appointment to the present level.

Academic Promotion

After the initial academic appointment has been received, there is a standard pathway and timeline for promotion that will vary between institutions. The typical time interval for promotion to Associate

Professor is 4–6 years and then an additional 6–8 years for Full Professor. Unlike the initial academic appointment, promotion will require demonstrating significant accomplishments and productivity in the chosen specialty or focus area. Although previously there was only one academic tract that applicants would follow for promotion, now most academic systems have several pathways that can be followed that focus on clinical activity, academic/research, or educational activity. Each of these pathways will have multiple criteria or demonstrated accomplishments that are required to be demonstrated for promotion to the next level. In general, these focus on a progression from local achievements, leadership positions, and reputation at your medical center to building a regional presence and reputation, and finally to a national presence and reputation. This is best achieved for the military surgeon by becoming active in local, regional, and national surgical organizations to build contacts and a reputation outside of the more insular military medical system.

Promotion to the Associate or Full Professor level will require a much more extensive and detailed application packet that demonstrates that the applicant meets all requirements in a number of areas. These areas typically include academic research and scholarly activity, teaching and mentorship, clinical activity, institutional service, and recognition at the regional and national/international levels. It is very difficult to produce all of this information and examples by waiting until the promotion packet is due and trying to reconstruct them from memory. We recommend creating a computer folder for academic promotion and copying any and all files or documents related to any of the above-listed areas. This includes making notations of all junior faculty and trainees that one has mentored, any educational programs or curriculum that the applicant has developed, all courses taught (such as ATLS), any honors/awards, and copies of all research publications. It is also critical to continuously update your CV with all new scholarly output, leadership positions with the organization, service on various hospital/university committees, and invited academic talks/presentations. Having these all collected in one location will greatly help reduce the time and effort required to put together the promotion packet.

A final common requirement that applicants often struggle with is the need for letters of support for the promotion from academic colleagues outside of their institution. This will include colleagues who know and have worked with the applicant and can attest to their qualifications, as well as several "arms-length" letters from surgeons or other academics who do not know and have never worked with the applicant but can review their packet and provide a recommendation about whether they feel the applicant meets promotion requirements. These letters are typically required to be from reviewers who are either at or above the academic rank that is being sought by the applicant. These letters can be solicited from colleagues who have been met through regional or national organizations, those with national reputations in the same area of study, or by recommendations from the applicant's colleagues and mentors.

The obvious way to meet promotion requirements is to conduct high-quality academic research, present this research at major national meetings, and publish the results in peer-reviewed high-impact factor surgical journals. However, alternative approaches that focus on clinical activity and reputation, or educational activity and scholarship are also now widely accepted. The interested surgeon should investigate the options for the best civilian academic societies to join and then should make all efforts to become an active member including serving on committees or task forces, serving as a military liaison for the organization, and working to achieve leadership positions such as Committee Chair and Board of Directors appointments. In addition to accruing accomplishments that will be critical for successful and early promotion, these are excellent opportunities to make a diverse network of civilian academic colleagues who can greatly help the military surgeon with academic aspirations. These colleagues will also be extremely valuable when you separate from the military and are searching for civilian job options at academic medical centers.

Local and National Leadership

As mentioned above, one criteria for academic success and promotion is the cultivation of a local and national reputation in whatever chosen area of research, education, or clinical activity the applicant decides to track on. This is most easily accomplished by joining several organizations focused on academic surgery and then being an active participant in activities that will frequently lead to leadership positions within the organization. These organizations may be specialty-specific (e.g., trauma surgery societies) or multi-specialty such as the Association for Academic Surgeons and the SAGES Military Committee. Most organizations have made this process much more transparent than in the past and will have posted information about how to volunteer for committees or other activities. Being an active and reliable committee member who takes on tasks and sees them to completion will then be positioned for selection to committee chairperson or other leadership position within the organization. In addition to building a reputation and "checking boxes" for academic promotion, these activities and the relationships that develop can be incredibly rewarding and create lifelong collegial relationships and friendships.

Conclusions

Becoming an academic surgeon requires focused effort, discipline, collaboration, and mentorship for all surgeons, but particularly for the military surgeon. By following the advice outlined above the military surgeon can successfully navigate these processes, develop an impressive academic portfolio that rivals their civilian colleagues at the same level and can help build lasting relationships with colleagues throughout their military and subsequent civilian career.

Military Research on a Global Scale

20

Diego Vicente, Tamara J. Worlton, and Joseph Caravalho Jr.

Historical Impact of Military Medical Innovation

The exigencies of austere environments and clinical severity of combat wounds have been key drivers of medical innovation. This phenomenon has been lauded from the time of Hippocrates to modern conflicts with innovations in triage, pre-hospital care, medical evacuation, resuscitation, surgical management, infectious disease, mental health, long-term care, and medical education [1, 2]. Today's routine examples of expedited care and management of severely injured trauma patients via ambulance and aeromedical evacuation may not have been developed in a timely manner without lessons learned from the horse-drawn wagons of the Napoleonic wars and the brave Huey pilots of the Vietnam War [3]. More recently, the medical providers in the conflicts in Iraq and Afghanistan revolutionized the concepts of blood product-based resuscitation and damage control surgery, and in concert with advances in pre-hospital care and infection control,

D. Vicente · T. J. Worlton
Uniformed Services University of the Health Sciences, Bethesda, MD, USA

J. Caravalho Jr. (✉)
The Henry M. Jackson Foundation for the Advancement of Military Medicine, Bethesda, MD, USA
e-mail: jcaravalho@hjf.org

A. T. Schlussel et al. (eds.), *The SAGES Manual for Navigating a Successful Military Surgical Career*,
https://doi.org/10.1007/978-3-031-88490-0_20

have improved the survival of battlefield injuries, as well as trauma patients at home [4–6]. Today, the lessons learned from centuries of providing medical care in unforgiving environments with limited resources, as well as the integration of military-civilian partnerships and translational research, continue to drive algorithmic and personalized care of the combat wounded and patients across the healthcare field [7].

Modernizing the Military Within the Human Domain

There are five or six (depending on how you think of the sea, namely, all-encompassing or separated by surface and subsurface maritime) warfighting, or military operational, domains. These reflect specific maneuver spaces within which warfare is conducted: land, sea, air, space, and cyber. As you can see, most are physical, with the latter being informational.

What's left in this construct (although not officially acknowledged in Joint doctrine), but impactful throughout the other warfighting domains, is the human domain. It doesn't fit nicely within this classification of where warfighting takes place, but it remains intuitive that all warfare reflects human endeavor.

This does not simply connote medical or health aspects, but, very clearly, health—whether its promotion, protection, maintenance, or treatment—is pervasive across the human domain. Other important domain considerations would include sociologic, anthropologic, economic, environmental, cultural, psychologic, and spiritual, along with the more intuitive man-machine interface and human performance topics, to name but a few.

The US Military, in its quest to remain the world's very best fighting force, places a premium on modernization, which, by its unique nature, involves a sophisticated research and development program. Military medical research aims to improve warfighter performance, survivability, and resilience in austere environments and under grueling conditions. The US Military should view these types of optimization studies as the way it modernizes within the human domain. As such, it should receive the same level of prioritization as do other modernization efforts applied within any of the current warfighting domains.

Collectively, these points should be used to justify the need for ongoing requirements-driven military medical research.

Strategic Importance of Military Medical Research

The 2022 National Security Strategy, the ultimate document that informs all subsequent security plans, continues to emphasize the US commitment for strengthening relationships with partners and allies [https://www.whitehouse.gov/wp-content/uploads/2022/10/Biden-Harris-Administrations-National-Security-Strategy-10.2022.pdf]. Health is mentioned as a core tenet of each geographic combatant command regional plan. The COVID-19 pandemic has highlighted the critical importance of the US military's impact on research, as well as the necessity for our efforts to have global reach. While there is a needed emphasis on bio-surveillance and the Global Health Security Agenda, the reality is that global surgical research will play a key role in the next conflict. Combat casualty care in the Indopacific theater will be a much different challenge than what was experienced in Central Command. Unique solutions will need to be researched to manage the surge capacity of casualties that could occur in a peer-to-peer conflict. In the FY23 Global Health Engagement Research Initiative (GHERI) grant, lines of effort for military and civilian integration for capability and capacity building was a key priority for five of the Combatant Commands [https://www.grants.gov/web/grants/viewopportunity.html?oppId=344833].

Tenets of Military Research

The basis of military medical research is to maximize operational readiness to improve the lethality of combat troops. With this goal, the tenets of military research include:

1. Requirements-driven
2. Distinct from private sector efforts
3. World-class effort

Efforts to maximize readiness are directed at promoting wellness, as well as prevention and treatment of injury and disease, with rapidly deployable and accessible means. Hence, the typical focus areas include:

1. Operational Readiness
2. Injury Prevention and Treatment
3. Rapid Deployment and Accessibility
4. Interdisciplinary Collaboration
5. Adaptation and Flexibility
6. Dual-Use Applications for Military and Civilian Needs
7. Ethical Considerations
8. Long-Term Health and Wellbeing
9. Data Collection and Analysis
10. Continuous Improvement

The means developed from these focus areas are then integrated across multiple arenas and levels of care by multidisciplinary teams, which can then adapt the means to deliver an optimal clinical outcome in the setting of the environment's limitations. Additionally, the military's Joint Trauma System and Military Health System's Data Repository give the opportunity to collect data and analyze the impact of these means on outcomes.

These seemingly impossible tasks are executed daily by our military service members and supported by civilian partnerships. A military researcher who has deployed to austere environments and cared for combat wounded brings a unique perspective to overcoming the barriers to improving patient outcomes [8]. We are frequently reminded that in the tents of Iraq and Afghanistan, medical providers honed blood product-based resuscitation and damage control surgery to improve the survival of injured troops to 92% despite increasing severity of injury. Few experiences in modern medicine can instill as much motivation as caring for combat wounded, and these situations truly reinforce that

"Necessity is the mother of invention." Hence, military researchers maintain a central role in the development of cutting-edge technology to maintain the medical readiness of the warfighter.

Medical Research Within the Military

In addition to research opportunities from medical societies, industry, and the National Institutes of Health available to the civilian population, military researchers have unique opportunities for database research, military-civilian collaborative projects, and directed DoD funding. These research and funding opportunities need to be balanced against operational requirements, which may interrupt research due to operational tempo, geographic separation, logistics, and connectivity. Furthermore, depending on leadership within the department, directorate, or operational command, one's billet may have a limited acknowledgment of requirements-driven research, and dedicating time to research activities may not be considered valuable for the command's promotion boards. Ultimately, in most billets, the choice to do research should be self-motivated and undertaken in the setting of limited support and understanding of your leadership, and in the interest of improving patient care.

The Defense Health Agency (DHA) has a Research and Engineering Directorate. Within this directorate is the Military Health System Research Branch and a Research Support Division. Their website has a list of DHA research resources as well as guidelines for conducting survey research, human subject research, and accessing military databases, as discussed below. Additionally, they have links to Army, Navy, and Air Force research oversight offices. One notable resource is the Clinical Investigator Program (CIP) which seeks to align Military Treatment Facilities (MTFs), graduate medical education (GME) and DHA research priorities. There is a CIP Young Investigator Competition that is conducted at the Society of Federal Health Professionals Annual Meeting (AMSUS).

Testing a clinical hypothesis, developing a novel database, or querying an existing database can be reasonably executed through the local MTFs Institutional Review Boards (IRBs). As noted in Table 20.1, examples of military specific databases include MHS Data Repository (MDR) (MHS Mart [M2] and KSA data available), DoD Trauma Registry, Naval Safety Center, and Maritime Surgery Quality Improvement Program. Information regarding these databases is readily available online, and database queries can be executed through local commands, as well as through centralized groups (i.e., Joint Trauma System). Of note, instructions on accessing these databases typically requires a common access card, authorization forms, and relevant trainings, given the sensitive nature of the information. Further, retrospective reviews of these databases should typically be done in conjunction under IRB protocol, and involvement with outside institutions will typically require a Data Sharing Agreement (DSA). Finally, the Center for Health Services Research at Uniformed Services University of the Health Sciences (USU)

Table 20.1 Examples of military medicine databases and associated resources

Military medicine databases	Data available	Website/resources
DoD Trauma Registry (DoDTR)	Trauma Infectious disease Traumatic brain injury Acoustic Military working dog	https://jts.health.mil/index.cfm/data/registries https://jts.health.mil/index.cfm/data/data_requests email: dha.jbsa.healthcare-ops.list.jts-data-enterprise@health.mil
MHS Data Repository (MDR)	MHS mart (M2) Knowledge skill assessment (KSA)	https://www.health.mil/Military-Health-Topics/Technology/Support-Areas/MDR-M2-ICD-Functional-References-and-Specification-Documents
Center for Health Services Research (CHSR)	n/a	https://chsr.usuhs.edu

offers trainings on accessing and utilizing the MDR with schedule available on website.

While independent research can be accomplished within the confines of MTFs and associated IRBs, the authors of this chapter have noted prolonged times in protocol development and approval compared to our civilian counterparts. Working closely with mentors with funded and established DoD projects that have clinical research coordinators, regulatory experts, and biostatistician support has been critical in the success of our DoD-based projects. Military surgeons should consider applying for faculty positions through the USU's Department of Surgery. These faculty appointments are an excellent way to access centralized resources, existing projects, and mentorship to help develop one's academic career.

Anecdotally, several researchers within the military may struggle to establish research projects despite sound hypotheses and methods. To this end, there are several training opportunities for enhancing a military researcher's potential as listed below. Examples of research training opportunities available in 2023 include the Association of Academic Surgery's Fundamentals of Surgical Research Course and Early Career Development Course, the American College of Surgeon's Quality Improvement Course.

Specifically through USU, surgical faculty have access to faculty development webinars through its intranet homepage. The Office of Research is also developing a USU faculty development seminar to cover networking, DoD funding sources, the language of DoD research, and how to align research with military readiness. Clinical trial development courses are also available through the Office of Research. Finally, centralization efforts within the military research network have made resources available to researchers outside of large MTFs, as well. These resources include regional IRB support and research resources, such as biostatisticians.

Access to distinct funding opportunities is also available to military researchers, as noted in Table 20.2. Information regarding these funding opportunities is available online, and partnerships with USU as well as civilian institutions may be a critical component of funding management and timeline adherence to mitigate operational constraints.

Table 20.2 Examples of funding opportunities for military researchers. The USUHS funding sources can be considered for surgical faculty

Program/organization	Program/funding	Resources
Defense Logistics Agency	Broad Agency Announcements	https://www.dla.mil/Strategic-Materials/Business/Broad-Agency-Announcement/
Uniformed Services University of the Health Sciences Adjunct Clinical-Research Faculty Opportunities	DoD Intramural	POM (Program Objective Memorandum) and Core Projects
	DoD Extramural	Congressionally Appropriated https://www.usuhs.edu/research/centers/tsnrp/research/funding-opportunities
	NIH	
	Industry	

Congressionally Directed Medical Research Programs (CDMRP)	Defense Medical Research and Development	https://cdmrp.health.mil/
	Specific Program Funding Opportunities	
	Medical Simulation and Information Sciences Research Program (JPC-1)	
	Military Infectious Diseases Research Program (JPC-2)	
	Military Operational Medicine Research Program (JPC-5)	
	Combat Casualty Care Research Program (JPC-6)	
	Radiation Health Effects Research Program (JPC-7)	
	Clinical and Rehabilitative Medicine Research Program (JPC-8)	
	Traumatic Brain Injury and Psychological Health	

(continued)

Table 20.2 (continued)

Program/organization	Program/funding	Resources
Combat Casualty Care		
Intramural Opportunities	U.S. Army's Telemedicine & Advanced Technology Research Center's (TATRC)	https://www.tatrc.org/www/
	U.S. Army Medical Research and Development Command	https://mrdc.health.mil/
	U.S. Army Institute of Surgical Research	https://usaisr.health.mil/
Extramural Opportunities	Medical Technology Enterprise Consortium	https://mtec-sc.org/
	Linking Investigations in Trauma and Emergency Services Trauma Clinical Research Network	https://www.litesnetwork.org/
	DARPA	https://www.darpa.mil/
Military Health System Research Program	U.S. Army Medical Research Acquisition Activity	https://grants.gov/

Beyond these military-specific opportunities, the authors recommend considering surgical society membership and reaching out to join committees and projects within these societies. Military member involvement is often welcomed by these medical societies, and active committee involvement is typically associated with promotions within these societies. One of the strengths of military surgeons may be a relatively more flexible schedule to accommodate society projects (i.e., position papers, review articles), and completion of these projects may help strengthen the researcher's network, as well as increase access to additional projects.

The Society of Gastrointestinal Endoscopic Surgeons (SAGES) was one of the first to establish a Military Symposium via the SAGES Military Committee, of which a main purpose is to highlight military surgical research, particularly that which may not fit well into traditional surgical conferences and often overlooked in military conferences [9]. Similarly, the Association for Academic Surgery (AAS) also has a distinct military committee with opportunities for research, mentoring, and civilian collaborations as well as national presentations for military-specific research. Beyond General Surgery societies, the Society of Military Orthopaedic Surgeons (SOMOS) meets annually and provides an excellent opportunity for military orthopedics residents and faculty to present their research. In addition to these symposiums, there are several military conferences that highlight military specific research. The Society of Federal Health Professionals, AMSUS, meets annually in Washington, DC, and has the only United States-based journal for military research, "Military Medicine." The annual Military Health System Research Symposium (MHSRS) provide excellent venues for military providers and research partners to share data and ideas. Biennial international conferences include the IndoPacific Military Health Exchange, IPMHE, which is co-sponsored by USINDOPACOM and a rotating country in that region. Special Operations Medical Association (SOMA) focuses on tip-of-the-spear medicine and conducts an annual meeting in coordination with multiple relevant groups, including Wilderness Medical Society and Deployed Medicine. Finally, the International Committee of Military

Medicine, ICMM, is a biennial conference that rotates host countries and has an associated journal, the "International Review of the Armed Forces Medical Services."

An annual opportunity for military residents and trauma fellows is the American Association for the Surgery of Trauma (AAST) and American College of Surgeons (ACS) Committee on Trauma Region 13 trauma paper competition, which includes a monetary award. The winners are announced at the Excelsior Society Symposium, the military organization that is now an official ACS committee.

Special Resources for Military Researchers (Access to Grant Submission/Award Management, Intrinsic Research Backbone of USU) and the Role of HJF

Congressional appropriations to the DoD are categorically time-limited. For the purposes of this discussion, medical research falls into the Research, Development, Testing, and Evaluation (RDT&E) category. These funds must be executed/disbursed (i.e., not simply obligated) before the end of the second fiscal year from federal appropriation. Delayed funding due to federally enacted Continuing Resolutions further shortens the time in which congressional appropriations must be executed.

Because most DoD medical research is funded through Congressional appropriations, military principal investigators (PIs) may elect to partner with civilian organizations (whether non- or for-profit) when conducting long-term research studies. Alternatively, short studies can be accomplished intramurally (i.e., without external partners).

A PI should select their implementing partner based on the value they provide. Consider the implementing partner's spectrum of offerings during both the pre- and post-award phases; scalability of support for large, widely dispersed studies; timeliness and responsiveness to both planned and unplanned requests; and reliability in meeting regulatory, compliance, and reporting requirements.

Specific offerings may include: (1) administrative and programmatic management services that enable PIs, research clinicians, and their partners in academia and industry to focus on the science; (2) assistance with formal agreements (i.e., contracts, grants, cooperative research and development agreements); (3) assistance with technology transfer activities, such as patents and licenses, clinical trials, financial and compliance reporting; (4) identifying pertinent funding opportunities and research partners within DoD, academia, and industry; and (5) technical assistance with preparing and submitting highly competitive proposals.

One such example of a non-profit partner is The Henry M. Jackson Foundation for the Advancement of Military Medicine (HJF), authorized by Congress in 1983 to support USU in conducting world-class research in support of its medical school mission. It is not the exclusive USU or DoD implementing partner, but HJF is the only entity explicitly named in federal statute to conduct such supporting actions. There are other specialized nonprofit organizations capable of providing implementation support to military medical research, such as the Military Health Research Foundation, Geneva Foundation, and Metis Foundation.

Finally, costs can seem daunting to the young military investigator. Charged rates are reviewed and approved by federal oversight authorities, so the PI can rest assured their rates are within an acceptable range for the military. Support costs are captured in both direct and indirect rates charged to the award, or in fees charged to the contract. These are not "taxes" levied on awards, but organizational costs needed to sustain the comprehensive services available to the PI.

Examples of Existing DoD Projects

As noted above, there are several databases unique to the military health care system that allow for real-time and retrospective analyses of innovations for DoD healthcare beneficiaries. Additionally, there are numerous military-civilian partnered projects working to develop cutting edge technologies. Specific to personalized medicine, we will highlight some of the one of the author's ongoing projects, including

USU's Surgical Critical Care Initiative (SC2i) and the Murtha Cancer Center's (MCC) Biobank, APOLLO (Applied Proteogenomics Organizational Learning Outcomes), and PROMETHEUS (PROject for Military and Toxin History Evaluation in US service members) projects. As a surgical oncologist with a background in trauma research and USU surgical faculty appointment, this author has capitalized on researching the relevance between the inflammatory pathways which drive poor outcomes in severely injured trauma patients and similar pathways which drive the neoplastic process.

The Surgical Critical Care Initiative (SC2i) is a military-civilian collaborative project that focuses on tissue and data acquisition to advance critical care management with clinical decision support tools. Analysis of integrated clinical databases and available tissue banks has allowed researchers to evaluate clinical outcomes with biomarker discovery and identify early markers for critical illness as well as potential for interventions to optimize clinical outcomes. Further, access to comprehensive data and various tissue types has led to discoveries in wound healing, activation of inflammatory cascade, and viral reactivation [10]. Projects analyzing multi-omics and novel biomarkers in these databases are ongoing and welcoming of researchers.

The DoD's MCC has extended collaborations across multiple MTFs, Veterans Affairs hospitals and civilian institutions to develop a clinical database and biorepository of neoplastic tissue samples eligible for advanced proteogenomic analysis (APOLLO). This combination of high-quality clinical data and multi-omics data will allow for comprehensive considerations of systemic and tissue biomarkers that may evolve both prognostic factors and predict responses to therapy. The creation of a "Big Data" repository, like the National Cancer Institute Cancer Research Data Commons (CRDC), will facilitate computational and pathway analysis that may also reveal treatment resistance mechanisms evolved in tumors and elucidate new molecular targets for intervention.

Beyond biorepositories, the MCC has also developed the PROMETHEUS through President Biden's White House Cancer Moonshot 2022 initiative as a Cancer Moonshot 2.0 Project. As has been well described in the PHASE 1-a—STUDY ON THE INCIDENCE OF CANCER DIAGNOSIS AND MORTALITY

AMONG MILITARY AVIATORS AND AVIATION SUPPORT PERSONNEL, published in February 2023, US military service members are at increased risk of cancer. The PROMETHEUS projects will be largely directed at considering the risks of military-relevant exposures and may include common exposures such as tobacco to military-specific environments such as burn pits and shipboard environments. Comprehensive questionnaires, with considerations for deployment and exposure history, as well as blood samples from the DoD's biorepository and prospectively collected blood samples from operation setting, may help shed light on the occult connection between military service and increased cancer rates. The MCC will be expanding these projects to multiple operational sites and MTFs and eager researchers should consider a partnership with these groups.

Impact of Military Medical Research on Civilian Healthcare

The authors' review of military medical research in this chapter is meant to provide both a perspective and a means for surgical residents and faculty to begin their research projects. The perspectives gained by military surgeons in austere environments have the potential to yield novel research questions as well as interventions and treatments in both trauma and non-trauma patients. While some of these projects may be executed in the domestic community hospitals or military academic centers, some projects may be completed in the international setting, onboard ships, or in a tent (e.g., the majority of this chapter was written on a laptop in a tent during a field exercise). We hope these perspectives inspire military researchers to be creative with their time and resources to further the research mission and ultimately improve the care for those in harm's way.

References

1. Scultetus AH, Leonel Villavicencio J, Koustova E, Rich NM. To heal and to serve: military medical education throughout the centuries. J Am Coll Surg. 2006;202(6):1005–16.

2. Rich NM, Burris DG. "Modern" military surgery: 19th century compared with 20th century. J Am Coll Surg. 2005;200(3):321–2.
3. Butler FK. Two decades of saving lives on the battlefield: tactical combat casualty care turns 20. Mil Med. 2017;182(3):e1563–8.
4. Pruitt BA Jr, Rasmussen TE. Vietnam (1972) to Afghanistan (2014): the state of military trauma care and research, past to present. J Trauma Acute Care Surg. 2014;77(3 Suppl 2):S57–65.
5. France K, Handford C. Impact of military medicine on civilian medical practice in the UK from 2009 to 2020. BMJ Mil Health. 2021;167(4):275–9.
6. Blyth DM, Yun HC, Tribble DR, Murray CK. Lessons of war: combat-related injury infections during the Vietnam war and operation Iraqi and enduring freedom. J Trauma Acute Care Surg. 2015;79(4 Suppl 2):S227–35.
7. Lee J, Roberson L, Garner R, Kim E, Glaser J, Choi P, Vicente D. Trauma and critical care military-civilian publications increased after the COVID-19 pandemic: a literature review. J Surg Res. 2023;292:97–104.
8. Grathwohl KW, Venticinque SG. Organizational characteristics of the austere intensive care unit: the evolution of military trauma and critical care medicine; applications for civilian medical care systems. Crit Care Med. 2008;36(7 Suppl):S275–83.
9. Lim RB, Ahnfeldt E, Wisbach G, Worlton T. Why the military committee is important to SAGES? Surg Endosc. 2023;37(1):774–9.
10. Vicente D, Schobel SA, Anfossi S, et al. Viral micro-RNAs are detected in the early systemic response to injury and are associated with outcomes in polytrauma patients. Crit Care Med. 2022;50(2):296–306.

21 Professional Education and Leadership Development on Active Duty

Mary O'Donnell, W. Bryan Gamble, and Rex E. Atwood

Introduction

Clinically active general and subspecialty-trained surgeons typically leave the military after completion of their initial active-duty service obligation (ADSO) or after achieving military retirement at 20 years in service. This corresponds to 5–8 years in residency/fellowship, 10–24 total years on active duty, and military retirement age as early as 46 years old. The age of 40–60 years is considered the "prime years" of an operating surgeon, which is why military service beyond 24 years is rare. In civilian academic surgical departments, a residency Program Director or the Chairman

M. O'Donnell (✉) · R. E. Atwood
Department of Surgery, Uniformed Services University of Health Sciences, Bethesda, MD, USA

W. B. Gamble
Department of Surgery, Uniformed Services University of Health Sciences, Bethesda, MD, USA

Trauma/Surgical Critical Care, Brooke Army Medical Center, San Antonio, TX, USA

A. T. Schlussel et al. (eds.), *The SAGES Manual for Navigating a Successful Military Surgical Career*,
https://doi.org/10.1007/978-3-031-88490-0_21

of Surgery is often an individual with 25–40 years of experience as an attending surgeon. As a result of the dearth of sagacious surgeons, leadership roles are acquired much earlier in a military general surgeon's career, often at the rank of O-5 or early O-6 and age of 37–45.

Traditionally, surgeons have spent more time deployed than their non-surgeon counterparts, and general officers rarely continue to be clinically active. This has led to the military having a gap of surgically trained leaders which are critical to our wartime success. With careful planning, surgeons can balance the PME needed for advancement with deployments and the rigors of an active clinical practice. This balance is crucial because the military needs surgeon leaders to train the next generation of surgeons, lead organizations with an understanding of surgical practice, and advise line commanders on the realities of surgical care in wartime.

In the operating room, the operating surgeon is the leader of the team, with the overall mission of a successful, safe, and efficient procedure for a patient. Graduate Medical Education (GME) is designed to train a physician in this role, and certification from the American Board of Surgery should verify completion and competence in this training. Professional development as a military officer typically corresponds to rank and is acquired through leadership opportunities with progressively increasing responsibility and completion of professional military education (PME). Due to the decade of post-graduate training necessary to become an independent general surgeon in the United States, the alignment of these two timelines for leadership development is distinctive in comparison to other medical specialties. For example, the first Army PME course available after basic training, Captain's Career Course (CCC), is difficult to take before completion of 5–6 years of residency training, when a general surgeon has already been selected for promotion to Major. The military leadership timeline of the general surgeon is unique in comparison to other servicemembers and other military physicians. This chapter serves to guide surgeons in this pathway and to describe numerous opportunities (often limited to the military) by which an individual can become a surgeon-leader in education, administration, strategic-level roles, and in the combat zone.

Education as a military surgeon beyond GME usually consists of real-life experience during deployment overseas, professional military education (PME), and attainment of leadership roles in the surgical department, GME, hospital, or military-wide. The chapter does not seek to describe a "checklist" to be completed to ensure promotion in rank, but rather describe recent promotion trends and pathways by which a military surgeon can pursue leadership. The chapter will list different educational opportunities in military medicine, describe leadership opportunities for the military general surgeon, and discuss how the traditional pathways of academic or organizational promotion might be applied toward military career growth.

Professional Military Education

Professional Military Education (PME) is a key part of officer and leader development. Although much of it is oriented toward the line and training for staff roles, it can be valuable for military surgeons. Understanding military systems, processes, and language can be immensely helpful for surgeons to effectively interact and communicate with line units and leadership. It also better enables surgeons to advocate for themselves and military medicine. These courses, particularly at higher levels, often offer exposure to the geopolitical climate and the role that we play within it. Some of the courses field versions specifically designed for medical personnel, both in subject matter and their length and provide an opportunity for networking beyond the military. While not always explicitly required to promote, PME a potential discriminator for promotion boards to consider.

The branches that train general surgeons, such as the Army, Navy, and Air Force, offer PME at each level of officer rank (Table 21.1). All three have a basic officer course that is to be completed prior to starting or during the summer months after first year of medical school since there are no available blocks of

Table 21.1 Professional military education

	O-1	O-3/O-4	O-4/O-5	O-5/O-6
ARMY	Direct Commission Course (DCC) Basic Officer Leader Course (BOLC)	Captain's Career Course (CCC)	Command General Staff College Intermediate Level Education (CGSC-ILE)	Army War College
NAVY	Officer Development School Basic Readiness Officer Course (BROC)	Advanced Readiness Officer Course (AROC), Intermediate Leadership Course (ILC)	College of Naval Command and Staff	Naval War College
AIR FORCE	Officer Training School-Abbreviated (OTS-A)	Squadron Officer School (SOS)	Air Command and Staff College	Air War College
JOINT/ DHA Joint Medical Executive Skills Institute	N/A	Joint Medical Executive Skills Institute (JMESI)—Healthcare Management Course	JMESI—Intermediate Executive Skills Course	JMESI—Capstone Course for Military Heath System (MHS) Leaders

time away from school/training until after residency. Below are the recommended minimum PME by service and the corresponding rank for when the course should be completed.

The respective services recommend that each course be completed as part of leadership development of the military officer. The completion of these courses does tend to correspond with a higher chance of promotion to the subsequent officer rank, but completion is not a mandate. For example, selection for Army promotion to O-5 in FY2021 was 92.9% for individuals who had completed CCC and 100% for those who had completed CGSC-

ILE. For officers who had only completed BOLC, it was 65.7%. However, failure of height/weight standards and physical fitness tests, poor officer evaluation reports, or lack of board certification can prevent promotion as well. Completion of residency training and successful passage of American Board of Surgery exams correlates positively to promotion from O-4 to O-5. Of Board-Certified Army officers in FY2021, 93.3% were selected for promotion to lieutenant colonel. In the Army, "proficiency designators" are added to the end of a surgeon's Area of Concentration (AOC) that reflect trainee status: fellow: 61J9F, intern: 61J9E, resident: 61J9D, completion of residency/board eligible: 61J9C, and board certified: 61J9B. A similar process exists for the Navy, in which a special designator of "K" is added to the end of the sub-specialty code in the Officer's Service Record to indicate board certification. In the Army, the 9A designator is awarded for expertise in one's field, typically as a LTC or COL. It requires demonstration of professional excellence across the academic, military, and/or operational domains. Some of the potential criteria include academic appointment of Associate Professor, GME leadership, publications, professional organization leadership, PME completion, and serving in senior roles within either the MHS or the operational force.

Finally, the Order of Military Medical Merit (O2M3) is awarded to "individuals who have clearly demonstrated the highest standards of integrity and moral character, displayed an outstanding degree of professional competence, served in the Army Medical Department (for a minimum of 15 years) with selflessness, and have made a sustained contribution to the betterment of Army Medicine. Any Active Duty, Reserve Component, civilian, or retired member of the Army Medical Department who, through dedicated application of talent, effort, and spirit, has made a significant contribution having an impact on the whole of the Army Medical Department (AMEDD), shall be eligible for induction into the Order" [1].

The Defense Health Agency (DHA) has combined service medical education courses into joint programs focused on DHA-specific policies and procedures for officers serving in DHA billets. Some services include these courses in promotion board records, while others do not. These courses are critical for acquiring competencies needed for executive medicine certification and executive and commanding officer (XO or CO) billets. Officers seeking promotion should consider these courses as both learning opportunities and ways to provide a signal to promotion boards that the officer is ready to lead at the highest level.

Pathways Toward Leadership

Strategic Level Medical Command

A unique aspect of military medical leadership is the differentiation of clinically active leadership from the strategic level leaders. A general surgeon who desires to command the hospital will have a difficult time managing this position and maintaining a busy surgical practice. Once achieving the rank of O-7, military physician leaders are typically not performing clinical work and no longer receive their physician specialty bonus. The significant pay cut with promotion to the general/flag officer ranks particularly hits surgeons harder than it does those in non-surgical specialties and disincentivizes such a pursuit for many. Because these positions are extremely competitive, a soldier, sailor, or airman physician must determine as an O-5 whether to pursue this track. PME at the highest level, such as JPME II or service specific War Colleges, is also recommended. In the Army and Navy, centralized selection boards consider candidates for command billets at the O-5 level and above. Interested parties generally must opt-in to the board for consideration. Broadening and joint assignments are often looked upon favorably. These may come through staff positions at the Pentagon, Defense Health Headquarters, and each service's respective medical command structures, among others. Inspiration to pursue these roles often begins during an operational deployment, where military operations and medical support functions intersect.

Organizational Level Medical Command

Operational Leadership

Leadership roles available for the military surgeons in operational units are within MTOE (modified tables of organization and equipment) or TDA (tables of distribution) units. Formerly known as a forward surgical team (FST), a forward resuscitative surgical detachment (FRSD) commander leads 10–20 soldiers at a Role 2 far-forward surgical capability. This is an excellent role for a surgeon interested in operational leadership, starting at the rank of Major. The larger Field Hospitals and Hospital Centers are typically commanded by Lieutenant Colonels and Colonels, respectively. Surgeons might also consider Division, Corps, and Command Surgeon assignments, serving as special staff to advise the commander on all health matters for the unit. In the Navy, Command Surgeon or Fleet Surgeon billets serve a similar purpose, providing medical advice to operational commanders. Navy-specific organizational level medical commands usually fall at the officer-in-charge (OIC) level and are reserved for officers in the grades of O-5/6. Roles that are occasionally held by surgeons include Commander, Amphibious Task Force (CATF) surgeon/Fleet Surgical Team (FST) OIC for surgical teams deploying on amphibious ships, as well as Casualty Receiving and Treatment Ship (CRTS) OICs for upgrading amphibious ships to Role II+ status. Expeditionary Resuscitative Surgical System (ERSS) OICs may also be surgeons. These positions allow command experience and the ability to deploy while still functioning in a clinical role. In the Air Force, medical personnel can pursue promotion and leadership through Flight Commander/Surgeon, Squadron and Group command, and surgeon billets within larger Air Force commands. These are roles not usually filled by surgeons or even physicians, but are served well having medical personnel fill them for realistic input related to patient care.

Clinical Pathways of Command

Clinical leadership positions within the hospital can be grouped into those related to surgery directorates, hospital committees, Accreditation Council for Graduate Medical Education (ACGME), and Undergraduate Medical Education (UME). There are opportunities for leadership throughout your military treatment facility, medical center, field hospital, hospital center, or deployed surgical teams to lead. These are often rewarding, and they demonstrate to others your interest in promotion and positions of greater responsibility. Upon arrival to your first duty station after residency or fellowship as an O-4, involvement can begin with membership in hospital committees for local improvement and oversight, American College of Surgeons (ACS)-recognized local groups such as the Commission on Cancer (CoC) and the Committee on Trauma (CoT), surgical department leadership, and GME leadership. The military encourages leadership positions early within the surgeon's career and even if not interested in a lifetime of academia or department leadership, the experience these positions provide are valuable. These roles also provide experience toward organizational leadership roles, such as Consultant to the Surgeon General.

An Example of Directorate of Surgery Career Pathway

Local committee involvement > Deputy Director of Surgical Services (DSS) > DSS > Director of Surgery (DoS) > Deputy Consultant to the Surgeon General > Consultant to the Surgeon General.

Medical Center (MEDCEN) or Military Treatment Facility (MTF) Leadership

At your home institution, it will be encouraged that the military physician become involved within and outside your department. From a military standpoint, this provides the military surgeon with medically relevant command leadership that's recognized hospital or base-wide. That scope of influence is reflected on yearly evaluation reports and ultimately promotion. Opportunities within your department include division chief or deputy division chief of general surgery. Outside your department, opportunities exist on credentialing committees, quality improvement committees, Commission on Cancer (CoC) committees, committees on trauma, and as CoC cancer liaison physician, trauma medical director, National Surgical Quality Improvement Program (NSQIP) champion, hospital DSS or deputy DSS. While the continued practice of clinical medicine improves one's ability to direct change and understand issues at the patient level, these leadership roles are an additional duty removing the surgeon from direct patient care.

Leadership as a Clinical Educator

A surgical educator often refers to the education of undergraduate medical students on their surgery rotations or of graduate-level surgical residents and fellows. Pursuit of the UME and GME educator pathways can often run congruently and complement each other at different stages of the surgeon's career (Table 21.2). In the military, the UME educator typically requires rotating medical students at the MTF. Starting as a senior resident, surgeons provide MS3 lectures, provide regular on-the-job instruction, and seek to inspire students with their passion for surgery. Surgeons should mentor MS4s applying to surgery residency. Leadership roles include the local MTF's MS3 Surgery Clerkship Coordinator or Associate Coordinator. With completion of educator coursework, increasing levels of UME leadership include: USUHS Surgery Clerkship Coordinator; the USU Advanced Clerkship Course Director; USU Core Surgery Clerkship Director (serving all military MTFs and MEDCENs); Associate Dean (many varieties); and USU Vice Chair of Education.

At the graduate level, the educator role requires a residency program at the MTF, but could begin with mentoring junior officers and new surgeon arrivals where there is no GME program. Rotation coordinator of a physician's assistant program or 68D

Table 21.2 Example career pathways

Directorate of Surgery	Local Committees	Deputy Director of Surgical Services	Director of Surgical Services	Deputy Consultant/ Specialty Leader	Consultant/ Specialty Leader
UME	USU Surgery Clerkship Coordinator	USU Advanced Clerkship Course Director	USU Core Surgery Clerkship Course Director	USU Associate Dean	USU Vice Chair of Education
GME	Local ACGME Committees	Core Academic Faculty	Associate Program Director	Program Director	

(medics, corpsman, etc.) education can give experience toward the educator role. An example of a GME educator pathway may be: ACGME Committees locally > Core Academic Faculty > Associate Program Director (APD) > Program Director (PD) of General Surgery Residency > APD or PD surgical fellowship. Curricula is available at USU in the Center for Health Professions Education (https://chpe.usuhs.edu/) to obtain skills as an advanced educator with certificates, master's degrees, and PhDs available [2]. A number of courses are available virtually for individuals who are not local. If pursuing the position of program director of a residency, the Association of Program Directors in Surgery (APDS) has a 2-day course, the *Program Directors Workshop*, for new APDs and PDs. The educator pathway serves the military surgeon well, allowing them to remain clinically active and achieve academic promotion.

Pathways Toward Academic Promotion

In parallel with clinical, educator, or research surgeons' careers, academic promotion in rank is attained through USU and often through their local partnered civilian university hospital.. From Instructor to Assistant Professor, Associate Professor to Full Professor of Surgery, the primary "tracks" for promotion may differ within the university but generally are: Teaching and Education, Clinical Expertise and Innovation, and Investigation. At USU, these tenure-ineligible tracks are: Clinician-Educator, Clinician-Investigator, Educator, and Research [3]. These academic ranks demonstrate achievement in each field and translate to civilian academic practice, so they are strongly recommended. More information can be found at the USU Department of Surgery: https://medschool.usuhs.edu/sur.

Additional Military Courses for Leadership Development

Courses offered by DHA or individual military branches promote professional development, broaden knowledge about military leadership, and may increase rates of promotion (Table 21.3). The description of the Iron Majors' Week (IMW) makes it clear why many of these courses are needed in the development during the O-4 to O-5 ranks.

PME such as the CCC and ILE Courses prepare officers with military unique skills focused on building tactical and operational competencies. The curricula of the Senior Service Colleges (SSC) focus on building senior leader conceptual competencies later in an officer's career, if at all. The five-to-eleven-year gap between ILE and SSC is a critical time in the lifecycle and promotion opportunities of an officer who is continuing to develop and broaden the skills necessary for senior leadership, or seek key and broadening or strategic billet type assignments. IMW enriches the officer's Professional Military Education portfolio by serving to close this critical educational gap, and it is especially important for those who will compete for future strategic billets. IMW also provides an Officer Record Brief unique identifier that Army senior leaders have grown accustomed to during competitive selection board processes [5].

Table 21.3 Leadership development courses

Course	Description
Junior Leadership Course [4]	The purpose of the JLC is to identify outstanding junior leaders who demonstrate the core Army Values and Warrior Ethos and who demonstrate the skills, attributes and potential required to become future AMEDD leaders. Over 5 days, 79 competitively selected Captains and Majors took part in roundtable discussions and briefs with senior leadership from Army Medicine, DHA, Training and Doctrine Command, and the Defense Intelligence Agency on various topics.

(continued)

Table 21.3 (continued)

Course	Description
Iron Majors Course [5]	Recognizes select Army Medical Department (AMEDD) Majors for both their accomplishments and identified potential to serve in strategic positions. Selected nominees attend a 1-week professional experience in the National Capital Region, designed to expose officers to concepts that help prepare them for strategic positions that involve critical joint, interagency and military-civilian relationships with a specific focus on emerging initiatives within the Army, AMEDD, Joint Health Services Enterprise (JHSE) transformation, Interagency and Military-Civilian relationships.
Female Physician Leadership Course [6]	Interactive leadership development opportunity for emerging and prospective mid-level female physician-leaders in the MHS. Provides an interactive leadership development opportunity addressing many of the 40 Core Competencies, specific goals of this course include: • Provide women with a greater understanding of leadership opportunities within their respective services and within the MHS. • Deliberate development and strengthening of military-medical leadership skills. • Emphasize the value of mentoring (whether receiving or providing mentoring to others) and networking as a component to sustainable success and culture change. • Provide assistance with working toward a work-life balance and prevent burn-out. • Introduce emerging leaders to the mechanics of Performance Based Management and effective Project Management • Identify emerging female physician leaders and equip them with the tools to be successful leaders in military medicine.
JMESI Healthcare Management Course [7]	This course is a Tri-Service event designed for first time clinical supervisors and provides them with the administrative tools to successfully manage their clinical areas. Topics include: • Civilian personnel • Contracting • Budgeting • Quality management • Tools available through the TRICARE operations center • Efficient scheduling and utilization management

(continued)

Table 21.3 (continued)

Course	Description
JMESI DHA Intermediate Executive Skills [8]	The Joint Medical Executive Skills Institute Intermediate Executive Skills Course provides education and training on leadership and management skills necessary to successfully serve in an intermediate-level leadership position within a DHA medical treatment facility. The course is designed to facilitate attainment of selected JMES core competencies as identified by a Tri-Service review board of MHS senior leaders. The course consists of 12 web-based training modules available through the DHA Learning Management System followed by a 4-day live, web-based video conference course hosted on MS Teams. The course goal/mission is to facilitate achievement of joint medical executive skills competencies expected of intermediate-level leaders within a DHA market or MTF. Graduates will demonstrate: • Understanding of the DHA mission and strategic plan. • Skills consistent with professional expectations required to serve in an intermediate-level leadership position within a DHA market or MTF. • Ability to communicate effectively, lead change initiatives, and manage resources.

(continued)

Table 21.3 (continued)

Course	Description
JMESI Capstone Course of MHS Leaders [9]	With the smaller class size, direct interaction with policy makers and military health care leaders, and its joint audience the Capstone Course has come to provide firsthand, real world, applicable knowledge/information for the attendees to incorporate into their day-to-day and future work in the MHS. Upon completion of the course the participants will: • Have an enhanced understanding of MHS policymaking dissemination and the legal basis for those policies. • Gain a deeper sense of TRICARE issues and policies that shape the delivery of DOD health care. • Become familiarized with information systems that support executive decision-making, and tools for evaluating quality assurance, customer satisfaction, and metrics. • Discuss issues of military retention/recruitment and national perspectives, financial and business matters related to MHS. • Share networking opportunities to include, but not limited to, the Surgeons General, members of other services serving in similar capacities, OSD leaders including Deputy Secretaries, the VA, civilian health program managers, and academia. • Become familiar with unique ways of dealing with human relations and gain a better appreciation for the way they are perceived by others. • Exchange ideas on current issues such as risk management, patient safety, Homeland Security, bioterrorism, war fighters (the line) and Reserve Forces. • Gain an enhanced appreciation for fiscal issues within the DOD.

(continued)

Table 21.3 (continued)

Course	Description
Medxellence [10]	USU's MedXellence Course provides current and aspiring Military Health System (MHS) leaders 40 h of continuing education credits and an unparalleled opportunity to expand their leadership and management skill sets, through its robust curriculum consisting of both lecture and hands-on small group exercises that are based on real-world MHS scenarios. Since its 1993 introduction, MedXellence has been praised by the thousands of MHS professionals as being highly relevant to their current leadership and management positions, and, just as importantly, to those positions that they will hold as they progress in their careers. Drawing on senior faculty and other highly knowledgeable DHS and Service Subject Matter Experts, this week-long course provides students in all disciplines with most powerful and most current information about today's, and tomorrow's, Military Health System. Curriculum involving both lectures and hands-on small group exercises bases on real-world MHS scenarios designed to give attendees unparalleled opportunity to build leadership and management skill sets.
Interagency Institute for Federal Healthcare Leaders [11]	The institute provides an opportunity for the seasoned, practicing federal health care executive to examine current issues in health care policy and management and to explore their potential impact on the federal health care system. The design of the course assumes a high level of conceptual knowledge and operating ability on the part of the participants. Given the intelligence and sophistication of these selected executives, the faculty maximizes the learning experience by presenting new materials resulting from research and experience, as well as examples and case studies from the contemporary national health policy decision-making process. Faculty members also seek involvement and interaction by the participants to stimulate understanding and communication across traditional agency boundaries.
Medical Strategic Leadership Program [12]	JSMLC is a 5-day, classroom-only course designed to enhance preparation of medical leaders (senior O-5 s to O-6 s) who have a high probability of being named as a Joint Task Force Surgeon, JTF senior medical leader, or occupy a senior medical planning position in a joint environment. In addition, the course would be valuable for those serving in senior departments, training and preparing forces for joint operations and deployment.

In addition to these courses offered by the military, standard civilian leadership and management courses can also be highly beneficial to one's career. For example, a Masters of Business Administration or Masters of Healthcare Administration covers approximately 50% of the core competencies needed for executive medicine certification prior to becoming CO or XO eligible. Many surgical fellowships, including those sponsored by the military, offer these degrees at no cost during the surgical fellowship years. Officers pursuing outside degrees, or those entering service with additional degrees should ensure that their service records are coded correctly to maximize visibility for promotion boards.

Additional Leadership Courses and Certificates

The American College of Surgeons has a cache of excellent courses for the development of the surgeon leader after GME training. The courses offer something toward each pathway of leadership: ACS Surgeons as Leaders Course, ACS Surgeons as Educators Course, and conferences such as ACS Leadership and Advocacy or the ACS Quality and Improvement Conference can offer professional development toward those leadership roles surgeons can hold in their hospitals. Within the military, USU offers a Masters in Health Professions Education, a Health Administration and Policy Certificate, a USU Faculty Development Certificate, and a Masters of Public Health in Global Health without incurring additional military obligation. If stationed locally, these may be completed without incurring an additional service obligation. If they require a permanent change of station, though, they will generally add to your obligation. Madigan Army Medical Center offers a Faculty Development Fellowship that also yields a masters level degree. The American Association of Physician Leadership has a Certified Physician Executive Course, and Stanford has a Faculty Development Center for Medical Teachers.

Key Challenges and Solutions for Scheduling Military Education

In 2019, the 7-week-long Army Officer Basic Course (OBC)/ Basic Officer Leadership Course (BOLC) was lengthened and expanded into two separate courses called DCC and BOLC. Since medical students only have unfilled time in their academic schedules prior to the start of medical school and potentially during the summer between first and second years, completing these courses has become a challenge. Some are now forced to complete these courses immediately following medical school graduation, delaying the start of their intern year and significantly complicating the academic schedules for many residency programs. Communication with incoming interns can help to schedule these courses to minimize disruptions. For direct accession surgeons, prior communication with the incoming duty station and detailer can help to ensure that adequate time is given to allow completion of these courses prior to starting one's first active-duty assignment.

Scheduling PME with a busy clinical schedule will continue to be challenging. However, prior planning can contribute to completing these courses with maximum efficiency. With the COVID-19 pandemic shuttering many in-person courses, many online courses have now become permanent options to finish requirements for service schools and PME. For example, JPME, which used to be a master's level course offered through each service specific war college, now is a certificate-level course which can be completed entirely online, in a blended environment, or as a fully dedicated 1-year master's at most War Colleges. Similarly, most of the Navy-specific advancement courses can be completed as a blended option, with the pre-class work being completed on the Joint Knowledge Online (JKO) website. Many courses, such as online JPME offered through the Air Force, are on a traditional academic semester schedule, allowing the officer to take a few classes at a time. Timing these courses around a PCS or deployment is often optimal, as lapses in credentialing or significant downtime can exist prior to restarting clinical practice. Surgeons should follow each course's calendar closely, as class spots often fill up very quickly, especially for courses seen as "required" for promotion. Additionally, it is often easiest to book courses at the start of the fiscal year when funds are guaranteed, especially if significant travel expenses are anticipated.

Conclusion

Leadership and professional development for active duty physicians goes beyond the role of an officer or traditional commander of units. The complexity and diversity of healthcare systems require leaders within GME, UME, medical research, clinical research, hospital executive management, and more importantly the future military needs well-rounded leaders. Numerous and often free educational opportunities, professional mentorship, and career growth pathways are widely available within the military. Motivated, talented, and self-effacing individuals have incredible opportunities to ascend in leadership roles, especially early in their careers, to influence the future of the military healthcare system.

Finally, leadership within the military, whether in the operational, academic, or institutional setting, can be used to bolster future career opportunities outside of active duty. As previously mentioned, military service allows officers to enter leadership positions usually reserved for more senior individuals in the civilian market, which allows officers to gain valuable experience that may help them obtain work outside of the military. While PME was previously considered at the certificate or correspondence course level, now many PME courses can be obtained that have Master's or higher level degree opportunities in fields such as leadership or education. Finally, many officers end their careers by transitioning to the reserves, allowing for dual leadership opportunities as a civilian and servicemember. Serving in a leadership role can have an impact on the officer's short- and long-term career goals while in the military and beyond.

References

1. AMEDD Center of History & Heritage. The order of military medical merit (O2M3). [cited 2024 Nov 10]. Available from: https://achh.army.mil/regiment/merit-o2m3
2. USU Center for Health Professions Education. Master in Health Professions Education (MHPE). [cited 2024 Nov 10]. Available from: https://chpe.usuhs.edu/graduate-programs/mhpe
3. Uniformed Services University (USU). School of Medicine policies for the academic administration of the faculty instruction 1110A. [cited 2024 Nov 10]. Available from: https://medschool.usuhs.edu/sites/default/files/media/documents/1100asigned22924acc.pdf
4. Lovelace CJ. Soldier, AMLC civilian attend Army Medical Department's 2023 Junior Leadership Course. Defense Visual Information Distribution Service; 2023 May 18 [cited 2024 Nov 10]. Available from: https://www.dvidshub.net/news/445009/soldier-amlc-civilian-attend-army-medical-departments-2023-junior-leadership-course
5. COL Jeffrey Oliver. Iron Majors' Week summary v2.pdf. 2019.
6. Schofer J. 2024 Female Physician Leadership Course (14–16 May) nominations – due NLT 02 Feb 2024. Joel Schofer's Career Planning Blog; 2023 Dec 31 [cited 2024 Nov 10]. Available from: https://mccareer.org/2023/12/31/2024-female-physician-leadership-course-14-16-may-nominations-due-nlt-02-feb-2024/
7. Joint Medical Executive Skills Institute. Healthcare Management Course. [cited 2024 Nov 10]. Available from: https://health.mil/Military-Health-Topics/Education-and-Training/LEADS/JMESI
8. Joint Medical Executive Skills Institute. Intermediate Executive Skills Course. [cited 2024 Nov 10]. Available from: https://health.mil/Military-Health-Topics/Education-and-Training/LEADS/JMESI
9. Joint Medical Executive Skills Institute. Capstone Course for MHS Leaders. [cited 2024 Nov 10]. Available from: https://health.mil/Military-Health-Topics/Education-and-Training/LEADS/JMESI
10. Uniformed Services University. About MEDEXCELLENCE. [cited 2024 Nov 10]. Available from: https://medschool.usuhs.edu/pmb/education/medxellence
11. Federal Health Care Executives Institute Alumni Association. Interagency Institute for Federal Health Leaders Course. [cited 2024 Nov 10]. Available from: https://www.fhceiaa.org/iiffhce-course
12. Defense Medical Readiness Training Institute. Joint Senior Medical Leaders Course. [cited 2024 Nov 10]. Available from: https://www.health.mil/Military-Health-Topics/Education-and-Training/DMRTI/Course-Information/Joint-Senior-Medical-Leaders-Course

Command Tract: How to Become a Flag Officer

22

Adam M. Robinson Jr. and Jemorie Teixeira

Introduction

How do you become a Flag Officer? This is an odd question because there is no formulaic answer. It is like asking how can you win a lottery or a game of chance. To avoid trivializing the position that Flag and General Officers assume in our nation's military, the question necessitates a different response. There is no formula or guaranteed method to becoming a flag officer that, when utilized, will provide assured success. Therefore, the topic of becoming a flag officer revolves around these thoughts and considerations.

What professional, character, and leadership attributes should one possess that would make them eligible to compete for selection as a general and/or flag officer?

First, there is a quick discussion regarding nomenclature.

What is a Flag Officer?

A Flag Officer is a commissioned officer in our nation's armed forces. Senior enough to be entitled to fly a flag to mark the position from which the officer exercises command.

A. M. Robinson Jr. · J. Teixeira (✉)
VA Pacific Islands Health Care System, Honolulu, HI, USA
e-mail: Jemorie.Teixeira@va.gov

A. T. Schlussel et al. (eds.), *The SAGES Manual for Navigating a Successful Military Surgical Career*,
https://doi.org/10.1007/978-3-031-88490-0_22

The essence of the concept of a Flag Officer then revolves around the concept of command. The essence of command is leadership. Leadership is defined in many ways. The essence: the ability to influence others to follow your guidance and direction.

> Nearly all men can stand adversity, but if you want to test a man's character, give him power
> —Abraham Lincoln

Leadership

Our personal responsibility to others as we travel through our lives.

Leadership is a topic that is written about by many, and I think it is understood by few. It is an instant way to garner attention, especially when it is placed in conjunction with a famous or historic character such as Presidents, Military Leaders, or other famous people.

It is rarely defined in any clear or concise way—but there are a number of defining characteristics that are used to explain it. For example, a leader is one who leads—this is a classic dictionary definition—but it does little to enlighten us about what leading is all about, and it does not help us answer: What is the essence of leadership?

We hear the term "leadership" in all its forms constantly—*leadership* traits, *leadership* skills, functional *leadership*, situational *leadership*—and let us not forget the age-old delineation between *leading* and *managing*.

First, let me define leader in my worldview. A leader is one who provides VISION for the group. VISION is the ability to set an "END STATE," which represents a destination in which all are benefited.

In contrast, management is EXECUTION of the VISION or the plan. Implementation becomes mostly a management function. Putting a finer edge on our difference: We *lead people*; we *manage inventory*. People are led; things are managed.

As Ross Perot cited in Anderson (2013): "Lead and inspire people. Don't try to manage and manipulate people. Inventories can be managed, but people must be led" [1].

What are the most frequently found characteristics of leaders—those traits that define successful leaders? The following are characteristics that I've compiled that provide a solid foundation from which to build and expand upon from a leadership perspective.

Defining Characteristics of Leaders

1. Vision Ability to communicate Discipline
2. Integrity
3. Dedication
4. Magnanimity
5. Humility
6. Openness
7. Creativity
8. Fairness
9. Assertiveness
10. Sense of humor

Vision, Ability to Communicate, Discipline—these are key foundational characteristics. Having a vision for yourself and those you lead, the ability to communicate it effectively, and having the discipline necessary to ensure it is executed are crucial.

Integrity—Outward actions/inner values. Your actions and behaviors display integrity more than words ever could.

Dedication—Spending the necessary time and energy to accomplish the task.

Magnanimity—Giving credit where it is due.

Humility—We are all equal. No one is better or worse on our teams.

Openness: Listen—to new ideas, and be flexible and open to considering them.

Creativity: The ability to think differently.

Fairness: Dealing with others consistently/fairly.

Assertiveness: Not aggressiveness-the ability to clearly state expectations.
Sense of humor: Vital to relieving tension and boredom.

> Where there is no vision, the people perish
> —Proverbs 29:18

Leadership is an introspective journey that allows us, through self-realization of who we are as a person, to cast a path for others whom we are privileged to guide or lead in our lives. All of us at times in our lives lead others—and we are simultaneously led. We must remain agile and flexible in thought and spirit to capture the full essence of our lives as followers and display our creativity and innovation as leaders. It is in these instances that we learn what kind of leader we want to (or don't want to) be. These lessons and experiences ultimately shape our leadership style. They come with ups and downs, like the shoreline ebbs and flows, falling back and pushing you forward to the next challenge. Not every lesson is painless. It is important to take the difficult and challenging lessons—the ones that may push you to almost breaking—to realize you can withstand more than you think.

Flexibility and composure are what will keep you from breaking when forces around you are challenging and intense. The spirit and courage to bend, not break, are what shape tomorrow's leaders. Every triumph and each failure build resilience and capability, like roots that lay the foundation for a sturdy and strong tree.

VISION requires introspection. Introspection allows us to focus and frame our DREAMS. Our dreams are a reflection of the thoughts, feelings, and yearnings of our heart and soul. When our love for others is brought into this calculus—and fulfilled—it allows us to be swept into a vortex of spirited connectedness and awareness that both permits and enhances our ability to be leaders.

The signs of a good leader are best reflected in their followers—the people who work for them.

Here are the questions I want to ask you:

- Are your followers reaching their potential?
- Are your followers learning?
- Do your followers achieve the results required for success in your department?
- Do your followers accept change with grace?
- Do your followers manage conflict well?

The answer to these questions will be the major way that you know that you are an effective leader.

Max De Pree in his wonderful and powerful book "Leadership is an Art", offers these characteristics of the leader and leadership:

LEADERS ENDORSE A CONCEPT OF PERSON.

Leadership is about knowing your people in all of their goodness and badness—but most importantly, it's about affirming your people and the special gifts which they bring to us—to you—everyday and in every situation.

We must understand and accept the gift of diversity in our followers: we must recognize their different talents and their different skills.

We must be ready to acknowledge that we cannot do everything ourselves—we need the help of committed and inspired followers in order to achieve our common institutional and personal goals.

Understanding this will lead us to understand our:

1. OPPORTUNITY/OPPORTUNITIES—in all situations and with all people.
2. EQUITY—it will allow equity in our decisions where fairness and consistency can prevail, and it will establish both our:
3. IDENTITY and PURPOSE—That is, who we are, and what we stand for.

These attributes of opportunity, equity, and identity allow us a more fundamental understanding of the difference between goals and rewards.

So what do teachers need to know?

I will give you three things which I feel are essential for successful leaders:

1. FIRST, *Leaders must define reality.*

   They must show us what is GENUINE.

   By doing this, they help to ground us and keep us from being duped or deceived by what is either artificial or extraneous.

   The *reality* of a situation changes with the circumstances, the people, the mission, the goals, and the rewards promised, but the effective and successful leader must be able to decide and define the reality for their followers.
2. Secondly, leaders must COMMUNICATE with their followers.

   In order for communication to be successful, there must be both the transmission of a message and the receipt of that message.

   Communication is key—it is the way the defined reality is passed from one to another.

   Effective communication can be accomplished by *word of mouth or by written word*, but the leader knows *how*, *when*, *where*, to deliver the message, and to whom he is speaking, for communication with different groups, requires different styles.

   But one thing that is always true for all groups: COMMUNICATION must be HONEST, SIMPLE, STRAIGHTFORWARD, AND SINCERE.

   Remember if you say it, and it was not understood, you have failed.

   If it was not believed, you have failed.

   If it was not appreciated—that is, your followers did not care to listen—you have failed.

   And lastly, if it was not heard, you have failed.

   Followers must
   (a) UNDERSTAND,
   (b) BELIEVE,
   (c) HEAR, and
   (d) VALUE what you say.
3. Finally, leaders must provide an environment in which followers have the *space and the freedom* to *expand their creativity and their gifts.*

Max De Pree states:

- We need to give each other the space to grow, to be ourselves, to exercise our diversity.
- We need to give each other space so that we may both give and receive such beautiful things as IDEAS, OPENNESS, DIGNITY, JOY, HEALING, AND INCLUSION.

So I think that the third characteristic of leadership is EMPOWERMENT.

My definition of empowerment is:

- ENABLING the gifts of our followers to be exercised.

I think that by empowering our followers, we also empower ourselves so that we can fully recognize and develop our own gifts.

So there you have it: Leaders, Leadership:

1. Defining REALITY
2. COMMUNICATING THE REALITY
3. EMPOWERING your FOLLOWERS TO FULLY DEVELOP AND DISPLAY THEIR TALENTS.

These are my top three attributes that must be practiced and perfected by the LEADER.

Leadership is ultimately an outward, practiced, and sincere expression of faith in our people.

It is the acknowledgment that institutions such as churches, universities, and even governmental and military organizations, EVEN OUR NAVY, are no more than the people—*you and I*—who serve in them, and who re-establish and perpetuate the values, goals, rewards, and mission.

Leaders are no more than servants to the servants.

Finally, leadership must be capable of having and knowing their individual ethical standards and boundaries before they are presented with ethical crises.

And these difficult times will call for clear engagement.

There are two important aspects that every person must address prior to assuming any leadership position.

First, there are times when the leader must establish fast and definitive action by those they are leading.

It is wonderful and desirable to have discussion, collaboration, and consensus in decision-making.

From an organizational development perspective this is the usual and desired method in setting course and direction.

But there are times when the leader must make a quick and decisive decision in which all must move without debate, resistance, or question.

These times are dependent upon the circumstances that exist and they are critical to the health, well-being, and often the survival of the group.

So the issue becomes the necessity to know, inform, and educate your constituency when decisions are made which must be obeyed quickly and without hesitation or deliberation.

Leaders are responsible for the well-being of the group both in good, normal times and also in times of urgency and crisis.

Group training and dynamics necessitate these responses must be addressed and learned prior to a crisis.

The ultimate goal is to have fast, decisive, and affirmative group response in order to survive.

The second critical issue that all leaders must address is to know and establish their moral and ethical boundaries before a crisis situation is encountered.

The time to establish your response to an ethical dilemma needs to be established prior to the situation arising.

It is often difficult, if not impossible, to decipher your position or to offer clear and credible responses to a moral or ethical situation without leader preparation and thought.

It is also desirable to share your ethos of leadership with the individuals/group being led in order to help them define the desired end states and to allay any anxieties or questions they may have regarding the moral boundaries of your leadership position and the group's desired end state.

Attempting to have these conversations in real-time, that is, in crisis, may be impossible and may result in less than desirable outcomes because of cloudiness of thought, delay in actions, and overall non-clarity of the position in the given situation.

An ethos and mode of operation based upon clearly defined ethical boundaries and standards is critical in order to make, or take, clear and decisive action.

Perfection is always desired, but usually not unattainable.

Clarity then becomes a standard for communication and execution of the plan.

> In matters of style, swim with the current; In matters of principle, stand like a rock
> —Thomas Jefferson

The great twentieth-century theologian and mystic Howard Thurman described in a short essay the three things that define what a leader must possess. In his book *Strange Freedom*, Thurman (1998) states that leaders must [2]:

1. Know themselves and be comfortable with who they are,
2. Be responsible for their actions, and
3. Be responsible for their reactions.

Leadership is *serving* others.

Leadership is *service* to others.

Leadership identifies our responsibility to ourselves and to our fellow human beings.

Leadership demands a thorough understanding of who we are. Before we can connect with and understand someone else, we must first connect with and understand ourselves. We must have a fundamental and truthful understanding of ourselves.

> Do not follow where the path may lead. Go instead where there is no path and leave a trail
> —Ralph Waldo Emerson

Self-realization demands that we come to terms with who we are. The inability to do this—the inability to be honest with ourselves—will not permit us to lead. We must know who we are in order to connect with and understand another person. Those characteristics that we dislike or even loathe in ourselves become the basis for criticism and disgust in others. Other people become the mirrors that reflect those things that we dislike in ourselves and despise in others. Our perception of others becomes the reflection of how we feel about ourselves. You can see why this is so important. Knowledge of your tendencies, your personal biases, your communication style, strengths/weaknesses, and more, become tools to build and expand your connections—with yourself and with those you will lead. It is less about using one technique or leadership style and more about being flexible and using these tools to shape what is needed to effectively lead others.

Our actions and our reactions to the currents and winds of our lives are dependent upon our ability to take responsibility for our lives.

Responsibility requires three things:

1. Maturity
2. Introspection
3. Integrity

We act because we make a decision to act.

We react because we make a decision to react.

Now, these decisions are not always made consciously. We are often not fully cognizant of why we do or say what we do. This does not eliminate or obviate our responsibility. However, it does inform us of the complexity of thought and action. We are fully capable of acting or reacting to the 'fumes' of our subconscious mind, which often guides us and forces us into uncompromising and uncomfortable thoughts and memories.

Often, our subconscious mind blocks our ability to remember by selective editing, blocking, and distortion of words or facts, both negatively and positively. That is, things are remembered in totally altered and erroneous ways to support the mind's ability to eliminate distress rather than facing it—adapting and overcoming it. Another word for this is denial. The basis of psychotherapy helps us overcome these mental obstacles and distortions, which can plague our ability to live fulfilling and complete lives.

Maturity allows us the time needed to more fully understand our situations. Maturity helps us by offering a capacity to discern the boundaries of our memories but not to distort the essence of the truth of our memories.

Introspection provides understanding based on our intellect, our life experiences, and our spiritual awareness. Placed in a frame of integrity and honesty, we become truth-tellers—someone who tells the truth about what is really happening in a situation [3] (Cambridge Dictionary, 2023).

Therefore, we return to this proposition:

We must know ourselves—and we must learn to be comfortable with who we are.

We are the responsible person in our lives, and we must always accept responsibility for what we do and how we act.

When we can do this, we are not only leaders, but we are also something more. We become the beacon for others as we display our vision of the end state. That end state is this: that our real purpose in this life is to help one another, to guide one another—to love one another as God loves us.

Finally, I would like to leave you with three additional things we must do in preparation for our life's journey and our lives of service and leadership:

1. **Professional Competence**

   Education is a foundational anchor of professional competence. To secure professional competence, we must become lifelong learners. It is necessary to connect to a course of continuous educational expertise and improvement. This keeps us fresh and combats both intellectual lethargy and contentment. New ideas and new ways of thinking are critical to remaining grounded in our professional thinking. It allows for innovation, creativity, and critical thinking and analysis. It does not matter what our chosen profession is. It only necessitates our active participation in a steady and lifelong course of seeking continuing educational exercises and achievement.

2. **Personal Readiness**

   Tunnel vision is a syndrome that we must avoid. Setting the aperture of our lives too narrowly provokes a shallowness of thought and experience. We are unable to see the innumerable possibilities of our possible directions and experience the depth and challenges of our lives. To lose this ability stunts our personal growth and our creative and innovative possibilities. To put a useful definition here, think of work-life balance.

   None of us can focus only on one thing in our lives if we are to be fully functioning. If we are only concerned with our work and professional conditions, success, and achievements, we are stilted and ill-formed. We are also at great risk of experiencing both the physical and emotional illnesses that occur when we are imbalanced in our lives.

   There is another equally serious effect to consider. Our health and well-being are directly reflected by our families. Additionally, their health and well-being can also suffer from our inability or neglect to balance our professional and personal lives.

   Personal readiness is that part of our lives that must include our families, however, we define them. They are an integral part of who we are and how we define and display ourselves and the structure of our lives. We must be both cognizant and sensitive to the necessity of balancing our work-life commitments.

   To paraphrase a familiar biblical reference: what does one accomplish to gain the world, yet lose our family? I recognize that soul and family are different. However, in many ways, our families bolster and sustain our souls. Proper adherence to personal readiness can prevent this tragedy.

3. **Spiritual Awareness**

   Often, when one hears the word "spiritual", there is a reflexive thought about religion. If this happens to you, don't stop reading. It may mean religion to you—it does to me. However, I ask you to consider this definition: something in our lives that is larger and more important than us.

We often think that we are the center of the universe—the most important thing in our world. My thought is very simple: we are not the center of the universe. The faster we come to understand and accept this fact, the faster we can learn what servant leadership is about and how we may begin to practice and experience its positive effects. When we can stop personalizing our lives around our thoughts, desires, and actions, and begin to reflect on the part that others play in creating the world in which we exist, only then can we make the necessary commitments to have respect and deep affection for those who help complete our world. This is what the beginning of servant leadership means to me.

Spiritual awareness comes into focus when we realize that our job is not to be served but to serve. This proposition was first formally espoused by Robert Greenleaf in his essay, *The Servant as Leader* [4]. Notably, Greenleaf credited his inspiration for this concept to a 1932 book, *Journey to the East*, by Herman Hesse, a 1946 Nobel laureate in Literature. In Greenleaf's formulation, the most important characteristic servant leaders must possess is the ability to be servants first—"to come for the needs of others around them, to ensure the growth of future leaders".

According to Greenleaf, two premises come from the servant leader mentality:

- I serve because I am a leader
- I am the leader because I serve

The first premise signifies the act of altruism. The Oxford Dictionary defines altruism as the belief in or practice of disinterested and selfless concern for the well-being of others [5].

The second premise (I am the leader because I serve) begins with a rooted ambition to be a leader.

Larry Spears, the author of several books on servant leadership, takes the servant leader construct and attaches Ten Traits of Servant Leaders [6]. Through these traits, he broadens and deepens the servant leader role and impact, and securely places it in both an ethical and spiritual realm.

Spears' Ten Traits include:

1.	Empathy
2.	Listening
3.	Healing
4.	Awareness
5.	Persuasion
6.	Conceptualization
7.	Foresight
8.	Stewardship
9.	Commitment to the growth of people
10.	Building community

My perspective on each trait is as follows:

Empathy—Placing yourself in the position of another.

Listening—Uninterrupted and nonjudgmental. Hearing to understand.

Healing—Where there is discord or hurt, initiate therapeutic resolution.

Awareness—Perceiving and discerning situations with understanding.

Persuasion—Convincing and coaxing to produce a basis of common belief.

Conceptualization—To consolidate ideas and build a mental construct.

Foresight—Predicting the future: what will be needed for the future?

Stewardship—Be responsible and caring for property, money, and resources with fidelity.

Commitment to the Growth of People—Be responsible for advancing the position, knowledge, education, capacity, and general benefit of the people serving with you. All should leave better and advanced from your care.

Building Community—Community represents the ability to share common attitudes, interests, and goals.

The Ten Traits broaden our understanding of servant leadership. It also deepens our responsibility in performing the servant leader role. This harmonization of people with mission is apparent throughout the servant leader concept.

Joe Iarocci's "Servant Leadership in the Workplace" lists three priorities [7]:

1. Developing People
2. Building a Trusting Team
3. Achieving Results

This is a concise listing, and although brief in number, his priorities parallel the Ten Traits of Spears.

Servant leadership is a leadership model that is both inspirational and contains moral safeguards.

In *Servant Leadership: A Systematic Review and Call for Future Research,* Mulyadi Robin and Sen Sendjaya (2019) [8] wrote that servant leadership serves as a holistic paradigm for leadership, as it not only is transformative and ethical but also engages workers in workplace spirituality.

A way of operationalizing servant leadership concepts into practice is given to us in this next section, which highlights Marian Wright Edelman, founder and President of the Children's Defense Fund—this is only one of many of her major contributions to our country reflecting servant leadership in action in our society's realms of law, social justice, and education—who wrote wonderful gems of wisdom and understanding in her book.

Edelman has provided for me true gems of wisdom and understanding in her book *Lantern: A Memoir of Mentors* [9]. She defines mentor as a trusted friend or guide, and for me, she has become a mentor and role model. She writes about many phases of her life and the people who have guided her through the years. She describes 25 Life Lessons—lessons that will help make us more complete. Lessons that will sustain us when the night falls and we need lanterns to find our way safely.

I want to share six of them with you. I hope you remember these words and the feelings which she describes:

- *Lesson 1*

  Always remember that you are God's child. No man or woman can look down on you, and you cannot look down on any man, woman, or child. Hold your head high, be yourself, and be happy being yourself.
- *Lesson 2*

  Don't be afraid to stick your neck out, to make mistakes, or to speak up. The only person who does not make mistakes is the person who does nothing. Take my advice: In this life, if you're doing the right thing, proceed until apprehended.
- *Lesson 3*

  Keep your word and your commitment. Remember that integrity—that is, adherence to a code of values—is the most important currency that human beings exchange between one another. Be as good as your word, and the richness of respect will always be yours.
- *Lesson 4*

  Don't let anybody or anything get between you and your education. Remember what luck is all about: preparation and opportunity. In addition, by the way, Education is preparation. It is a treasure trove of possibilities, which is yours for the taking. With education, be greedy.
- *Lesson 5*

  Take responsibility for your behavior. Don't make excuses, blame others, point fingers at 'others', or hide behind "everybody's doing it." Accountability is the operative phrase. Maturity is the way to attain independence. These actions—responsibility and accountability—are what make you ready to contribute to our world.
- *Lesson 6*

  Possessions and power do not make the person; principles, character, and love do.

These are lifelong lessons to learn, demonstrate, repeat, and pass on.

These lessons are not automatically known; they must be taught. Therefore, my charge to each of you is to teach these lessons to all those you know, including those whom you have the honor of leading and teaching. Because when you teach someone, you too have a chance to learn again. And again, the knowledge upon which our humanity renews itself.

Marian Wright Edelman operationalizes what servant leadership can be.

> If your actions inspire others to dream more, learn more, do more, and become more, you are a leader.
> —John Quincy Adams

When I was a young officer, there was a common question that was asked. What is most important: Mission or People? I think this may be a question still asked. For a long time, I thought mission was the imperative—mission being the greatest good. I now know that this is incorrect. People are our goal. People are the greatest good because people are the elements that execute or accomplish the mission. No matter what the mission may be or how well or how poorly it has been developed or planned, people will execute the mission and accomplish the plan.

The supported people who are trained, resourced, and affirmed can successfully execute a poorly planned mission. Conversely, the nonsupported people, poorly trained, resourced, and not affirmed will not be able to execute the best planned mission.

The servant leader ethos will produce teams that have the desire, capacity, and resilience to conquer any obstacle and execute any mission again and again. People are our most treasured assets.

Conclusion

I was asked during a recent talk what two things that my life in medicine and the military taught me:

1. Service—Military

   The military emphasized and heightened my understanding and the critical importance of leadership.

2. Medicine—Humanity

   Practicing medicine enhanced my discernment that the love of humanity is critical to the success of caring for another.

This is truly the lesson of leadership and a practical guide to living. Most of all, it is an affirmation that we are not placed in this world as isolated, self-sufficient beings. The English poet, scholar, and solider John Donne [10] had it right: we must always strive to make a difference in service to others. We can only do this if we first serve ourselves. Only then can we realize that God's overarching plan for us is based on his all-consuming love for us. This is the love we must share with others in truth, in spirit, and finally, in deed.

While this chapter is less of a "how-to" guide on becoming a flag officer, the focus is on the foundational and key characteristics of what it truly means to lead others effectively.

You must build and secure your foundations and place them upon sturdy platforms. To be successful, you must also take charge of yourself and become the pilot of your vision and course.

I think that William Ernest Henley's poem *Invictus* expresses how we should meet the triumphs and accomplishments, and the failures and disasters in our lives. Henley charges us in an affirmative way to understand that the choices we make determine our life's goals. Remember, we make the choices, and thereby set the directions of our lives.

INVICTUS

Out of the night that covers me
Black as the Pit from pole to pole
I thank whatever gods may be
For my unconquerable soul.

In the fell clutch of circumstance
I have not winced nor cried aloud.
Under the bludgeonings of chance
My head is bloody, but unbowed.

Beyond this place of wrath and tears
Looms but the Horror of the shade,
And yet the menace of the years
Finds and shall find me unafraid

It matters not how strait the gate,
How charged with punishments the scroll,
I AM THE MASTER OF MY FATE,
I AM THE CAPTAIN OF MY SOUL.
—William Ernest Henley [11]

VADM Robinson Recommended Book List

Donne J. The major works: including songs and sonnets and sermons. Oxford University Press; 2009.

Edelman MW. Lanterns: a memoir of mentors. Beacon Press; 1999.

Gates HL. Speaking of race, speaking of sex: hate speech, civil rights, and civil liberties. New York University Press; 1994.

Gates HL. The trials of Phillis Wheatley: America's first black poet and her encounters with the founding fathers. Basic Civitas Books; 2003.

Gates HL. Stony the road: reconstruction, white supremacy, and the rise of Jim Crow. Penguin Press; 2019.

Greenleaf R. The servant as leader. The Greenleaf Center for Servant Leadership; 2012.

Iarocci J. Servant leader in the workplace. 2023.

Robin M, Sendjaya S. Servant leadership: a systematic review and call for future research. Leadersh Q. 2019;30(1).

Spears LC. Character and servant leadership: ten characteristics of effective, caring leaders. J Virtues Leadersh. 2010;1(1):25–30.

Thurman H. Strange freedom. Beacon Press; 1998.

References

1. Anderson AR. Good leaders are invaluable to a company. Bad leaders will destroy it. 2013. Available from: www.forbes.com/site/amyanderson/2013/01/14/good-leaders-are-invaluable-to-a-company-bad-leaders-will-destroy-it/
2. Thurman H. Strange freedom. Beacon Press; 1998.
3. Truth-Teller. In: Cambridge advanced learner's dictionary & thesaurus. Available from: https://dictionary.cambridge.org

4. Greenleaf R. The servant as leader. The Greenleaf Center for Servant Leadership; 2012.
5. Altruism. In: Oxford English dictionary. 2023. Available from: https://www.oed.com
6. Spears LC. Character and servant leadership: ten characteristics of effective, caring leaders. J Virtues Leadersh. 2010;1(1):25–30.
7. Iarocci J. Servant leader in the workplace. 2023.
8. Robin M, Sendjaya S. Servant leadership: a systematic review and call for future research. Leadersh Q. 2019;30(1):111.
9. Edelman MW. Lanterns: a memoir of mentors. Beacon Press; 1999.
10. Donne J. The major works: including songs and sonnets and sermons. Oxford University Press; 2009.
11. Henley WE. Invictus. A book of verses. New York: Scribner; 1893.

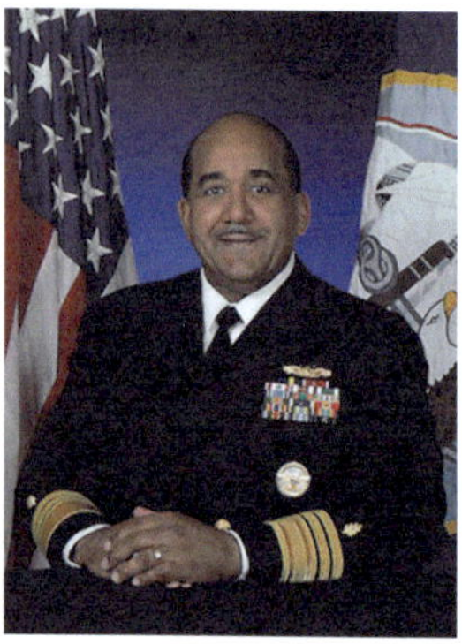

Adam M. Robinson Jr., MD, MBA, FACS, FASCRS, CPE, Vice Admiral (Retired), MC, 36th Surgeon General U.S. Navy is a native of Louisville, Kentucky. He entered the naval service in 1977 and holds a Doctor of Medicine from the Indiana University School of Medicine, Indianapolis, through the Armed Forces Health Professions Scholarship Program. Following completion of his surgical internship at Southern Illinois University School of Medicine, Springfield, he was commissioned.

Robinson's first assignment was as a general medical officer, Branch Medical Clinic, Fort Allen, Puerto Rico, before reporting to the National Naval Medical Center, Bethesda, Maryland, in 1978 to complete a residency in general surgery. His subsequent duty assignments included staff surgeon, US Naval Hospital, Yokosuka, Japan, and ship's surgeon, USS *Midway* (CV 41).

After completing a fellowship in colon and rectal surgery at Carle Foundation Hospital, University of Illinois School of Medicine Affiliated, Campaign-Urbana (1984–85), Robinson reported to the National Naval Medical Center, Bethesda, as the head of the Colon and Rectal Surgery Division. While there, he was called to temporary duty in 1987 as ship's surgeon in USS *John F. Kennedy* (CV 67) and in 1988 as ship's surgeon in USS *Coral Sea* (CV 43).

Robinson reported to Naval Medical Center Portsmouth, Virginia, in 1990 as the head of the General Surgery Department and Director of the General Surgery Residency Program.

He was appointed acting medical director for the facility in 1994. While at Naval Medical Center Portsmouth, Robinson earned a master's degree in Business Administration from the University of South Florida. In 1995, Robinson reported to commander, Naval Surface Force, US Atlantic Fleet, as the force medical officer, serving in that capacity for 2 years. Following that assignment, he reported to Naval Hospital Jacksonville in 1997 as the executive officer. In January 1999, as Fleet Hospital Jacksonville commanding officer, Robinson commanded a detachment of the fleet hospital as a medical contingent to Joint Task Force Haiti (Operation New Horizon/Uphold Democracy).

In August 1999, Robinson reported to the Bureau of Medicine and Surgery (BUMED) as the director of Readiness and was selected as the principal director of Clinical and Program Policy in the Office of the Assistant Secretary of Defense for Health Affairs in September 2000, where he also served as the acting deputy assistant secretary of Defense for Health Affairs, Clinical and Program Policy. Robinson was assigned as commanding officer of US Naval Hospital Yokosuka from September 2001 to January 2004, after which he received assignment back to BUMED as deputy chief of BUMED for Medical Support Operations with additional duty as acting chief of the Medical Corps. In July 2004, Robinson reported as commander, National Naval Medical Center, Bethesda,

MD. He assumed the duties as commander, Navy Medicine National Capital Area Region in October 2005. Finally, he served as the 36th surgeon general of the Navy and chief of the Navy's Bureau of Medicine and Surgery.

As the Surgeon General, Dr. Robinson served as the principle Tricare Health Plan representative for active duty Sailors and Marines, their families, and Navy and Marine Corps retirees and their families, numbering over 2.5 million people. Dr. Robinson led a team of 63,000 Navy Medicine personnel in over 220 health care facilities located worldwide with an annual budget of $3.5 billion. This included three tertiary care medical centers located in geographically diverse parts of the United States that provided the single largest source of residency-trained health care providers for the Navy medical department.

Upon retiring, Robinson was appointed as the Chief of Staff of the Veterans Affairs Baltimore Health Care System in 2014. He was then appointed Executive Director of the Veterans Affairs Baltimore Health Care System in 2015. He also served as the acting Executive Director of the Washington DC VA Medical Center in 2018. Robinson was appointed Director of the VA Pacific Islands Health Care System in 2020.

Robinson's personal decorations include the Distinguished Service Medal (two awards), Legion of Merit (two awards), Defense Meritorious Service Medal (two awards), Meritorious Service Medal (three awards), Navy Commendation Medal, Joint Service Achievement Medal, Navy Achievement Medal, and various service and campaign awards.

Preparing for Deployment 23

Jason S. Radowsky and Zachary W. Brown

Introduction

Preparing for your first deployment can be a daunting prospect. However, as a wise high school biology teacher I was fond of said: Proper Prior Planning Prevents Poor Performance! By proceeding in an organized fashion using the suggestions in this chapter as a guideline, you can embark on your deployment with confidence that you have addressed both professional and personal requirements, with only the myriad variables of an operational environment lying in wait.

J. S. Radowsky (✉)
Department of Surgery, Walter Reed National Military Medical Center, Bethesda, MD, USA

Department of Surgery, Uniformed Services University of the Health Sciences, Bethesda, MD, USA
e-mail: Jason.s.radowsky.mil@health.mil

Z. W. Brown
Department of Surgery, Naval Medical Center, Portsmouth, VA, USA

A. T. Schlussel et al. (eds.), *The SAGES Manual for Navigating a Successful Military Surgical Career*,
https://doi.org/10.1007/978-3-031-88490-0_23

When to Deploy: Timing (Can Be) Everything

Preparation for deployment should begin LONG before you are actually selected to go. You may even consider volunteering for a specific cycle, which has numerous, tremendous benefits, not least of which is life-planning. One all-too-frequent gripe about deployments is when "short-fuse" notice is given. Though last-minute changes to the personnel of a deploying team are always possible, you can largely avoid being the selected replacement if you are already slated to deploy for another mission. By employing this strategy, you will not only earn bonus points with your detailer, but you may be able to select a deployment that aligns with a pre-existing professional schedule (such as board exams or the start date of a fellowship) or improves your ability to plan a special event like a wedding or the birth of a child.

However, even if you are selected for a deployment which overlaps an important date, do not despair! Communicate with your consultant team, specialty leader, and/or the commander of your medical platform to determine if you can shift your deployment timeline slightly to accommodate a special need. Be extremely judicious in the nature of your request and how it is presented—aggressive, entitled demands are considered far less favorable than humble entreaties. Also, remember that there are many reasons why your request may be denied, and almost none of them has to do with you as an individual, so do not take a refusal personally.

Finally, deployments are also an excellent opportunity to set yourself apart from your peers at promotion boards. A recent Fitness Report (FITREP)/Officer Evaluation Report (OER) with meaty impact statements achieved in a combat environment and an accompanying impact award make a significant impression on board members and can be pivotal for selection in competitive cycles. Consider this, especially if you are a year or two from falling in your promotion zone for the first look at your next rank.

Communication: Share the News!

Remember the adages "Don't be the senior man with a secret" or "Bad news doesn't get better with time?" Both are quite applicable when you receive notice that you'll be deploying. For your military family, make sure that you immediately notify your chain of command, both at the organizational (hospital) and local (surgery department) levels. Do NOT assume that they have been made aware! Your hospital leadership will be responsible for funding much of your training, so bringing them into the loop helps with their financial planning. Your surgery department will also need to start planning for your departure by adjusting both your schedule and that of your colleagues so the call and caseloads can be redistributed and you have the necessary time to attend mandatory pre-deployment training. You will also need to find people to cover your collateral duties, including committee assignments, leadership positions, and academic requirements such as medical education or research. The hospital Institutional Review Board (IRB) will require any deploying Principal Investigators (PIs) to appoint a new PI for the duration of their absence; you can still be an Assistant Investigator (AI) without issues. If you are a rater or senior rater for fitness reports, you will likely have to find a replacement, as deployments of more than 90 days' duration require such a change. This situation may necessitate writing OERs/FITREPs before you deploy on personnel for whom you are the senior rater. Additionally, at least for the Army, you will require an OER to be completed before deployment if your last one was done more than 90 days in the past.

Your family may also be interested in learning about your upcoming international field trip! This conversation can actually be quite complicated depending on your family situation; hopefully, it is not the first time the topic has been brought up. Some variables which may require special attention include the number of people for whom you are responsible and their health. Do you care for a family member with significant health issues or a child with special needs? If so, make arrangements for that care to continue in your absence. For Exceptional Family Member Program (EFMP) planning, engage with the healthcare team to let them know that making appointments might be more difficult for a time and that there will be added stressors for the duration of the deployment. Do you have a spouse who is pregnant and scheduled to deliver while you are away? If so, make sure preparations for the addition to your family are complete prior to your departure. Keep it fun and positive! Many of these activities can help you and your partner bond over your future child, a connection that will pay dividends while you're gone. Do you live far from family, or maybe you recently moved and haven't yet established close friends in the area? If so, you need to develop a plan for how your family will be supported while you are gone. Some people choose to temporarily relocate to be closer to their family or friends while a partner is deployed (or have those family/friends come to them). If that isn't an option, consider helping connect your partner with other deployed servicemembers' families. There is definitely some truth to "misery loves company," and there is no replacement for having someone to be a helping hand, not just in the case of emergencies but for day-to-day assistance who is sharing a similar experience. Finally, though commands generally assign an ombudsman to share deployment information with families, it may be wise to consider this as a backup rather than a primary means of providing updates. Construct a plan for communication with your family while deployed. Depending on the location and security levels, your phone and email access may not be continuous. Sharing that possibility with your family helps them to accept those periods of unplanned communication blackouts as part of the experience rather than a reason to panic.

Legal and Financial: Failing to Plan Is Planning to Fail

In order for your family's life to run smoothly while you are away, you need to help provide them with the tools to complete any tasks that you normally manage. This can be accomplished with Powers of Attorney (POA), which your legal department can assist you with completing. In the past, a broad, durable POA was an option. However, the current practice is establishing more limited POAs for specific authorities. For example, you may draft a POA giving a family member authority to conduct a financial transaction on your behalf, such as buying a car or selling a house. It may seem tedious to have to create multiple POAs but remember that the current system exists to both help AND protect you. It is also worth mentioning that some financial institutions will not honor a POA, and you should consider reaching out to your bank, credit card companies, and other such entities to ask them what their policies are and what documentation they require for someone else to conduct business on your behalf.

Thinking about worst-case scenarios isn't pleasant, but it is a necessary task. Schedule time with your family to explicitly discuss your wishes in the event of injury or death. Do not put them in the position of having to guess or extrapolate what you want, especially during the already stressful period after receiving unexpected bad news. This conversation, though important, does not replace the legal codification of those plans. Your legal department can help you complete both a Will and a Medical POA.

Another legal consideration involves contracts. Depending on the length of your deployment, you may be able to use your orders to break financial contracts such as rental housing or a vehicle lease. This can be particularly financially helpful if you are single, a geographic bachelor, or otherwise live alone. For that same group of individuals, you may need to enlist the help of others to take care of specific responsibilities like caring for a pet or storing personal property. If you set up an arrangement like this, consider formalizing the agreement with a contract, even if no money is being exchanged. A contract helps to establish the terms for both parties so expectations are clear, and there is a path to recourse in the case of a poor outcome. It's great to have a friend agree to watch your car for free, but it's frustrating to return to a vehicle with a dead battery and flat tires because you didn't specify that they needed to start the car every so often and drive it around the block!

Your military pay will likely increase while you are deployed. How much depends on myriad factors, which will be discussed shortly, but it can be significant. There is a temptation on deployment, especially when income increases, to feel justified in spending more. However, deployments are also a potentially wonderful time to make the most of your financial gains, whether it is paying down past debts or investing for your future. Which of these options (or both!) is right for you can only be determined if you plan ahead, which starts with getting a rough idea of how large your financial windfall will be.

If you are deployed in a combat zone, some of your income may be tax free. This can be important for the timing of certain bonuses, such as Retention Bonuses, as a portion of them may also become tax-free. There are some bonuses you will earn just by virtue of being deployed, such as Family Separation Pay if you and your dependents reside at the same address. You may also receive additional bonuses, such as Hostile Fire or Imminent Danger, if your location rates them. Your command should be able to inform you which bonuses you will receive, the amount of those bonuses, and whether you are expected to be deployed in a tax-exempt zone (and for how long). This should help you calculate a ballpark monthly deployment income.

With that approximate value in mind, now you can talk with your family, financial planner, and accountant to develop a plan. Consider long-term strategies you may not have used in the past, such as the Thrift Savings Plan (which cannot be recommend enough, especially the Roth TSP). There may also be deployment-specific investment opportunities, such as the Savings Deposit Program (10% interest on $10k maximum), which are worth investigating. Funds deposited in TSP while deployed are tax-exempt, and the overall amount that can be placed in the fund also increases. If your deployment will overlap tax season, consider requesting an extension early to eliminate the stress of trying to compile your documents and file remotely. Finally, remember that Murphy's Law is alive and well globally, and electronic communication is guaranteed to fail at the most inconvenient times! With that in mind, schedule recurring financial transactions through automatic direct deposits and save your credit score from accidentally missed payments.

Prior to deployment, discuss with your unit or the individual you are replacing what fees might be encountered on your upcoming adventure. Some locations do not have provided meals, which will require cash purchases on your part, either as a weekly lump sum or for each meal. Wardroom or MWR fees may also be encountered. Internet is also sometimes a cash purchase rather than something that can be done through a credit card. Added up, this can sometimes result in thousands of dollars of cash that you need to take with you for a 6-month deployment. Locations requiring this much outlay by you generally come with high per-diems, so be sure to acquire documentation of your presence as well as unavailable amenities, which will help with the submission to finance on your return. ATMs are sometimes available at your destination, but they often run out of cash. Fees can be generally reimbursed on your return through DTS.

Professional Training: The Medical

Preparing for the medical aspect of your deployment will arguably be your most important and time-consuming set of requirements. The good news is that most of the material you will cover will be just a review of things you learned and practiced during surgery residency. So grab a copy of "Top Knife" and start re-honing your trauma skill sets!

There are many acronym courses that you already maintain as a surgeon: Basic Life Support (BLS), Advanced Cardiac Life Support (ACLS), and Advanced Trauma Life Support (ATLS) are a few notable examples. It is worth noting that the expiration date of these certifications must be valid through the end date of your deployment. These three can generally be found at military hospitals without the need for specialized funding applications.

However, military surgeons are required to take additional courses before heading downrange. These requirements include the military version of Advanced Surgical Skills for Exposure in Trauma, also known as ASSET+, for general surgeons and Combat Orthopedic Trauma Surgery, or COTS+, for orthopedic surgeons. The ASSET+ course uses human cadavers for training and includes not only instruction on REBOA (the focus of the Basic Endovascular Skills for Trauma, or BEST, course) but also modules for ENT, orthopedic, and neurosurgical trauma, as well as obstetric emergencies. ASSET+ and COTS+ are offered several times yearly at Walter Reed, Naval Medical Center Portsmouth, and Brooke Army Medical Center. The current requirement is that military surgeons attend these courses every three years; however, depending on your comfortability with managing trauma, you may want to take the course every two years for skill sustainment.

You may also want to consider attending the Advanced Trauma Operative Management (ATOM) course, which teaches operative trauma techniques on a live porcine model, or Fundamentals of Critical Care Support (FCCS), which may be beneficial depending on mission requirements.

Prior to deployment, you may be tasked to go to a training platform with the unit to which you will be assigned. This is especially true for those who will be with the unit at the beginning of their tour. There are multiple such trauma training centers and will be specific to your service branch. For the Army, this is typically at Ryder Trauma Center at Jackson Memorial Hospital in Miami, where the Army Trauma Training Center (ATTC) is co-located. Another location is Joint Base San Antonio, where the Strategic Trauma Readiness Center (STaRC) has a course with similar objectives. For the Navy, this is typically at LA Trauma in Los Angeles, where the Navy Trauma Training Center (NTTC) is co-located. For the Air Force, this is typically at the R Adams Cowley Shock Trauma Center in Baltimore, one of the C-STARS locations. This program is usually 2 weeks in duration and incorporates simulated trauma lanes for the unit as well as didactics and courses such as ASSET+. Your team will also take call at the trauma center under supervision of their trauma staff. Of note, this course should be entered into your service record as it reflects the additional trauma training you have completed.

Finally, though this is not a formal requirement, it would be wise to acquire the Clinical Practice Guidelines (CPGs) published by the military's Joint Trauma System, which can be found at www.DeployedMedicine.com. These well-researched and frequently updated instructions were written by and for deployed physicians. Not only are they a treasure trove of information presented in a high-yield format, they also represent the benchmark of patient care expectations against which you will be evaluated. While even the authors recognize that the CPGs are not meant to replace your clinical judgment, you should be prepared to defend deviations from the standards after every patient encounter. Patients will be discussed at weekly multidisciplinary conferences in which you will be expected to participate. Downloading them prior to deployment, rather than relying on internet connections, which might be temperamental, is recommended.

Professional Training: The Military

As you are not only a physician but also an officer, your respective service branch will have some military-specific training to accomplish. Some of this will be online training similar in structure, format, and production quality as you complete annually for your General Medical Training requirements. Some of it will be classroom-based training, such as learning how to communicate in an operational environment via radio. Some of it will be field training, such as how to survive and escape a convoy vehicle rollover. You will likely have to complete weapons training on both pistol and rifle and possibly additional weapons systems. As the training requirements for service branches may not be the same, and some training elements will be specific to the environment into which you are deploying, a universal list of what to expect is not possible, and the rule of "Semper Gumby" applies.

There are two ways to approach this training: positive or negative. As much of this training will not be done as an individual but rather as part of the team with which you will deploy, be cognizant of the effect of which path you choose. As a surgeon, you will likely be one of the more senior members of the team. Your enlisted and the other officers will take their cues from your behavior, which can set the tone for the entire deployment. The training will be completed whether you like it or not, whether you believe it is necessary or not, and regardless of the amount of complaining you do along the way. However, your standing among the team as a trusted leader may be damaged if you choose to act as an entitled diva rather than an equal participant.

Team Turnover

Just as you must communicate with your local command, family, and friends about your upcoming deployment, it is equally important to reach out to the surgeon whom you will be replacing. S/he will have an ENORMOUS amount of useful information that can help shape your expectations across the personal and professional spectrum. Details concerning such mundane subjects as laundry and shower facilities can make significant differences in how you pack for your deployment. Inquire about housing and rooming arrangements, gym facilities, dining (or lack thereof), MWR presence, and internet availability. If there is no wi-fi, ask what their team did for communication and whether they recommend bringing specific hardware or if it is better to acquire it when you arrive, either from them or a local vendor. Discuss uniform requirements. While the dress code is usually dictated by the base commander, individual units do have some leeway in the uniform posture. Some deployments always require uniforms, including at the gym. For others, especially in support of Special Forces, civilian attire is appropriate. Finally, ask specifically about the local and regional command structure to identify who has Administrative, Operational, and Tactical Control (ADCON, OPCON, and TACON) of your team, as those three organizational functions will dictate who is responsible for nearly every aspect of your deployment.

As the medical mission is the primary focus, make sure to thoroughly understand the situation into which you will settle. For your local medical facility, this should include discussions of equipment, availability of blood and blood products, sterilization equipment, supply chain, and the quality of your provided translator(s). In particular, identify items you will need to bring with you that they have been unable to obtain through their supply chain. It is also essential to identify roles and collateral duties on the team you are replacing so you can identify who among your people will be most appropriate in those jobs and to facilitate turnover between the outgoing and incoming personnel. Finally, learn about the presence and capabilities of other medical assets (United States, Coalition, and civilian) in the region and how your team functions in the system. However, you may wish to defer review of specific MEDEVAC/CASEVAC platforms and procedures until you arrive.

After talking with the surgeon, contact the regional medical commander. Discuss your anticipated role and the mission. Establishing these parameters prior to deployment can avert issues with leadership later. Their expectations of uniforms, educational activities, work-day tempo, and lines of communication should be delineated. Your commander may be remote from your location and may delegate some command authority to you. Others desire a more formal structure running through their executive officer. The regional medical commander has significant, if not complete, control over much of your mission; signs your Fitness Reports and (most) deployment awards, and keeps you informed and functioning throughout the deployment. Make a good first impression!

Packing

After you have squared away your required gear list (ALWAYS talk to an experienced senior enlisted or officer with deployment experience before autonomously deciding not to pack something you were issued but you think you won't need), make sure you make room for some essential items to include: two pairs of gym/running shoes, extra batteries for whatever electronics you are bringing, three combination locks, foreign power adaptors, and a travel pillow. Though not mandatory, an inexpensive laptop with a CAC reader and external hard drive with movies and books will provide good entertainment options while consuming minimal additional space.

For any comfort items you want beyond these basics, consider shipping directly to your deployment site in a Tuff Box (or something similar) or waiting until you arrive to assess your needs. As discussed above, the team you are replacing will have provided you with what sorts of amenities are available at your deployment site. They will also likely be willing to give you or sell at a very reasonable price some of their comfort items, including internet access devices that may be regionally specific (aka PUCKS), mattress toppers, etc. Also, life is much easier in the era of Amazon and modern mail service, and it usually does not take long (with the exception of the holiday season) to get deliveries of things that are not available at your nearest exchange.

Focusing on the necessities and keeping your packs as light as possible is important because you will be responsible for transporting your own gear wherever you go. Since your previous experience with travel likely involves pulling a wheeled suitcase into an airport over smooth ground, it is helpful to understand that this in no way resembles deployment travel. You may have to move your gear long distances over sand and uneven terrain, often in the dark and likely at least once in extreme heat. You will have to do this at each stop to and from your destination. It is possible you will have to relocate multiple times during the deployment, particularly if you are with a small Role 2 surgical team. Staying light and agile will help you get through these moves with fewer head (and back) aches. If you are deploying from a CONUS Replacement Center (CRC) try to find someone you know at that post to hold in their garage some items that you will not need for the duration of your deployment. Be sure to give them a nice gift to lighten your load.

Conclusion

You got the call: it's time to deploy! This is one of the main reasons for your existence in military medicine, and you are about to have a unique experience that will be among the most rewarding you experience in your career. Share the news with your command and family. Make appointments with your financial advisor and military legal office. Attend to your training obligations. By understanding how to prepare financially, legally, personally, and professionally, you can lessen anxiety leading up to the time you step off, optimize your and your family's ability to perform at your peak while you are gone, and set yourself up for a successful transition when you return. Now pack right, pack light, and go support the fight.

How to Avoid Pitfalls of Deployment

24

Suzanne Gillern and Erik Roedel

Introduction

Deployment is one of the most stressful but rewarding aspects of a military surgical career. While many service members with other military occupational specialties may go their entire career without the opportunity to deploy, surgeons will continue to have a high deployment tempo while our fellow military members serve abroad in high-risk environments. The goal of this chapter is to review some basic tips based on the authors experiences deploying in multiple environments with many different teams during the era of the Global War on Terror. While this chapter won't cover every possible scenario, it should give the reader some key concepts to make deployment more successful.

S. Gillern
Tripler Army Medical Center, Honolulu, HI, USA

E. Roedel (✉)
Madigan Army Medical Center, Tacoma, WA, USA

A. T. Schlussel et al. (eds.), *The SAGES Manual for Navigating a Successful Military Surgical Career*,
https://doi.org/10.1007/978-3-031-88490-0_24

Start Strong: Mindset/Perspective

It may sound overly simple or reductive, but having the right mindset is one of the most important keys to success on deployment. As surgeons, we are taught that the decisions we make have life and death consequences. In addition to making difficult decisions, we are expected to lead the clinical team in the care of some of the most complex and critically ill patients. This creates an inherent conflict in the deployed environment. As opposed to the clinical leader role surgeons are used to in the hospital, the deployed environment is often more hierarchical. Unit commanders may be equal or junior in rank to the surgeon, and most of the time, they will be less clinically experienced. It is critical to remember that you are not in the hospital environment, and maintaining a professional and humble mindset can make a huge difference in your success as a team member. The hard reality is that most of your time deployed will not be clinical.

One of the key differences between the US Military and other countries is our commitment to each individual volunteer service member. Part of that promise is that when the US sends someone into harm's way, there is a surgical team ready to care for them in their time of need. The cost of this promise is that the majority of surgeons currently deploying will not perform many, if any, trauma surgeries during their time away. This can be one of the most difficult things for a surgeon to grapple with while struggling with the hardships of deployment. When boredom and frustration begin to creep in, remember to focus on the promise. Don't forget that even if you never use your hard-earned surgical skills, your presence in theater gives our nation's finest an extra layer of reassurance that can help them perform their dangerous mission.

Don't Be Embarrassed to be Comfortable

Just because you are going to be deployed does not mean that you need to live without some comforts of home. These small things can go a long way for improving your mental health. When preparing for your deployment, key practical things to ask the surgeon you are replacing include: will you be wearing uniform or civilian clothes, can you work out in civilian clothes, will you have your own living space, and what is the bathroom/showering situation. Pack light for your travels to include only the things you will need for two to four weeks. We recommend packing the following: headlight/flashlight, swiss army knives, combination locks, just enough personal products to get you through your travels, shower shoes, work-out clothes/shoes, a few pods/drying sheets (in case you get access to laundry during travels), and your own sleeping bag and pillow (or get army issued sleeping bag). Approximately one month before you depart we recommend sending a package to your deployment destination with your personal comforts such as: mattress pad (this may seem super bougie, but no matter what type of location you are going to, you want to be able to sleep comfortably and a mattress pad is very helpful), sheets, good blanket, good pillow, comfortable civilian clothes (pending location), room freshener (your living space will likely smell awful), books to read for pleasure, text books/surgical exposure resources (ie. ASSET), and hygiene products to last the entirety of the deployment. Give your address out, mail is incredible morale booster. The sooner you give your address to friends and family the sooner you will get care packages. The key thing to remember is that you should not be embarrassed to be comfortable.

Clinically Integrate with the Team

When you arrive in theater, it is important to remember to make a good first impression with your team. One of the challenges with deployment is that you may have had limited opportunity to meet or work with your team prior to your arrival. This can be extra challenging because there is no way to know when your surgical skills will be needed, and often you will be the sole general surgeon in your team. As you are preparing to integrate with your team it is also important to understand how your rotation fits in with the unit's overall deployment. Because some services acknowledge that surgery is a highly perishable skill; many deployments that are four months or longer may split the deployment into two surgeon rotations. Keep this in mind as you are preparing to meet your team. Covering the front half of the unit's deployment gives you the benefit of establishing practices and setting a good example from the start. This rotation may also give you the opportunity to participate in the unit's pre-deployment training and validation. While traveling for the extra pre-deployment training can add a significant burden in time away from your surgical practice and your family, it can also be vital for assessing your team's clinical experience in a low consequence environment.

If you are covering the back half or a later portion of the deployment this can bring its own set of challenges. In this circumstance, you cannot control what precedent the surgeon before you set whether it be positive, negative, or just different from your style. Also, remember to stay humble and know that other team members may have a significantly longer deployment than you. It is human nature that the stress of deployment takes its toll over time. Burnout will often set in at the three-to-four-month mark just as you are arriving. Don't take this personally. Use your arrival as an opportunity to reinvigorate the team and bring positive energy to a group that may be struggling personally with the distance from loved ones. It is also critical to remain humble in this environment and acknowledge that surgery is an art and not always black and white. The team may have developed great pride in their protocols or practice patterns prior to your arrival. If your first interactions are too critical or it is perceived that you are trying to discredit the prior surgeon, you are likely setting yourself up for a tough deployment.

Regardless of whether you are covering the front or back half of a deployment, it is critical to learn how to work as a team clinically. The lesson of humility applies in both scenarios. Even if you arrive in theater with your team, you will likely be participating in a relief-in-place (RIP). This is again where it is important to listen more than speaking. Allow the outgoing team (or your existing team if you are covering the second half) to share their lessons and experiences without your immediate injection of, "good ideas." Unless you see something that is truly unsafe, take a breath, and work toward building the relationship first, then work to refine processes. If there is not already a scheduled patient drill, exercise, or MASCAL politely request one. Remember your attitude shouldn't be that the team is proving themselves to you, you are requesting to learn from them, and see how you can integrate with them. Also remember that in this environment clinical competency and knowledge is currency. It is highly likely your team may never see you perform surgery. That is why teaching classes and participating enthusiastically in training is how you develop your credibility. If you see an area for improvement, take the time to read, prepare, and offer to teach on the subject. Give each team member an opportunity to shine. Ask questions about their area of responsibility, ask for them to teach to their expertise.

Part of integrating with your team clinically is understanding the limitations of your equipment and supplies. One of the hardest things for many military surgeons on deployment is adapting to low resource or austere medicine. It can be an extremely difficult mental transition to go from training in an academic medical center with a focus on the highest quality of care for each patient with every resource available; to performing austere damage control surgery and resuscitation typically without even basic diagnostic tools. That is why it is essential that as soon as you arrive in theater you begin to get briefed on what equipment, supplies, blood products, and expertise is in your group. When working in small teams such as a role two in a forward location, you will not have the support team you are used to having in the hospital. You won't have a respiratory therapist to run the vent, an extra nurse to set up the pump, and your scrub tech is also your sterile processor, your mechanic, and maybe even your electrician at the same time. That is why it is vital for you to learn your equipment and know the basics of how to operate and troubleshoot it when needed. One way to be methodical regarding review of your supplies is to bring some of the more critical surgery preference cards from your home institution (ex-lap, bowel resection, vascular bypass) and then review the supplies on hand and then think through how you could adapt for what is missing. You would be surprised with the random collection of sterile supplies that are in a mature theater. You will also be surprised by how much is expired, damaged, or missing. Thinking about these things prior to a sick trauma patient showing up in your triage area can be lifesaving.

As you are getting to know your team and setup, it is also critical to learn about the trauma system you are a part of. While it is easy to feel isolated, especially when you are the sole surgeon of your specialty in your location, you are not alone. You will be part of a large trauma and medical evacuation system. Often, there is a wealth of different sub-specialists throughout the theater. I would strongly recommend reaching out to the Theater Trauma Medical Director (TMD) when you arrive. The Theater TMD has situational awareness of all the surgical capabilities in your system and can offer advice, mentorship, and if they can't answer your specific question, then they will connect you with someone who can.

Finally, regarding integration, your relationship with your unit command and the medical command in theater can make or break your experience. Because of the long training pipeline to become a surgeon, it is not uncommon for the surgeon on the team to be of the same or higher rank than the commander. Most likely, you are also the most clinically experienced and knowledgeable team member when it comes to managing traumatic injuries. However, the commander has a burden of administrative responsibilities that as a surgeon you may never experience. The operational environment is also very different than the hospital. To keep it simple, when the command looks good, you look good. When the command looks bad, you look bad. Choose your battles, be professional, and try to focus on quality patient care. Try not to apply your surgeon brain to "fix" every non-clinical problem and burn all your capital.

Keep Yourself and Your Team Ready

As you develop your relationship with your team, remember every deployment is different and will have different operational tempos. It can be very frustrating if you are not busy clinically and operatively. Even if not clinically busy, it is important to always be ready. As the surgeon, you are the clinical team leader, and it is up to you to make sure your team is ready for the next casualty. Establish a weekly training/simulation schedule. In addition, have a lecture schedule and keep the whole team engaged. Go through the clinical practice guidelines as a team and have a plan on how your team will implement them. Do your best to make it fun, it is very easy for the team to become complacent, especially if they are not busy, but this can be very dangerous. It is also very important to integrate with pre-hospital and base/FOB resources. Offer to give lectures/training to other medics on the base. Perform mass casualty exercises so the whole base is prepared. Often you will have local nationals on base with you. Integrate them in your training. Not only will this provide professional fulfillment, it will help keep your team well-prepared.

Another way to keep the team engaged is to capitalize on every patient care experience. While you may be surprised at how little trauma you see, you will often be surprised by the other strange and complex non-battle injury pathology that makes it into theater. Indulge your own academic curiosity and take time to read about the pathology in each patient care experience and use it as a prompt for your own education. Then expand this to the rest of your team. Nothing helps people retain information better than a patient experience where there is a human face to associate with the knowledge. If your operational tempo allows, try to coordinate your team's education calendar to participate in the Joint Trauma System conferences. This is another area your Theater TMD can help coordinate and prepare you for if you will be presenting patients.

Avoid Boredom

The biggest pitfall of deployment is boredom. Depending on the operational tempo at your location, you may be doing little to no surgery. This can lead to significant frustration. The best way to avoid this frustration is to avoid boredom. The key is to establish a routine. Prior to leaving on your deployment make a list of personal/professional goals you wish to achieve on deployment. Goals can include personal health, clinical and academic development, and Military professional development.

Personal Health

One of the biggest advantages of deployment is the ability to routinely work out. Set personal fitness goals for your deployment. This may include training for a race, starting a weight lifting routine, or achieving a weight loss goal, to name a few. Set the goals early in your deployment and hold yourself accountable.

Also, utilize this time on deployment to catch up on sleep. Get in habit of getting 8 h of sleep/day and build in a nap time. Sleep debt is a real thing, and this is a wonderful time to start to make up for all of the sleep debt that goes along with surgical residency and a career as a General Surgeon.

Deployment provides a unique opportunity to dedicate time and engage in a new hobby or work on a new skill. This is great for your mental well-being and a way to feel fulfilled even if not surgically busy. Some examples include learning a new language, learning a new musical instrument, and/or reading more books for pure pleasure.

Clinical and Academic Development

Deployment is also very useful to have dedicated time to enhance your clinical knowledge and work on your academic career. Before deployment, choose a list of articles you would like to read while away to help keep you engaged with your specialty and remain current. Perhaps set a goal of certain chapters of a text book that you would like to read and review. Consider purchasing SESAP prior to your departure and make it your goal to complete the entire program while you are away. SESAP, which offers over 150 Category 1 CME, and other similar professional question banks are a great way to both stay current and obtain all of the CME needed for hospital and board certification CME requirements. It also means one less thing for you to worry about when you are home and focusing on your clinical practice and loved ones.

If you are interested in an academic career, deployment serves as a great time to write and edit manuscripts. Another good use of one's time is to prepare lectures. These lectures can be used while deployed but also it is helpful to build a library of lectures on topics that interest you that can be used in the future for medical students, residents or colleagues when you return. This again is a good way to use your time to prevent you from stressing about these tasks when you have other pressing matters at home.

Military Professional Development

Another way to make your deployment productive is to work on Military Leadership training. For example, in the Army, the first portion of Captains Career Course is online and deployment is a great time to get this done. In addition, Distance ILE is offered, and deployment is an ideal time to get through the majority of this course. The key for both of these courses is to start working on your enrollment process 3 months prior to your deployment so that you are ready to start the coursework as soon as your deployment begins. ILE has three different sections, and to move on to each section is limited by the course director's grading. Nevertheless, it is very possible to get through at least two of the three sections in a 3 or 4 ½ month deployment. There are also options to enroll in the Naval Command and Staff Program & JPME Phase I (https://usnwc.edu/college-of-distance-education/Online-Program/JPME-Phase-I) and the Air Command and Staff College (IDE) Distance Learning Program (https://www.airuniversity.af.edu/GCPME/ACSC/), based on your service branch and rank.

Support Your Loved Ones

There is no perfect way to prepare for leaving your spouse, children, and/or other loved ones. It is important that you go into your deployment understanding the following three things:

1. It will be hard on you—missing milestones/memories
2. It will be hard on your partner—carrying the burden of a household or sole childcare
3. It will be hard on children—differences depending on age (and often harder on you)

There is not a perfect recipe to overcome these hardships. These are some tips that have worked for other physicians in your position. Try to facetime every day at a consistent time as operational tempo allows. This works better for older kids, but know that attempting to facetime young children, it will be hard to keep their attention. Consider calling it a "work trip" reinforcing to your children that it is temporary. Also, remind them that communication can be unpredictable and that they shouldn't worry if you miss a call or if your call drops out. If possible, try to have your family travel to visit extended family or arrange for lots of visitors to your family. This allows your children to get additional love and support and can provide emotional and physical assistance to your partner. A fun idea is to set up a jar of Hershey kisses with the number of days of deployment. Each day, your child gets one kiss (representing a kiss from you) and is a way to count down the days until your return. In order to help out your spouse, there you can consider setting up a weekly DoorDash to allow at least one night a week without meal prep.

When dealing with your family, understand they will have bad days and frustrations with you being gone. Specifically, remember that often, your spouse or loved one just wants someone to listen to their challenges, not to solve them. Avoid being "the good idea fairy" for problems you can't fix. Also, be graceful with yourself. You will have bad days. Let yourself be homesick. The important thing is not to allow yourself to stay in a funk for too long. Try not to use your limited time communicating at home only to address conflicts or vent your frustrations. Try to find fun things to discuss, plan trips, and talk about the things you miss doing and what you are excited to do with your family and friends when you return.

Finally, set realistic expectations for your loved ones. Deployment is unpredictable. Traveling in and out of the theater is complex, with many moving pieces that can make your return unpredictable. To be safe, try not to plan anything that cannot be canceled or postponed for 3–4 weeks after your projected return date. The final month of deployment is often the hardest mentally, and there is nothing more demoralizing than getting extended another week or two when you took your departure dates as gospel. Even worse than dealing with your disappointment, is breaking that bad news to your family. It is safe to generally add at least two weeks of "fudge factor" to the duration of your deployment when setting expectations. Coming home earlier than expected is always a win; coming home later than expected is always a loss. If you do have major events that can't be moved, be open and transparent with your leadership. This is where being a good team member from the beginning will pay dividends. Remember, other members of your team often will deploy longer than you and don't understand the challenges of your training, practice at home, and the sacrifices your loved one has made for you to become a deployable surgeon.

Last But Not Least: Have Fun

As crazy as it may sound, use this time to have fun. Stay engaged with your team. Avoid spending all of your time alone. Alone time is definitely good, but try to eat your meals together and participate in group activities. It will help with team cohesiveness, which is very important for work purposes, but will also help the time go faster. Try to establish a game night or a day where you play a group sport such as volleyball, cornhole, or ping pong, pending what is available to you at your location. Interact with non-medical personnel on the base. This is a unique time to integrate with all different types of people with different life experiences and skill sets. In addition, there is an opportunity to work with local nationals, get to know them, and understand their culture. All of these things will help time pass and make the deployment a fulfilling experience.

Conclusion

The most important thing to do during deployment is to maintain a positive attitude. This is definitely hard at times, but it will keep you in a much better head space and will have a positive effect on those around you. Appreciate the unique opportunity you are in and the privilege of being trusted in your position. Remember the promise.

In summary, the key tips to avoiding the pitfalls of deployment are:

- Positive attitude
- Surgery is the easy part
- Have an open mind
- Teach
- Have a set of personal goals
- Be social and try to have fun

The Challenges of Redeploying

25

Jeremy W. Cannon, Margaret M. Morgan, and Robert M. Rush

Introduction

The deployment/redeployment cycle represents a hallmark of every military surgeon's career. Although this process is nearly universal, it can prove exceedingly stressful, particularly during a surgeon's first deployment. There are so many unknowns as you transition from "business as usual" at your home station civilian or military hospital to a foreign area, perform your mission, and then transition home again. In many cases, young surgeons have

J. W. Cannon (✉)
Division of Traumatology, Surgical Critical Care and Emergency Surgery, Department of Surgery, Perelman School of Medicine at the University of Pennsylvania, Philadelphia, PA, USA

Department of Surgery, F. Edward Hébert School of Medicine at the Uniformed Services University, Bethesda, MD, USA
e-mail: jeremy.cannon@pennmedicine.upenn.edu

M. M. Morgan
Division of Trauma and Acute Care Surgery, UCHealth Memorial Hospital Central, Colorado Springs, CO, USA

R. M. Rush
Trauma and Acute Care Surgery Service, PeaceHealth St Joseph's Medical Center, Bellingham, WA, USA

Division of Healthcare Simulation Science, Department of Surgery, UW Medicine, Seattle, WA, USA

A. T. Schlussel et al. (eds.), *The SAGES Manual for Navigating a Successful Military Surgical Career*,
https://doi.org/10.1007/978-3-031-88490-0_25

just started their home station "in-garrison" practice just prior to deploying and may be uncertain of the usual timelines one should expect for winding down this practice pre-deployment and then ramping back up post-deployment. In addition, surgeons may feel inhibited in asking for support from their colleagues as they return to their in-garrison practice. Thankfully, over the past 20 years, we have learned a lot about the norms of the deployed experience (at least as they relate to asymmetric warfare in Operation Iraqi Freedom [OIF], Operation Enduring Freedom [OEF], and other more recent insurgency combat operations). Our objective in this chapter is to summarize our lessons learned from the process of returning home from a deployment, termed *redeployment*, and to provide practical tips on how to make this process as smooth and stress-free as possible.

Getting Ready to Return

No matter the deployment, planning for your redeployment back home should begin prior to your actual deployment. Why? Starting at your home duty station or at a deployment readiness center, there are many people and places you will ultimately encounter again upon your return. So remember these people/places, take some notes, listen carefully, and *always* be humble and kind as this approach will greatly enhance the speed of your *redeployment* process. Then, when you are downrange, in general, preparation for your exit from theater should start in earnest at about the halfway point for shorter deployments and at about the 3 months prior to your final out for longer deployments. Over the course of your down ramp process, many administrative, logistical, family, professional (leadership and clinical), health, and emotional activities will require attention (Table 25.1). Recall that military movements are classified events (SECRET at a minimum); so communicating your redeployment schedule and itinerary to your family must be done cautiously. We advise that you come up with some phrases or keywords prior to deploying that let them know you are changing location and/or redeploying.

Table 25.1 Summary of pre-redeployment activities

Category	Examples
Administrative	Complete evaluation reports for yourself and ratees
	Submit awards for yourself and your team
Logistical	Ensure accountability and serviceability of your equipment
	Identify returnable vs non-returnable items
	Clear all hand receipts
Professional	Map out potential clinic and OR schedules (with flexibility)
	Identify academic conferences to attend in the months after redeployment
Personal	Share appropriate pictures/media with teammates
	Beware of social media posts/discuss with PAO
	Take caution in communicating your redeployment schedule
	Mail home anything you do not absolutely need in-transit
	Avoid making firm plans for trips outside the local area soon after returning

Return Activities

Military Duties: Redeployment Checklist and CRC

During redeployment, prepare yourself mentally for another round of checklists including an out-processing checklist from your deployed location and another checklist at your home duty station. In the Army, you will follow one of three redeployment pathways:

1. If you deployed with a unit, stayed the entire deployment with that unit, and redeployed with the unit you will travel to that unit's home station for your redeployment processing and reintegration. If you are stationed elsewhere, you will then proceed to your home station and re-process there as well. If the latter occurs, the redeployment processing at the unit's home station is very short (usually 1–2 days).
2. If you deployed through a Continental US (CONUS) Replacement Center (CRC), all redeployment activities will

occur at that same center. Upon returning to your home station, you will have further in-processing and reintegration activities there as well.
3. A combination of the above is also possible, as are other nuances.

In the Navy, Active Duty medical personnel generally deploy as a unit and Ops/Admin work through the deployment/redeployment checklists. Historically, the Navy Reserves required a four-week Expeditionary Combat Readiness Center (ECRC) for post-deployment physicals and debriefs to ensure a smooth transition from active duty back to reserve duty. This process is undergoing a transition to more local mobilizations to minimize prolonged family separation before and after the actual deployment.

The Air Force tends to deploy medical personnel individually with redeployment activities conducted at the home station. The timeline for these activities and the post-deployment limits on travel outside the local area likely vary. For all services, the best approach for the deploying surgeon is to check your ego at the door (you may be important to patient care, but the Army/Navy/Air Force and the larger mission does not revolve around you) and remain highly flexible as the details of the redeployment process change often.

Domestic Duties: Family Life

Remember that during your deployment, life for your family (immediate and extended) and friends continued essentially as normal, albeit without your contributions to the family dynamic and workflow. Modern deployments allow for much better communication than in decades past, but you are still absent. In this void, your spouse and family have been forced to adapt and go about life to the fullest extent possible. If you have school-age children, they continued to attend school and engage in all their extracurricular activities. Your spouse or significant other went to work and ensured that things around the house and involving your family's finances continued as usual, likely with minimal interruption.

Because your family adjusted to your absence, remember that everyone—you and those you love and live with—will need to adjust once again upon your return. In many ways, your absence was likely much more challenging for them than it was for you—the uncertainty of your safety, the need to maintain a sense of normalcy, and the loss of companionship all take their toll. Work together to reintegrate into their lives as they reintegrate into yours by carefully yet intentionally navigating that fine line between patience and passiveness.

As a word of caution, you will likely be tempted to make plans for a family trip outside the local area. This is very natural and completely understandable whether it's a family reunion with extended family members you have not seen in a long time or that once-in-a-lifetime trip to an exotic locale. These trips can be extremely enjoyable and rewarding, but in our experience they are best enjoyed long after your redeployment. Squeezing in this type of travel shortly after your return can add significant unneeded stress to you and your family due uncertainty about your exact return date and the risk of disrupting the planned trip. The best approach we believe is to focus on re-integrating locally early after redeployment. Avoid making any travel plans outside the local area until you arrive home and then target a time frame that will allow you to comfortably and fully return to your normal home and work routine first.

Box 25.1

The end of one of my deployments was fast approaching in the early spring. For many years, my extended family had traveled to Colorado for a ski trip during our boys' Spring Break. I had missed two prior trips and was determined to join the family for this one to decompress and enjoy the beautiful spring Colorado air. Unfortunately, the timing of my return was such that I had to request special permission from my commander to take the trip (which he graciously approved). I thought we were home free! I had just made it

(continued)

Box 25.1 (continued)
and was starting to breathe a sigh of relief. But then my younger son was injured while playing soccer. He complained of wrist pain for two days, right before our planned departure. After spending weeks planning this trip and barely making it home, I was reluctant to take him in for medical attention. I performed a cursory exam and told him to just suck it up. Thankfully my sensible wife insisted I take him in for an exam and x-rays. Sure enough, he had a distal radius buckle fracture. My orthopaedic surgical colleague casted his arm…and we were still able to make the trip, cast and all (with a plastic bag to wrap around the cast during his ski lessons). So, although this worked out in the end, my inflexibility in planning this trip added significant stress and led me to miss a distal radius fracture in my own son. Don't make this same mistake!—Jeremy Cannon

Surgical Duties: Return to Work

The lifecycle of a military surgical practice can be characterized as shown in Fig. 25.1. Closing and then re-opening one's practice represent significant administrative tasks required of military surgeons. Generally, this cycle requires about 3 weeks pre-deployment and then about 7 weeks post-deployment [1]. Prior to returning home, start to map out a rough return to work timeline and share this with your team. Be careful to leave enough buffer time before your first clinic and OR cases to allow for the uncertainty in your return date. You can use any unfilled time upon your return to work to double scrub cases with colleagues in your practice.

Your early clinics can be filled with established continuity patients that you engaged with or operated on prior to your deployment. For new patients, although legislation passed after Gulf War I officially protects military physician practices during deployment (particularly aimed at deploying guard and reserve military members) [2], referral patterns may have shifted during your deployment. These will need to be re-established as you return to practice and re-populate your OR pipeline.

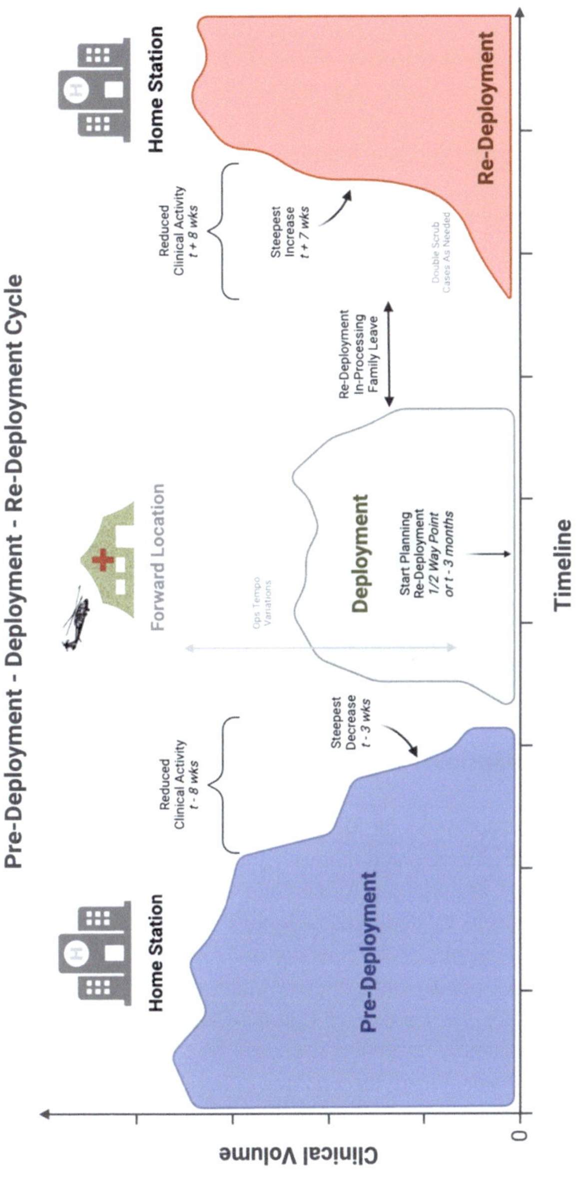

Fig. 25.1 Typical life-cycle and clinical experience during a deployment. Timeframes presented here are suggested by Hall et al. [1]

Skills decrement represents a significant concern for all military physicians returning from deployment. Downrange clinical responsibilities often diverge significantly from in-garrison practice. Medical specialists and pediatricians focused on combat casualty care during deployments face an even greater challenge returning to practice than many surgeons [3]. For general surgeons and surgical specialists, the number of patients and operative procedures varies greatly. Sometimes you and your team are extremely busy, mostly with open penetrating trauma cases. Of late, most deployments have very little clinical volume; so surgeons return feeling rusty. Deployments with low clinical volume and limited/absent laparoscopic or robotic procedures accentuate this feeling; however, objective analysis of basic laparoscopic skills demonstrate no detectable decrement relative to predeployment [4].

Do not be surprised if your practice requests some sort of focused proctoring plan and do not be afraid to ask for that yourself, especially if you have been out of the hospital and out of your practice for 6 months or longer. Depending on your practice, your group may be eager to have you back and will just assume you can pick up as you were prior to your deployment. Pay attention to your own skill set and advocate for what you need.

Academic Duties: Research, Conferences, Writing

Deployment represents an ideal time to think, formulate proposals, and write abstracts and manuscripts. Some journals including the Journal of Trauma and Acute Care Surgery make their entire journal available to deployed surgeons. Organizations like the Eastern Association for the Surgery of Trauma (EAST) maintain repositories of deployment-relevant manuscripts. The American Association for the Surgery of Trauma (AAST) recognizes military members and conference attendees who have deployed over the previous year during the opening ceremony with a challenge coin and a group photo.

Returning to your home station presents an opportunity to present talks about your deployed experiences to a wide range of audiences. The authors have given such talks at local, regional, and national meetings: Uniformed Services University Trauma Day; Missouri Chapter of the American College of Surgeons Annual Meeting; Pennsylvania Trauma Systems Foundation John P. Pryor Lecture; American Trauma Society, Pennsylvania Chapter. These talks represent an ideal opportunity to reflect on the course of your previous deployment(s) and to cement clinical, administrative, and leadership lessons learned that you can then disseminate for the benefit of civilian surgeons and other military surgeons who may deploy in the future.

Joining national societies with a strong support infrastructure and network for military surgeons can greatly enhance your military career. A strong ethos of a shared mission can lead to lifelong friendships, new academic collaborations, and mentoring relationships. Examples include the Excelsior Surgical Society of the American College of Surgeons, the SAGES Society of Military Surgeons, and the AAST Military Liaison Committee.

Cautionary Tales

Redeployment represents a disruptive time in your career, by definition. We recommend taking time to take stock of your deployed experiences, say the things that often go unsaid as you prepare to leave theater, and then stay alert for some classic behavior patterns that can emerge as you return to your in-garrison routine. These are summarized in Table 25.2.

Table 25.2 Cautionary Messages

Category	Key messages
The Wind Down	Thank the members of your deployed team Re-connect with key team members after deployment Actively process deployed experiences in-theater and at home
The Bag Drag	Pare your personal items down to 2 duffels and a backpack
Moral Injury and Distress	Surgeons can experience moral distress or even moral injury during deployment
Too Eager to Return	Give yourself ample time after redeployment before considering volunteering to deploy early

The "Wind Down"

As your deployment comes to an end, you will have worked with some of the finest professionals in the business of combat casualty care. Make sure to take time to thank them for their dedication to the mission, for their service to the team, and for their comradery as you say goodbye. All the authors of this chapter regret not spending enough time doing this for each of our teammates as we prepared to leave the theater.

You undoubtedly will also experience both patient care and leadership scenarios during your deployment that are rarely seen in the US. Take time to reflect on these experiences in the way that you find most meaningful. This can be a rightly emotional activity – at least it was for the authors of this chapter. Take time to wind down in theater (at the right time) either alone or with a group or trusted partners. Plan to spend ample time on the return side of your journey processing these experiences with your immediate family and your closest friends. They will all want to know "what it was like." Verbalizing your experiences can also serve to help you process not just the actual events but the meaning and the substance and the effect of these events on you as a military surgeon, a spouse, a parent, and a human being. We also advise taking time down the road to connect with key people whom you deployed with. The military societies mentioned earlier can serve this purpose through their military working groups and annual meetings. Likewise, teaching pre-deployment classes such as the ASSET+ course run by Col (Ret.) Bowyer function as mini-reunion opportunities. Some deployed surgeons have even formed their own social groups such as the "BADASS" group that meets in Las Vegas on a regular basis. These experiences add to the richness of one's military surgical career while supporting resilience and mental, emotional, and spiritual stability amidst the incredible challenges of a deployment-redeployment cycle.

The Bag Drag

The volume of "stuff" that one accumulates over the course of a deployment can be quite surprising. All those creature comforts! Fortunately, most media-related items like books come in electronic format these days. For physical items, donate them to the deployed unit (e.g., DVDs and video games), give them to someone remaining in theater, or mail them home ahead of time until you have your personal items down to two duffels and a small to medium-sized backpack. Beware, though, that mail services can be somewhat inconsistent. For example, items sent from a ship may be significantly delayed and may also be damaged due to the constraints of the environment. Ultimately, you must be able to carry everything in one trip or "drag." When redeploying through a theater clearing facility, it may take days before there is room on your flight out of theater, yet you still have to "show" for each potential flight. Then, the flight might be full, canceled, or repurposed, and back you head to lodging with your stuff in tow to get another room for the night (or multiple nights until the next potential flight) after already checking out earlier that day. Travel light in and out of theater!

Moral Injury and Distress

A recent mixed methods analysis of 20 surgeons who had deployed to Role 2 facilities in Iraq and Afghanistan explores the topic of moral injury and distress (MID) for the first time in military surgeons. Surgeons expressed concern over team members whom they felt were unqualified for their role and in settings with poor team cohesion and communication. The devastating injuries, unique patient populations (injured children, pregnant women, and US military members), and medical rules of engagement (MROE) all contribute to feelings of MID [5]. Physician leaders in a deployed setting are often involved in the interpretation of MROE situations. The decision to withhold treatment due to MROE or to direct an injured patient to a local healthcare facility where the outcomes are likely suboptimal or even terminal lead to feelings of extreme guilt. The response to such feelings can vary widely from mild distraction to incapacitating anguish. Consider confiding in a trusted colleague or seeking professional mental health support if you feel your response to such feelings is impeding you professionally. Further work in this area is also needed to better quantify MID among military physicians and to define the most effective strategies from prevention to treatment.

Box 25.2

During one of my deployments to Afghanistan, I served as Deputy Commander of Clinical Services. In this role, I fielded innumerable calls for medical consultation. Sometimes we were able to accept the patients to our Role 3 facility, but during times of increased operational tempo, this was not possible. One such scenario was captured by a reporter for the Atlantic, Brian Mockenhaupt [6]. I still tear-up when reading this article. Upon returning from Bagram they asked me if I had killed anyone. I answered "yes" on that question. That got some attention, of course, and the process that was in place in 2009 was thorough and welcomed by me – just the reassurance that I had done the right things.—Rob Rush

Over-Eager to Return

Hollywood makes much of the emotional aspects of the "deceleration injury" that occurs on returning (as in Hurt Locker). The mission and culture of a deployed setting are quite different from your in-garrison mission. In most deployed settings, the mission drives the culture. You have one job: to take care of American and coalition forces, as well as enemy combatants and civilian casualties in accordance with the Geneva Convention and MROE. The purpose is clear (most of the time, except for occasional unusual cases of MROE interpretation). The regulatory and administrative encumbrances shrink to a relatively small element of the experience making this like a surgical sabbatical. Upon redeploying, the numerous competing priorities and agendas and the regulatory burdens all come rushing back.

Some surgeons respond to this post-redeployment re-entry back into the seemingly routine and mundane practice by seeking back-to-back deployments. This mission-first approach is truly laudable. However, it can come at a steep price to the surgeon personally and professionally. For commanders, the specific deployment tempo for an individual surgeon must also consider the role that surgeon plays in the home unit, the military and academic advancement goals for that surgeon, and their family's ability to sustain repeated deployments. Finally, and perhaps most obviously, deployments carry an inherent danger, even for medical personnel who are relatively protected from direct fire. Loss of life or career-ending injuries represent infrequent but real possibilities that must be weighed when considering the compelling desire to jump the line to join the fight again.

Box 25.3

I deployed five times between 2006 and 2009, each time as a flight surgeon and most of the time as a Role II augmentee. My plan at the start of all those deployments was to return for an ENT residency, but halfway through my tour in Al Taqaddum, Iraq, I decided on trauma surgery and never looked back. I left active duty and completed residency and fellowship in the Reserves. I then proceeded to volunteer for every single deployment that came my way thereafter because all I wanted to do was go back. When I had deployed previously, I had the training of an intern and was only able work in the ED or at most, first assist in the OR. After my trauma fellowship, I finally felt that I could now contribute to the mission to my fullest potential as a trauma surgeon. This also gave me a break from the grind of inner-city

(continued)

Box 25.3 (continued)
ivism made me feel like I was failing to truly rescue my patients even after "great saves." Joining a forward-deployed surgical team allowed me to provide the level of care I couldn't provide over the previous decade and allowed me to serve those protecting our freedom.—Meg Morgan

Conclusions

In this chapter, we sought to unpack redeployment to help younger surgeons learn from our experiences—both good and bad. By understanding a typical pre-deployment and redeployment timeline and the many associated challenges, we hope this process will ideally progress along smoothly for you or that at the very least you will know what to expect. In the end, a humble, flexible, and positive approach will allow you to make the most of the life-changing and enriching experience of a surgical deployment.

References

1. Hall A, Qureshi I, Vasquez M, et al. Military deployment's impact on the surgeon's practice. J Trauma Acute Care Surg. 2021;91:S261–6.
2. Gates SM, McGovern G, Waggoner I, et al. Supporting employers in the reserve operational forces era. 2013. Available at: https://www.rand.org/content/dam/rand/pubs/research_reports/RR100/RR152/RAND_RR152.pdf. Accessed September 1, 2024.
3. Deering SH, Rush RM, Lesperance RN, Roth BJ. Perceived effects of deployments on surgeon and physician skills in the US Army Medical Department. Am J Surg. 2011;201:666–72.
4. Deering SH, Kavanagh LB, Chinn MK, et al. Objective evaluation of the effects of deployment on laparoscopic skills: the simulation and deployment laparoscopic skills study. Mil Med. 2016;181:1058–64.
5. Ryu MY, Martin MJ, Jin AH, et al. Characterizing moral injury and distress in US Military Surgeons deployed to far-forward combat environments in Afghanistan and Iraq. JAMA Netw Open. 2023;6:e230484.
6. Mockenhaupt B. The Doctor's war. The Atlantic. 2009:1–5. Available at: https://www.theatlantic.com/magazine/archive/2009/10/the-doctors-war/307659/

Global Health Engagement, Humanitarian Assistance, and Disaster Response

26

Joseph Aryankalayil
and Tamara J. Worlton

Introduction

An integral part of military surgery is the flexibility to operate beyond borders and out of the conventional operating room. Military surgery has responded to domestic and international disasters, worked shoulder to shoulder with our international partners, and saved lives during wartime. For many, the opportunity to provide selfless service has drawn them to join military medicine.

Working with our allies and partners is a fundamental part of our National Security Strategy. Global Health Engagement (GHE) emphasizes the fundamental link between health and security by conducting health related missions under security cooperation.

Disclaimer: The opinions or assertions contained herein are the private ones of the author/speaker and are not to be construed as official or reflecting the views of the Department of Defense, the Uniformed Services University of the Health Sciences or any other agency of the US Government.

J. Aryankalayil
Department of General Surgery, Walter Reed National Military Medical Center, Bethesda, MD, USA

T. J. Worlton (✉)
Center for Global Health Engagement (CGHE), Uniformed Services University of the Health Sciences, Bethesda, MD, USA
e-mail: tamara.worlton@usuhs.edu

A. T. Schlussel et al. (eds.), *The SAGES Manual for Navigating a Successful Military Surgical Career*,
https://doi.org/10.1007/978-3-031-88490-0_26

The Department of Defense (DoD) provided its first instruction and definition of GHE, Department of Defense Instruction 2000.30, in 2017 (Fig. 26.1). GHE has since continued to be a formal component of Joint Health Service Support Planning and Operations, as outlined in Joint Publication (JP) 4.02 "Joint Health Services" as of 29 August 2023. Of the vast array of programs and missions that are under GHE, several are pertinent to the military surgeon. These include building partner capacity and interoperability, humanitarian and civic assistance (HCA), disaster preparedness, humanitarian assistance and disaster relief (HADR), subject matter expert exchanges (SMEE), and international military education and training (IMET). With the formalization of GHE, various courses and professional tracks have been established (Table 26.1).

The Air Force boasts the longest-standing specialist program in GHE, known as the International Health Specialist (IHS) program, established in 2000. This program is an opportunity for

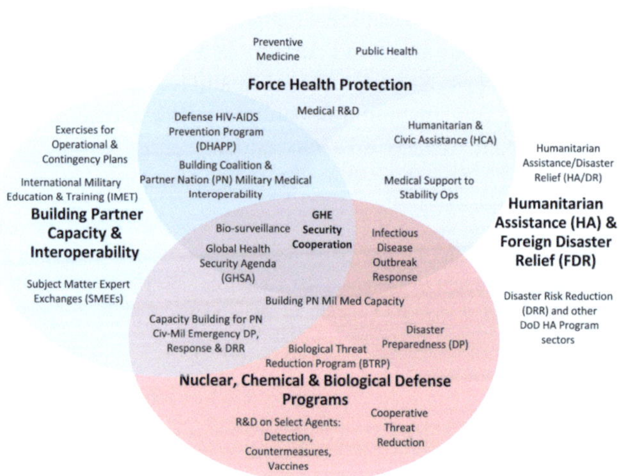

Fig. 26.1 Global Health Engagement Framework. From *DoD Instruction 2000.30 on GHE Activities (July 2017)* "The appearance of US Department of Defense (DoD) visual information does not imply or constitute DoD endorsement"

Table 26.1 Courses and professional tracks established for global health engagement

Military course	Where to enroll
Fundamentals of Global Health Engagement	cghe-education@usuhs.edu
Global Health Strategies for Security	cghe-education@usuhs.edu
Military Medical Humanitarian Assistance Course	**mmhac@usuhs.edu**
Global Health Engagement Orientation Course (formerly IHS Orientation Course)	Usaf.pentagon.af-sg.mbx.ihs-program-office@health.mil
Humanitarian Assistance Essential Course (Joint Humanitarian Operations Course)	dha.jbsa.dha-metc.mbx.jmop@health.mil (jhoc@usaid.gov)

Non-Military course	Where to enroll
Stanford University. Humanitarian Surgical Skills Course	https://globalhealth.stanford.edu/programs/international-humanitarian-surgical-skills-course/
The American College of Surgeons. Global Health Competencies for the Surgeon: Cognitive and System Skills	https://www.facs.org/for-medical-professionals/conferences-and-meetings/clinical-congress-2023/education-program/postgraduate-courses/didactic-courses/
United Nations. Global Surgery Learning Hub	https://www.surghub.org/
Geneva Foundation for Medical Education and Research. Global Health Curriculum	https://www.gfmer.ch/surgery/course-overview.htm

officer and enlisted medical personnel of all career fields, from the Active Duty, Air National Guard and Air Force Reserve components, to achieve a Special Experience Identifier (SEI) for experience and training related to GHE. There are more than 60 active duty IHS assignments supporting GHE at Combatant Commands, Air Force Component Commands and other organizations. Subsequently, the Navy introduced its own Global Health Specialist Program (GHSP) in 2017. For specific assignments, prerequisites such as Additional Qualifying Designator (AQD) 68M for GHSP and the IHS Special Experience Identifiers (SEI) are essential. These qualifications are particularly relevant for billets in organizations like the Defense Institute for Medical Operations (DIMO) and GHE specialists for Combatant Commands, among others. Despite the Army having a substantial presence in GHE, it currently lacks a Service-wide formalized training and qualification pathway, although the Army Veterinary Corps has a GHE Special Identifier.

Regardless of the branch, this chapter will explore the field of global health within the context of a military surgical career. GHE missions have significant value for diplomatic and strategic purposes, and as such will continue to have a permanent place within the military toolkit. Surgeons should ensure they have familiarity with GHE best practices, humanitarian principles and the relevant stakeholders in global health, to engage with and steer these GHE missions so that they meaningfully enhance international relationships through goodwill and capacity building, but also make long-term contributions to the advancement of partner-nation (PN) medical systems.

History of Military Medicine and Global Health

In 1898, the US engaged in the Spanish-American war and although it lasted for only 10 weeks, there was a remarkable disparity in attributable deaths between infectious disease and combat. Less than 400 soldiers were killed in combat, but more than 2000 died from yellow fever [1]. Through US military support, physicians identified the mosquitos as the vector of disease, allowing effective use of sanitation and vector control efforts [2]. Within a year of this discovery, yellow fever deaths were zero, facilitating economic development and stabilization in the region. Previous French attempts at forging a trans-oceanic passage through Central America were impeded by disease outbreaks. However, because of the medical progress made by US military efforts in the region, the Panama Canal opened in 1904 which supported US economic and military advancement in Central America. Tropical medicine and infectious disease efforts within military GHE efforts have continued to be a priority. Now, there are numerous bio-surveillance and research labs across the globe, working to protect the military force and inform pandemic preparedness.

Vietnam War era utilization of medical personnel demonstrated a marked shift from prior efforts aimed at force sustainment to utilization as a policy instrument by US political and military leadership. During lulls in conflict the US armed forces carried out several medical programs in support of South Vietnamese civilians through Medical Civic Action Programs (MEDCAP). The best record of these programs is from Dr. Robert Wilensky in his book "Military Medicine to Win Hearts and Minds: Aid to Civilians in the Vietnam War" [3]. This conflict ushered in a plethora of programs. Medical civic action program (MEDCAP) I was designed to use medical care to bolster confidence in the local government by training and equipping local health care providers. Later, MEDCAP II was used to gain the cooperation of the populace in areas controlled by the US by us offering direct patient care, bypassing the local system. During this time, US military physicians had just shy of 40 million health encounters with Vietnamese civilians. The impetus of these programs seems multifactorial, from genuine humanitarian desire to relieve suffering to swaying local opinion as a counterinsurgency method.

Many of these MEDCAPs involved an unannounced short-term engagement to a rural village where medical teams mainly provided care to children and the elderly. Physicians performed symptom management of immediate complaints because they were inadequately supplied and lacked the ability to schedule regular follow-up or longitudinal care of chronic diseases. The most impactful work done during these short-term engagements came in the form of immunizations for the pediatric population. Minor surgical procedures and ocular procedures were performed aboard Naval Hospital Ships. More complex surgeries and seriously ill patients were referred to local Vietnamese provincial hospitals, however the rural population was distrustful and hesitant to leave their homes, and without local providers to engage in the transfer of care these patients were often forgotten. Without standardized reporting, explicit analysis of the outcomes is difficult. Overall, there was uniform agreement among physicians that although single-visit engagements saved lives and trained some exceptional Vietnamese medics, there was very little done to advance medical care in the country. This was especially true without the support and involvement of local Vietnamese health officials.

From a strategic level MEDCAPs were designed to assist the Government of the Republic of Vietnam in their efforts to win over "hearts and minds" of the rural populace and to resist attempts of the North Vietnamese government to reunify Vietnam under a communist party. From this political objective, MEDCAPs failed to garner local populace support for their own government. When US personnel engaged in MEDCAPs with only a Vietnamese interpreter they undermined national capability and confidence. Villagers preferred to be treated by US medical teams and even traded US medicine on the black market due to the high regard over local therapies. This was compounded by the Vietnamese army who very infrequently engaged in civic actions, but when they did, often diverted supplies and food to their own families who were in more dire straits than the civilians they were tasked with helping. US direct action in the medical sphere hurt the psychological objectives of the mission in building up confidence in the Republic of Vietnam. Medical intelligence was another objective of MEDCAPs. Large numbers of civilians gathered around the location of the MEDCAPs, which provided an opportunity to identify changes in disease prevalence such as a new strain of malaria but also tactical intelligence from wounded civilians and soldiers. Reports from MEDCAPs noted that the wounded often readily disclosed the locations of mines and health of POWs. But this information was dealt with at the local unit level, and the link to strategic intelligence such as enemy troop movements or plans was never reported. Review of intelligence reports did not mention intelligence from medical sources or MEDCAP teams. The most successful strategic objective was seen back in the US in the form of hometown reporting of US military medical personnel helping the Vietnamese which garnered support for continued US involvement in the region.

The use of medical engagement to function as stability operations or counterinsurgency continued into Operation Iraqi

Freedom and Operation Enduring Freedom. Here it was noted that not only did these engagements have limited oversight and focus, but they lead to a plethora of unintended consequences, similar to the experience of the MEDCAPS in Vietnam. These included creating expectations of continuous health care from the United States, reduced public opinion of the capability of local doctors, displacement of local health infrastructure leading to brain drain, and infringement into the humanitarian space placing civilian aid workers at risk [4, 5]. This lack of a coordinated effort matched with measures of effectiveness led to the creation of the DoDI 2000.30. Under this, the priorities of GHE are to maintain trust and influence through activities that build PN capacity, bolster civilian confidence in their own government, and lower PN susceptibility to destabilizing influences.

The concept that GHE bolsters goodwill toward the US is widely acknowledged but difficult to quantify. It is certainly true that aid dollars in general increase positive opinions of the donor government. The foundational report from Terror Free Tomorrow documents opinions toward the US in Indonesia and Bangladesh after the USNS Mercy visited in 2006 [6]. Nationwide surveys reported increases in favorable opinions of the US and decreased support for Osama Bin Laden. This had waning durability over a 6-month period. A more scientific approach was conducted in Peru which noted that humanitarian and civic aid program positively impacted local opinion of US military and US government [7]. They more clearly demonstrated that this effort decreases over time and thus sustained engagement, both longer and more frequent missions, are ideal for diplomacy objectives.

The Field of Global Surgery and the Civilian Actors Involved

As demonstrated in the theaters of Iraq and Afghanistan, there is overlap in DoD health activities and what the civilian humanitarian community provides. Thus, it is important to understand the civilian context in which the field of global surgery exists. The Lancet Commission defines global surgery as the study, research, practice, and advocacy that seeks to improve health outcomes and achieve health equity for all people who need surgical and anesthesia care, with a special emphasis on underserved populations and populations in crisis [8]. This field of medicine seeks to alleviate the burden of 5 billion people who do not have access to safe, affordable surgical care when needed [9, 10]. Many civilian actors are involved within the field to meet the staggering need for surgical care, including academic groups and non-governmental organizations (NGOs). Estimates note more than 300 NGOs are involved in delivering surgical care to low- and middle-income countries [11].

The use of humanitarian assistance to support military aims during conflict is regarded by many NGOs as a threat to the humanitarian principles of neutrality and independence (Table 26.2). As such, many of these organizations have looked to establish separate operational channels so that they are not perceived as part of the military toolkit. However, there are spheres of global surgery which align well with both civilian and military objectives during peacetime and disaster response. Surgical system strengthening is one such area that facilitates cooperation with civilian entities. Investments in training, infrastructure, and processes fosters sustainable and self-directed growth within a

Table 26.2 World Health Organization Guidelines on Civil-Military Coordination for Humanitarian Activity (adapted from Civil-military coordination during humanitarian health action ver Feb 2011 Position Paper Inter-Agency Standing Committee Global Health Cluster)

1. The roles of civilian-humanitarian and military actors should be clearly separated
2. Preserve the civilian character and humanitarian principles of operations even if military assets are involved
3. Do not use military and civil defense assets of forces actively engaged in combat to support humanitarian activities
4. If military assets are deemed needed, the request must come through the Humanitarian/Resident Coordinator
5. Military assets should be used with a limited timeframe and a clear exit strategy
6. Generally, humanitarian convoys should not employ armed or military escorts

country. A strong health system underpins economic development and trust in the government, acting as a protective factor from radicalism and unrest. In the setting of trauma related morbidity, road traffic injuries are the most common cause of disability adjusted life years in men ranging from an age of 10-24 years old [12]. Building a strong trauma system to conserve the health of the military-age population also has implications for a country's national security. Recent COVID-era events have also highlighted how a strong surgical system can help pandemic preparedness and response due to availability of oxygen and personnel who can intubate critically ill patients [13]. Through these types of engagements military surgeons can cooperate with civilian colleagues to meaningfully improve quality and access to surgical care within another country.

These efforts to assist PNs in health systems strengthening allows US military personnel to understand the local context for care, build partnerships, and improve interoperability. In 2017, the Secretary of Defense directed military medical leadership to collaborate with the UAE to deepen and expand military ties with this key regional partner [14]. One of the initiatives focused on building a joint military trauma and rehabilitation center within the UAE. This culminated in the establishment of the Trauma, Burn, and Rehabilitative Medicine program (TBRM) within one of the UAE's largest hospitals. The program aims to build a robust and enduring trauma, burn, and rehabilitative medicine capability in the UAE, while also establishing an intra-theater military readiness platform to support combat casualty care. This model of PN global health engagement, capacity building, and civilian-military cooperation profoundly improves regional medical readiness. Due to integration within the UAE civilian sector, this program is self-sustaining.

More globally, the US government (USG) is slowly recognizing the importance of surgical care in its designated funding [15]. It was just in the past few years that surgery was even mentioned in a US Congress appropriations bill. To put this in perspective, trauma alone kills more people globally than HIV, malaria, and tuberculosis (and COVID-19) combined [16]. However, the USG funds the President's Emergency Plan for AIDS Relief (PEPFAR)

Table 26.3 Global surgery organizations

Organization/committee	Information
SAGES Go Global	https://www.sages.org/projects/go-global/
ACS HOPE (Health Outreach Program for Equity in Global Surgery)	https://www.facs.org/for-medical-professionals/membership-community/acs-hope/
AAS Global Affairs Committee	https://www.aasurg.org/leadership/committee-objectives/
Association of Academic Global Surgery	https://www.academicglobalsurgery.org
Global Surgery Student Alliance (GSSA)	https://www.globalsurgerystudents.org
G4 Alliance (surgical, obstetric, trauma, and anaesthesia care)	https://www.theg4alliance.org

at 6.9 billion USD in 2023 and the President's Malaria Initiative (PMI) at 1 billion USD. There is a lot of work ahead for surgeons to advocate and educate about the importance of surgical conditions to the global burden of disease and the indivisibility of surgical systems within national health systems strengthening [17, 18]. There are multiple national organizations and committees that engage in global surgery for the interested regardless of level of training (Table 26.3).

Ongoing Surgical GHE

Every year and in every CCMD, there are multiple GHE opportunities. The most consistent GHE that involve direct surgical care are described below.

Indo-Pacific Command

Pacific Partnership: The USNS Mercy responded to the 2004 Tsunami and subsequently, the diplomacy mission, Pacific Partnership was born in 2006. The initial positive goodwill results as mentioned above, really paved the way for all future ongoing endeavors of this type. Some aspect of direct surgical care has been a consistent theme [19–22].

Southern Command

Continuing Promise: Starting in 2007, USSOUTHCOM has had ongoing direct patient care missions in their area of responsibility. Although the hospital ship USNS Comfort is typically associated with this mission, other ship platforms will conduct medical and surgical engagement as well as associate fly in and fly out missions. There are multiple papers documenting the surgical footprint from Continuing Promise and the hospital ship missions [23–28]

Joint Task Force-Bravo: Established in 1984 by the request of the Honduran government, this joint Army and Air Force task force is the longest one in military history. The Medical Detachment engages in short-term surgical missions within Honduras and supports the Hospital Escuela, which is the largest center providing public services in the country. There are two ongoing projects here: Military Unique Curriculum in Honduras (MUCH) and Military Emergency Skills in Honduras (MESH). The unique environment of high-volume penetrating trauma and resource constrained setting makes this international engagement an ideal one to study the efficacy of maintaining military readiness. These are primarily Emergency Medicine programs but are expanding to a surgical component.

Resolute Sentinel: This annual joint exercise began in the mid 1980s as New Horizons, then Beyond the Horizon, in USSOUTHCOM. Although medical is not the central theme, there is typically a short-term surgical component within each of these missions [29, 30].

Africa Command

While not a direct surgical care GHE, African Peacekeeping Rapid Response Partnership (APRRP) is an ongoing capacity building program that began in 2015. This highly successful program which recently transitioned from CGHE to USAFRICOM has equipped and trained multiple countries' militaries to deploy UN Level 1 and/or UN Level 2 medical facilities. UN Level 2 hospitals have damage control surgery and resuscitation capabilities.

Uniformed Services University (USU)

The medical school has a Global Surgery Interest Group which has recently become a chapter of the Global Surgery Student Alliance (GSSA), which is the largest medical student global surgery in the US. USU also has an MOU with Harvard Medical School's Program for Global Surgery and Social Change (PGSSC) since 2020. This MOU allows for USU students to attend their intensive Introduction to Surgery Health Services Research program. Additionally, through this MOU, there is an annual opportunity for a military research resident to be a PGSSC Global Surgery Research Fellow.

Humanitarian Assistance Disaster Response (HADR)

Globally, natural disasters are increasing as a result of climate change [31]. The primary USG agency to respond to foreign disasters is the Bureau of Humanitarian Assistance (BHA) under USAID. The role of the DoD within the USG response is typically minimal and is covered in the Joint Humanitarian Operations course listed on Table 26.1. Unless there is a specific capability that only the DoD can provide, it is much more cost effective to use other organizations to respond to disasters. Additionally, there is the aspect of a country's sovereignty to consider as sending a military response without an invitation from the country is considered an invasion.

Although BHA is the USG primary response, the international response comes from the United Nations Office for the

Coordination of Humanitarian Affairs (UNOCHA). Following the Haiti earthquake, guidelines were developed for the role and coordination of military elements in disaster response via the UN Civil-Military Coordination (UN CMCoord) [32]. The areas of responsibility within a disaster response are divided by the cluster approach [33]. The World Food Program (WFP) is in charge of logistics and emergency telecommunications and therefore is the one to most likely coordinate with military entities [34].

Within the HADR missions conducted by the military, surgery is typically not needed DoD capability. The medical footprint in these responses have grown less over the years with the exception of the hospital ships when they are deployed for disaster response. In the initial few days of a disaster, the medical emphasis is on understanding what capabilities persist in the local healthcare system and assisting with triage [35, 36]. Orthopedic injuries are the primary needed surgical response within the first few days. As the disaster response continues, the medical response shifts to chronic conditions that are unable to be treated due to the disrupted healthcare system. A key lesson learned from previous DoD HADR responses to the 2005 earthquake in Pakistan and the 2010 earthquake in Haiti is that there needs to be a defined endpoint for the US military mission.

Best Practices During Direct Patient Care

There are also nuanced factors and considerations that need to be addressed during direct patient care [37]. One such consideration that will be increasingly prevalent is the dissimilarity in training between surgical trainees from high-income countries and lower- and middle-income countries. Training in the US has become increasingly focused on minimally invasive approaches. As a consequence, US surgical residents were found to be unprepared for the typical caseloads in an international hospital [38]. Surgeons have a duty to reflect on their scope of practice and training before engaging in surgical missions. Without the appropriate technical, cultural, and health context knowledge, deployment of undertrained trainees and surgeons can lead to mistrust and fractured international relationships.

Furthermore, preparation goes beyond intraoperative care to include preoperative and postoperative planning. When possible, early engagement and collaboration with host-nation (HN) physicians also plays an essential role in the preoperative environment. HN physicians can provide valuable information regarding specific challenges related to population characteristics, such as comorbidities that may impact the technical components of the surgery itself and the anesthetic risk. Postoperative considerations such as handling of specimens for pathology should be considered and discussed as well. Ideally, the HN surgeon should be operating side by side with the US team.

Often in surgical GHE, the surgeon is brought into the planning phase late which can complicate meeting mission objectives while also doing no harm [39]. The vast majority of these types of GHE are under two weeks, therefore any complications may not be present while the US team is still there, and the host-nation (HN) may not have the capability to manage the complication. Establishing an adequate follow-up plan is part of the mission preparedness to provide equitable care for the target population that extends beyond the operating room.

However, when a complication inevitably arises, we must rely on lessons learned from past experiences and the recommendations of HN surgeons, who have had to help manage them. The following recommendations are tailored to the military context where surgical teams have limited time in the country and hospital ships sail away to another port with limited communication capabilities. Recommendations include: (1) sharing accurate and descriptive operative reports with HN physicians so that an appropriate differential can be made depending on where difficulty was encountered. (2) The operating surgeon should give a detailed and standardized handoff to the HN surgeon that will oversee the patient's postoperative course. (3) A reliable method of communication should be disseminated to HN physicians overseeing postoperative care so that the surgeon of record can be contacted and involved in the management of their complications. (4) A treatment and contingency plan should be created and agreed upon between HN and US military parties before engaging in patient care.

The intersection of surgical expertise and global health initiatives introduces a unique set of challenges and opportunities, prompting a need for strategic insights and best practices. A critically important article by military surgeons, Welling et al., provides a list of seven areas of concern that are common and continue to challenge humanitarian medicine [40]. Although as we noted earlier, GHE is distinct from humanitarian missions, the pitfalls outlined in the article are still applicable to military surgical missions—especially considering the authors of the articles are esteemed military surgeons. The "seven sins" of humanitarian medicine are (1) Leaving a mess behind. (2) Failing to match technology to local needs and abilities. (3) Failure of involved parties/organizations to cooperate. (4) Failing to have a follow-up plan. (5) Allowing politics, training, or other distracting goals to trump service, while representing the mission as "service". (6) Going where we are not wanted or needed. (7) Doing the right thing for the wrong reason (publicity/advancement in academia).

Conclusion

Lessons learned from MEDCAPs in Vietnam, civilian care in Iraq and Afghanistan, highlight the need to clearly define objectives before engaging in GHE. Successfully orchestrated GHE missions have centered around building up capacity and capability of ally nation medical systems. The results of these types of missions have a much more profound ability to reduce the burden of disease within a country, impact interoperability, and improve/sustain diplomacy. Investment in the understanding and improvement of HN medical system capabilities can eventually even be leveraged to support US medical forces.

In the face of evolving and unpredictable global conflicts, increased ferocity of natural disasters, and the looming crisis of unmet global surgical disease, US military medicine has a unique role in answering these challenges.

Acknowledgments
Col Elizabeth Erickson, MD MPH
Chief, Global Health Engagement Branch & International Health Specialist Program
CAPT Danny Shiau, MD MPH
Director, USU Center for Global Health Engagement

References

1. Reid BH. The Spanish-American war: Land Battles in Cuba, 1895–1898; 2014. Published online February 25, 2014. p. 37–58. https://doi.org/10.4324/9781315036717-3.
2. Alexandra Minna Stern. Yellow Fever Crusade: US Colonialism, tropical medicine, and the International Politics of Mosquito Control, 1900-1920. In: Medicine at the border. Disease, globalization, and security, 1850 to the present; 2007, pp. 41-59.
3. Wilensky RJ. Military medicine to win hearts and minds. Aid to civilians in the Vietnam War. Published online 2004. Accessed November 27, 2023. https://books.google.com/books/about/Military_Medicine_to_Win_Hearts_and_Mind.html?id=eR25rVQVyIsC
4. Health Initiatives and Counterinsurgency Strategy in Afghanistan | United States Institute of Peace. Accessed November 27, 2023. https://www.usip.org/publications/2010/03/health-initiatives-and-counterinsurgency-strategy-afghanistan
5. Daniel JC, Hicks KH. A report of the CSIS Global Health Policy Center Sharpening a Key Tool for the Department of Defense. Global Health. Published online 2014.
6. Terror Free Tomorrow. Unprecedented Terror Free Tomorrow Polls: World's Largest Muslim Countries Welcome US Navy.
7. Flynn ME, Machain CM, Stoyan AT. Building trust: The effect of US troop deployments on public opinion in Peru. Int Studies Quart. 2019;63(3):742–55. https://doi.org/10.1093/ISQ/SQZ028.
8. Dare AJ, Grimes CE, Gillies R, et al. Global surgery: defining an emerging global health field. Lancet. 2014;384(9961):2245–7. https://doi.org/10.1016/S0140-6736(14)60237-3.
9. Meara JG, Leather AJM, Hagander L, et al. Global Surgery 2030: evidence and solutions for achieving health, welfare, and economic development. Lancet. 2015;386(9993):569–624. https://doi.org/10.1016/S0140-6736(15).

10. Meara J, Hagander L, Leather A. Surgery and global health. Lancet. 2014;383:12–3.
11. Ng-Kamstra JS, Arya S, Chung TE, et al. Mapping the playing field—a novel web-based strategy to identify non-governmental actors in global surgery. Lancet. 2015;385:S55. https://doi.org/10.1016/s0140-6736(15)60850-9.
12. Abbafati C, Abbas KM, Abbasi M, et al. Global burden of 369 diseases and injuries in 204 countries and territories, 1990–2019: a systematic analysis for the Global Burden of Disease Study 2019. Lancet. 2020;396(10258):1204–22. https://doi.org/10.1016/S0140-6736(20)30925-9.
13. Bouchard ME, Sheneman N, Hey MT, Hoemeke L, Abdullah F. Investments in surgical systems contribute to pandemic readiness and health system resilience. J Public Health Policy. 2021;42(3):493. https://doi.org/10.1057/S41271-021-00292-Z.
14. John SK, Berge AI, Bishop JM, et al. Independent study of force mix options and service models to enhance readiness of the medical force. Published online 2023.
15. Korn J, Sheneman L, Hoemeke L. Five billion reasons for ramping up global surgery | think global health. Published June 15, 2022. Accessed November 27, 2023. https://www.thinkglobalhealth.org/article/five-billion-reasons-ramping-global-surgery
16. Rossiter ND. Trauma-the forgotten pandemic? Int Orthop. 2022;46(1):3–11. https://doi.org/10.1007/S00264-021-05213-Z.
17. The U.S. President's Emergency Plan for AIDS Relief (PEPFAR) | KFF. Accessed November 28, 2023. https://www.kff.org/global-health-policy/fact-sheet/the-u-s-presidents-emergency-plan-for-aids-relief-pepfar/
18. The President's Malaria Initiative and Other U.S. Government Global Malaria Efforts | KFF. Accessed November 28, 2023. https://www.kff.org/global-health-policy/fact-sheet/the-presidents-malaria-initiative-and-other-u-s-government-global-malaria-efforts/
19. Gaidry AD, Lizardo RE, Prieto JM, et al. An analysis of essential pediatric surgical cases encountered during a decade of large-scale military humanitarian aid missions. Mil Med. 2020;185(11-12):E2143–9. https://doi.org/10.1093/MILMED/USAA177.
20. Reichl A, Schutt R, Walsh J, et al. Challenges in oncologic preparedness: a retrospective review of incident surgical cancers during pacific partnership missions, 2008–2016. Mil Med. 2022;187(1–2):E76–81. https://doi.org/10.1093/MILMED/USAA488.
21. Lagrew J, Lujan E, Nelson SC, et al. Pacific partnership 2010: Anesthesia support aboard the USNS Mercy humanitarian civic assistance. Mil Med. 2012;177(8):939–46. https://doi.org/10.7205/MILMED-D-12-00044.

22. Sykes AG, Brill JB, Wallace JD, et al. Trends in surgical case volume during pacific partnership missions onboard USNS Mercy. Mil Med. 2023;188(7–8):e1690–6. https://doi.org/10.1093/MILMED/USAB500.
23. Walk RM, Glaser J, Marmon LM, Donahue TF, Bastien J, Safford SD. Continuing promise 2009--assessment of a recent pediatric surgical humanitarian mission. J Pediatr Surg 2012;47(4):652-657. doi: https://doi.org/10.1016/J.JPEDSURG.2011.09.063
24. Chadwick JL, Sridhara S, Goodrich J, Mitchell AO, Gessler EM. Humanitarian otolaryngology: a navy hospital ship experience. Otolaryngol Head Neck Surg (United States). 2014;151(6):960–2. https://doi.org/10.1177/0194599814549159.
25. Fluke LM, Restrepo RD, Pryor HI, Duncan JE, Mann KE. The surgical experience aboard USNS COMFORT (T-AH-20) during Operation Continuing Promise 2015. Am Surg. 2018;84(8):1307–11. https://doi.org/10.1177/000313481808400842.
26. Hartgerink BJ, Chapman LE, Stevenson J, Donahue TF, Pagliara C. Utilization of surgical resources during the USNS COMFORT humanitarian mission to the Americas, June to October 2007. Mil Med. 2010;175(9):638–46. https://doi.org/10.7205/MILMED-D-09-00162.
27. Norris EA, Johnson MS, Mann KE, Pryor HI. Evaluation of surgical caseload aboard the USNS COMFORT (T-AH 20) during enduring promise 2018. Mil Med. 2020;185(3–4):325–7. https://doi.org/10.1093/milmed/usz416.
28. Worlton TJ, Gunasingha RMKD, Atwood R, Johnson M, Uber IC. A decade of surgery aboard the U.S. Naval Ship COMFORT (T-AH 20). Mil Med. 2023;188(7–8):e1802–7. https://doi.org/10.1093/milmed/usac278.
29. Lucha PA, Wallace D, Pasque C, et al. Surgical wound morbidity in an austere surgical environments. Mil Med. 2000;165(1):13–7. https://doi.org/10.1093/MILMED/165.1.13.
30. Charron BL, Dengler KL, Nguyen BT, Coggins A, Massengill JC, Tomkins TJ. Gynecologic SURGRETE, New Horizons Guyana 2019: an experience of a lifetime for global health engagement and medical readiness. Mil Med. 2023;188(5-6):120–2. https://doi.org/10.1093/milmed/usaa169.
31. How can climate change affect natural disasters? | U.S. Geological Survey. Accessed November 28, 2023. https://www.usgs.gov/faqs/how-can-climate-change-affect-natural-disasters
32. Civil-military coordination | OCHA. Accessed November 28, 2023. https://www.unocha.org/civil-military-coordination
33. What is the Cluster Approach? | Humanitarian Response. Accessed November 28, 2023. https://www.humanitarianresponse.info/en/coordination/clusters/what-cluster-approach

34. Military commanders learn about civil-military coordination at WFP | WFP Executive Board. Accessed November 28, 2023. https://executive-board.wfp.org/military-commanders-learn-about-civil-military-coordination-wfp
35. Arnaouti MKC, Cahill G, Baird MD, et al. Medical disaster response: a critical analysis of the 2010 Haiti earthquake. Front Public Health. 2022:10. https://doi.org/10.3389/FPUBH.2022.995595.
36. Worlton TJ, Shwayhat AF, Baird M, et al. US Navy Ship-based disaster response: lessons learned. Curr Trauma Rep. 2022;8(3):138–46. https://doi.org/10.1007/S40719-022-00227-3.
37. Alayande BT, Riviello RR, Bekele A. How to maintain ethical standards of global surgery practice and partnerships. In: Global surgery. Springer International Publishing; 2023. p. 21–37. https://doi.org/10.1007/978-3-031-28127-3_3.
38. Lin Y, Dahm JS, Kushner AL, et al. Are American surgical residents prepared for humanitarian deployment? A comparative analysis of resident and humanitarian case logs. World J Surg. 2018;42(1):32–9. https://doi.org/10.1007/s00268-017-4137-x.
39. Younger A, Worlton TJ, Wallace S, Allan Steigleman W, Ortiz-Pomales Y. Ethical considerations for surgical planners from the lessons learned on USNS COMFORT (T-AH 20) deployment 2019. Mil Med. 2021;186(5):117–20. https://doi.org/10.1093/milmed/usaa407.
40. Welling DR, Ryan JM, Burris DG, Rich NM. Seven sins of humanitarian medicine. World J Surg. 2010;34(3):466–70. https://doi.org/10.1007/S00268-009-0373-Z/METRICS.

Operational Assignments 27

Matthew D. Nealeigh
and Linda C. Benavides

Introduction

Operational assignments truly provide a crucible for surgeons. You are often isolated professionally and personally, yet expected to perform in some of the most intellectually, emotionally, and physically demanding situations you will ever face. The independence of thought and action required unveils many strengths you may not have known you had; sometimes weaknesses, too, are found, but—once found and addressed—these may become areas of quick and lasting growth.

Recurring themes emerge throughout this chapter around leadership, ownership, collaboration, and independence. This is a unique opportunity for true, multifaceted leadership. Here, the surgeon invokes the full meaning of "medical officer." The

M. D. Nealeigh (✉)
Uniformed Services University, Walter Reed National Military Medical Center, Bethesda, MD, USA
e-mail: matthew.nealeigh@usuhs.edu

L. C. Benavides
Madigan Army Medical Center, Tacoma, WA, USA

A. T. Schlussel et al. (eds.), *The SAGES Manual for Navigating a Successful Military Surgical Career*,
https://doi.org/10.1007/978-3-031-88490-0_27

deployed surgeon (as every operational billet is preparing for, executing, or learning from a deployment,) holds a unique role in the medical and military worlds. "[S]He who wishes to be a surgeon must go to war" holds true more than 2000 years after Hippocrates first uttered the phrase. For many, this role is why we joined the military—to fulfill our sacred commitment to the patients, as we have been entrusted with America's sons and daughters, each of whom have put their lives on the line for our country. Rarely is this more strikingly evident than on deployment.

Your Mission

In the operational assignment, your role as a medical officer requires you to find success in each lane of a tripartite mission: direct patient care, team and unit leadership, and support of the line commander's mission. Your primary mission is the safety and health of your patients, but the unit's mission is dictated by national policy and the theater commander's intent. The local unit commander's focus, therefore, will be on that intent, and they rely on you to keep their people safe and in-the-fight. Setting yourself up for success includes knowledge and appreciation of the commander's mission. Read and understand the doctrine guiding the mission so you can "speak the language" when needed. Emergency situations are suboptimal settings to make your introductions to the unit or battlespace commander, so establishing your "street credit," or at a bare minimum, an office call discussing your credentials, should be set up as early as practically feasible in your assignment. Cultivating a personal relationship with the executive officer and operations officer should be among your early priorities as the leader of your team.

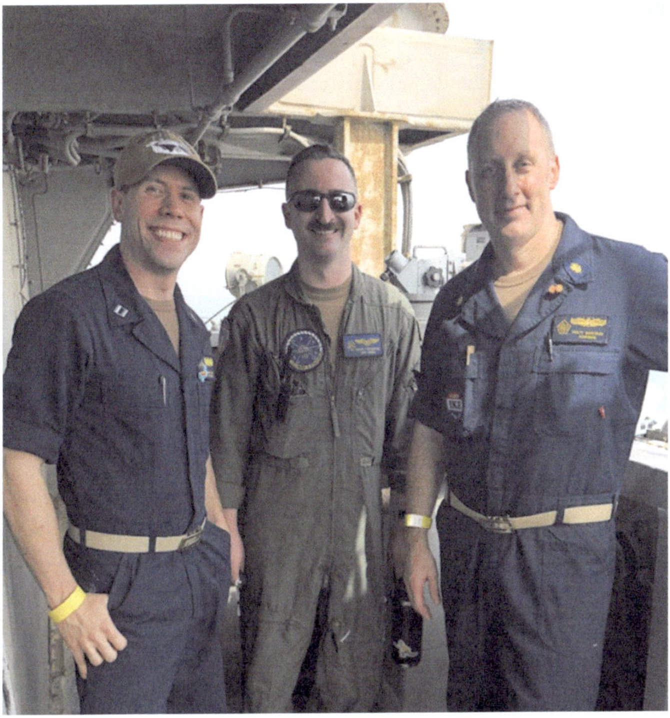

LCDR (Dr.) Matt Nealeigh (right) as Ship's Surgeon, with Ship's Psychologist LT Brendan Finton (left) and LT Brian Patterson, operations (center).

Your commander needs to trust both your skill and your judgment. Your counsel to the line and medical leadership should be based on evidence and easily supported. Understand that your medical opinions and the patient's needs may sometimes conflict with the commander's expectation or mission. Be prepared to "speak truth to power," respecting the chain of command while still advocating for the care of your patients.

Framing Your Success

As foreshadowed above, successful operational assignments begin in garrison with your personal, honest, needs and skills assessment. "Assessment" here means critically evaluating your personal clinical and leadership skills, those of your team, the intent of your immediate and higher commanders, the physical and metaphorical environment of your assignment, the logistics situation, and a myriad of other ancillary components that contribute to your future success.

Any needs assessment [1] begins with understanding the mission. Find the current incumbent for the assignment to get "boots on the ground" input for the purpose of you and your team. If no incumbent exists for this assignment, then talk to your next higher medical unit or the combatant commander's (COCOM) surgeon about their expectations; your service's consultant is also available to help guide you. Review after-action reports from prior iterations of this assignment, as these will be highly enlightening for the successes, failures, and frustrations of those who went before you; this may be the best starting place to frame your needs assessment. The Global War on Terror provided rich literature on combat casualty care [2–7]; small investments in reading the available data will yield great returns for your teams.

Imposter syndrome, a psychological phenomenon characterized by feelings of inadequacy, self-doubt, and a fear of being exposed as a fraud, despite having achieved success, frequently visits the isolated surgeon [8]. Remember, you are the most qualified surgeon on the team, often because you are the only surgeon on the team. In medical and surgical matters, you will have influence above your rank, but this must be earned and justified. There is no place for bravado—remember, the patient assumes all risk for any of your decisions.

Surgeons—in direct partnership with the anesthesia provider—should frankly discuss personal and team capabilities with medical and line leadership, including consideration of what could (or could not/should not) be handled with intrinsic capabilities of the team. These discussions can help build training schedules for the team to train and cross-train individuals.

Team Development & Training

Once you clarify your mission, your task list becomes quite pragmatic (Table 27.1). What can you do prior to the operational assignment to prepare? Clinical courses like the American College

Table 27.1 Task list by time block

Pre-deployment orientation and training	Identify mission, location, platform/facilities Establish command relationships Contact incumbent surgeon, review AARs Evaluate team (including who will be around) Training needs assessment and plan; examples include: ASSET: https://www.facs.org/quality-programs/trauma/education/advanced-surgical-skills-for-exposure-in-trauma/ ATOM: https://www.facs.org/quality-programs/trauma/education/advanced-trauma-operative-management/
Immediate pre-deployment	Check supplies Receive mission updates from command, surgeon
On arrival	Check supplies (including blood products) Confirm equipment status Establish/refresh command relationships Establish roles Establish MROE Update MEDEVAC plan, refresh theater/global medical contacts Initiate training plan
Routine (weekly, bi-weekly, monthly staff meeting)	Mission updates Morale check-in Training plan updates Supply/Pharmacy/Equipment/Maintenance updates MROE updates MEDEVAC options and capabilities updates Administrative topics (performance evaluations, awards, AAR)
Prior to returning	Administrative topics (finalize awards, evaluations, AAR)

MROE Medical rules of engagement, *MEDEVAC* medical evacuation, *AAR* after-action report

of Surgeons' ATOM and ASSET+, the Defense Medical Readiness Training Institute's Emergency War Surgery course, familiarization with Joint Trauma System (JTS) Clinical Practice Guidelines (CPGs) and other ad hoc training like point-of-care ultrasound can better prepare you. All of these will begin molding your skills for the test to come.

Operational medicine, especially surgery, really boils down to preparation for trauma and mass casualty care. An excellent place to start your training plan is reviewing the JTS CPGs with your whole team. What could happen? What happened in the past? What's the most devastating operational threat? What would overwhelm your capacity and capabilities?

One side note here is to remember that any medical person in the area (flight surgeons from an embarked air wing; physicians from a local Humanitarian and Civic Affairs (HCA) unit, etc.,) should be invited to bolster your ranks in the event of a mass casualty incident and incapacity of one of your team's members. These trainings and rehearsals may help identify gaps in your supplies (as one of the authors fell in on a surgical team who had no supplies for managing vascular trauma like Fogarty catheters, heparin, vascular shunts) capacity/capability, or evacuation chain.

Dr. Rick Jadick's book, On Call in Hell [9], provides raw, pragmatic examples through his deployment supporting the Marines during the Battle of Fallujah in 2004. He details training—even small tasks, like knowing where supplies are, must be drilled—and logistics, including participating in line unit planning meetings to ensure casualties could be evacuated. Establish protocols, roles, and expectations. Who will be the triage officer? Who has access to narcotics (and who is responsible for them)? Talk through traumatic scenarios with your team. Rehearsing events with as much realism as possible (to include appropriate timelines, placing IVs, drawing blood and running labs (iSTAT), practicing ultrasounds, movements of patients between ER/OR/ICU, documentation of care, etc.) will focus everyone's mind and let training kick in when adrenaline tries to evoke panic. If your team is not ready for the 100-patient mass casualty event, start small. What if you suspect diverticulitis in a patient, and there's no CT scanner within 500 miles? Pick a scenario and run the drill.

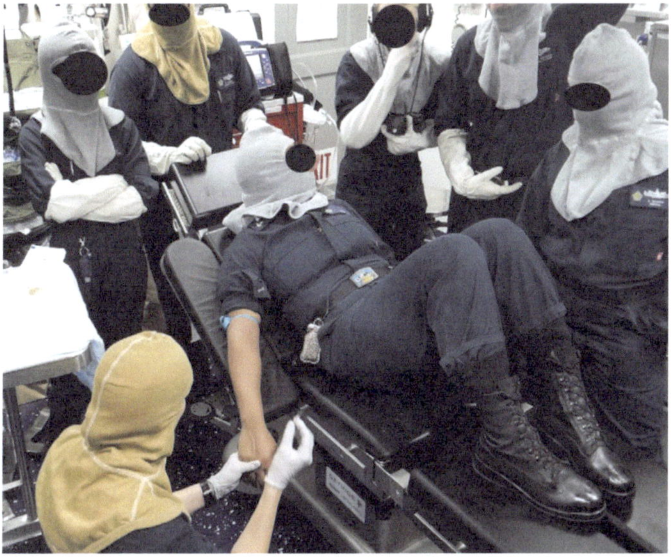

CRNA LT Liz Gallegos, NC, USN, demonstrates IV placement to a group of corpsmen during a General Quarters exercise while at sea aboard a U.S. Navy aircraft carrier.

Recognize that your teams, especially the enlisted members, will frequently be pulled in different directions, metaphorically and sometimes literally, during the deployment. Maintenance requirements loom. Facility improvements, sand bag details, or watch tower guard details must be filled. Throughout all of these "good idea fairy" scenarios, you must always be a leader, remembering that you lead a volunteer medical team who are feeling the same inadequacies that you do, and who have much less training than you. Many of them have never seen someone die, and almost certainly have not seen their friends *in extremis*. Those who have will be a valuable resource for context and development, as these are often senior enlisted personnel or line fighters who will crystallize the mission for your team. After patient care events (to include rehearsals), it is essential to conduct debriefings to improve for the next time and help members of your team process what just happened to prevent the emotional injury of Second

Victim Syndrome. This occurs when a healthcare provider experiences psychological and emotional trauma following an unanticipated adverse patient event [10].

Always know who you can call on for help. In-theater, this may be the Trauma Czar or theater's senior surgeon at the Role 3. In remote areas, this may require telehealth (like when you have a weird dermatology problem that you cannot figure out). This can also be surgeons back at your home hospital or those whom you trained with or under. The Advanced Virtual Support for Operational Forces program, or ADVISOR, is also a resource for deployed surgeons. This program offers global, on-demand access to a comprehensive range of medical tele-consultation services for emergent and urgent care. It supports providers in austere environments with limited to no local specialty assistance, delivering live help in 13 different medical specialties, including emergency care, critical care, infectious disease, and toxicology. Providers worldwide can call 1-833-ADVSRLN (1-833-238-7756 or DSN 312-429-9089). Other resources like *Top Knife* and the ASSET+ exposure book are crucial to have on hand when the internet is down, or you are trying to remember the incision for an upper extremity fasciotomy (both authors keep that book in the OR for this very reason).

Blood Bank & Resuscitative Medicine

What do you have and what can you do? This question requires more investigation than it may seem. Leading the blood bank, or blood program, sometimes doctrinally falls to the surgeon. Other situations direct that role to a dental officer, medical logistician, or others in leadership or administrative roles. However (other than the patient), surgeons and our anesthesia partners are certainly the most affected. You must have direct involvement in, and take ownership of, the blood program.

Land-based operational commands will vary widely with blood storage capabilities. If downrange with a full complement of staff you may have warm and/or cold storage capabilities, and whole or component therapy available. Enjoy this luxury, but keep well-updated on expiration dates for blood and the associated supplies, as well as the theater's ability to refresh your supply. This includes knowing the lead time required between sending the order and realistic expectations for having a blood product unit in-hand.

Conversely, smaller mobile teams may have very limited or no storage, period. Certain missions may require mobility with only a cooler of damage control transfusions if stored units are even accessible (Fig. 27.1). Often, this also occurs afloat, with amphibious assault ships and their embarked surgical teams carrying limited supplies of frozen blood which must then be carefully thawed before use—not a great solution during audible bleeding. Aircraft carriers, not doctrinally staged to receive mass casualties, almost exclusively rely on the walking blood banks detailed below.

Unfortunately, when a real blood bank is inconvenient or unavailable, the doctrine calls for the "walking blood bank"

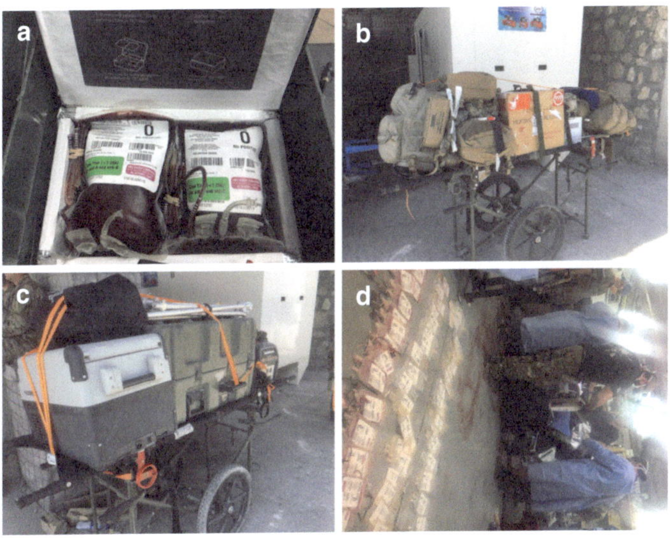

Fig. 27.1 Golden Hour Box for Point of Care Administration (**a**); Collins Box for blood transport (**b**); Cooler for blood transport (**c**); (**d**) Tracking blood transfusions in an austere environment

(WBB). This satisfies a check block in the planning process but fails to address what will be a critical need when required. In austere missions, this will be your only access to lifesaving transfusions but is meant for the "break glass in case of emergency" situations. Even the best-drilled WBB, with motivated personnel, would be lucky to have a transfusable unit ready in <15 min after activation; 30–45 min should be your pragmatic expectation. Obviously, this is too long for those who need blood the most. PRACTICE! Even though some line commanders will seem annoyed by pausing their operations, or by adding what they may deem a non-essential evolution to their already full training plan, you must convey the absolute necessity of success so WBB training is accomplished.

Earn some "street cred"…talk to the line team, to the local commanders, to the senior enlisted leaders. Make sure they know your face and your dedication to their people. Talk to their line medics and wrap them into your drills and operations regularly so emergencies can focus on medical care, not introductions, process questions, and how to help.

Logistics

> "Professionals talk logistics".

That familiar adage, uttered by General Omar Bradley, reinforces the central role supply plays in any successful operation. You are only as good as the gear you have. Check the gear! You need to know…BEFORE YOU GO…what you do and do not have, and what you might need to "acquire" or hand-carry with you. This may be painful for your team, as it takes time and effort, especially if you are opening sterile sets that must be re-sterilized and re-packaged. Finding out your chest set does not contain a rib spreader is good to know before you perform a resuscitative thoracotomy when this problem can be remedied. However, the investment is worth the pain so that you and your team are familiar with your gear when a pressurized moment arrives (Fig. 27.2).

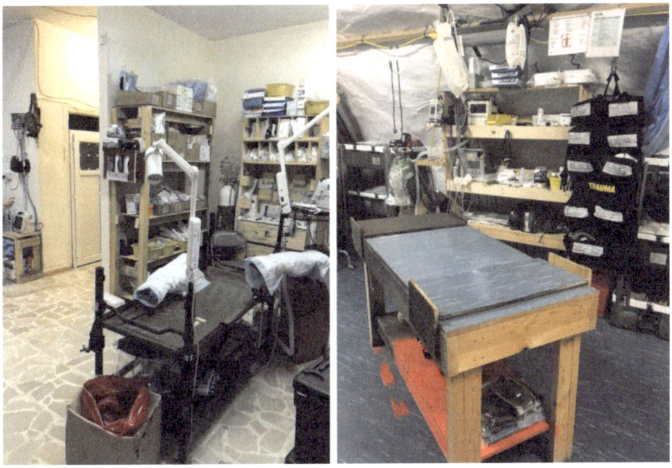

Fig. 27.2 Examples of a ground-based austere operating room

You, as the surgeon, will likely not be ordering supplies directly, but you need to be directly involved. Resupply while deployed is not as simple as calling the stapler rep to drive a new device to your hospital before your afternoon case. Discuss realistic resupply timelines with your logistician, and establish "red/yellow/green" supply levels among your team with these timelines in mind. "Spot checks" of your team's work should be conducted regularly. Too often the expiration date was read incorrectly, or—as happened to one author—the box of 200 electrosurgery pads reportedly in the storage room magically disappeared while deployed literally in the middle of the ocean, even though the supply team checked it "just two days ago." Remember, your patient assumes all of the risks of any choice you make. Do not let the minor inconvenience of opening a surgical set or double-checking your supply team supersede the patient's need for their surgical team to be confident and familiar with the gear. The same principle applies to your anesthesia teammate's equipment, the pharmacy (even if your "pharmacy" is a pelican case of meds), and your ward or other patient holding facility.

Relatedly, what if your gear never arrives? While this may seem an excessively hypothetical, doomsday scenario, even the best-planned military operations go through hiccups. Our colleagues in Afghanistan recently succeeded in a high-visibility mass casualty scenario, WITHOUT THEIR GEAR because they anticipated this scenario, showed incredible resiliency and teamwork, literally saving lives directly due to their dedication and ingenuity [11]. What can you—and your team—carry in backpacks for emergency situations?

Logistics also means medical transport and medical maintenance (Fig. 27.3). Most operational teams include a Medical Administration Officer (MAO), logistician, or other medical service corps professional who also functions as the medical evacuation (MEDEVAC) planner for both inbound and outbound patients, in conjunction with the local aviation or ground or sea assets. Once you establish your intrinsic medical capabilities and

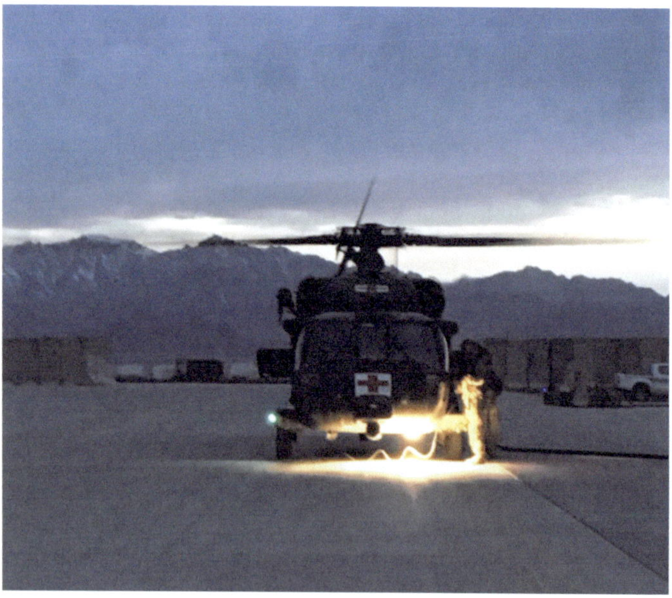

Fig. 27.3 Medical evacuation Black Hawk helicopter

capacity, prioritize connections with the local, regional, and global assets who are your immediate backup. For example, where is the nearest neurosurgeon? CT scanner? medical maintenance unit? Can you MEDEVAC local nationals or only enemy combatants and partner forces? Updates regarding these links should be a regular part of staff meetings and rehearsals. Understanding MEDEVAC capabilities and Medical Rules of Engagement (MROE) proves particularly poignant for Navy teams assigned afloat as this may change on a weekly basis—sometimes even daily or hourly, depending on the ship's movement, or ground units where evacuating patients requires crossing borders which change eligibility for care of patients.

For afloat or austere surgical teams, professional isolation is an ever-changing specter. Prepare for time periods, particularly in trans-oceanic crossings or severe weather events, where NO MEDEVAC IS POSSIBLE. You will quite literally be in the middle of the ocean, too far from land for inbound or outbound patient transfer. Even when close to land, sometimes operational requirements restrict your ability to send or receive patients (e.g., while transiting the Suez Canal). Weather and safe transport (i.e., "air superiority" or ground "route clearance") impact evacuation options just as much as geography when deployed with a ground-based unit. As mentioned above with supplies, close coordination with the larger line unit, and frequent communication within the medical team, isolation should never be a surprise. The Ukraine–Russia conflict of the early 2020s illustrated that air superiority—and air evacuation—cannot be presumed.

A note on medical administration: Like death and taxes, paperwork is inescapable, even when deployed. Medical documentation grows in importance downrange. Injured patients are about to embark on an epic international journey across multiple levels of care. No one know that patient better than you, and it is your responsibility to clearly communicate the patient's injuries, interventions, and needs. Think of how many questions arise in daily signout…and now inject hemispheres of travel, presumptions of anatomy and operative intent, and the game of telephone quickly escalates. Contact the next echelon of care directly, and when possible, include the entire multi-level chain of care. Identify from the incumbent surgeon how you will be documenting care, whether it be Tactical Combat Casualty Care (TCCC) cards, paper charts, legacy electronic health records (i.e., Theater AHLTA), or MHS Genesis. Participation in the weekly Joint Trauma System Combat Casualty Care Conference allows for patient follow-up as they progress through the system toward recovery.

Thought should also be given to several other important, though less urgent, administrative tasks. Regular (weekly, bi-weekly, or at least monthly) attention to content for evaluations, awards, training, and situation reports (SITREP) or after-action reports (AAR) will ease the looming administrative burden at the end of your assignment.

Summary

Operational assignments are the epitome of military surgery. Establishing your mission, training your team, and caring for your personnel will be incredibly rewarding. The personal and professional bonds you form while deployed will last a lifetime. Your leadership as a surgeon and military medical officer will ensure the growth of your team and safe care for those who volunteer to wear the uniform to defend freedom and democracy around the world.

Recommended Reading

Department of Defense Joint Trauma System Clinical Practice Guidelines: https://jts.health.mil/index.cfm/PI_CPGs/cpgs

Articles

"Saving the Military Surgeon: Maintaining Critical Clinical Skills in a Changing Military and Medical Environment" (Edwards & Shackelford, et al., PMI (PMID 27185158)

"Surgery at Sea" (Nealeigh & Rodriguez, et al., PMID 30952458)

"The Isolated Surgeon" (Nealeigh & Meyer, et al., PMID 33461780)

"Combat casualty care and lessons learned from the past 100 years of war" (Bradley & Rich, et al., PMID 28595716)

"US Navy Ship-Based Disaster Response: Lessons Learned" (Worlton & Tadlock, et al., PMID 35529774)

"Between the devil and the deep blue sea: A review of 25 modern naval mass casualty incidents with implications for future Distributed Maritime Operations" (Tadlock & Acosta, et al., PMID 34324471)

"How to maintain the readiness of forward deployed caregivers" (Tadlock & Galante, et al., PMID 33405471)

Books

- *Top Knife*
- *The Shock Trauma Manual of Operative Techniques*
- *Emergency War Surgery*
- *On Call in Hell*

References

1. Chen BY, Hughes MT, Kern DE, Thomas PA. Curriculum development for medical education: a six-step approach. 3rd ed. Baltimore: Johns Hopkins University Press; 2016. https://doi.org/10.1353/book.44600.
2. Edwards MJ, Edwards KD, White C, Shepps C, Shackelford S. Saving the military surgeon: maintaining critical clinical skills in a changing military and medical environment. J Am College Surg. 2016;222(6):1258–64. https://doi.org/10.1016/j.jamcollsurg.2016.03.031.
3. Nealeigh MD, Kucera WB, Bradley MJ, Jessie EM, Sweeney WB, Ritter EM, Rodriguez CJ. Surgery at sea: exploring the training gap for isolated military surgeons. J Surg Educ. 2019;76(4):1139–45. https://doi.org/10.1016/j.jsurg.2018.12.008.
4. Bradley M, Nealeigh M, Oh JS, Rothberg P, Elster EA, Rich NM. Combat casualty care and lessons learned from the past 100 years of war. Curr Problems Surg. 2017;54(6):315–51. https://doi.org/10.1067/j.cpsurg.2017.02.00433461780.
5. Worlton TJ, Shwayhat AF, Baird M, Fick D, Gadbois KD, Jensen S, Tadlock MD. US Navy ship-based disaster response: lessons learned. Curr Trauma Rep. 2022;8(3):138–46. https://doi.org/10.1007/s40719-022-00227-3.
6. Tadlock MD, Gurney J, Tripp MS, Cancio LC, Sise MJ, Bandle J, Cubano M, Lee J, Vasquez M, Acosta JA. Between the devil and the deep blue sea: a review of 25 modern naval mass casualty incidents with implications for future Distributed Maritime Operations. J Trauma Acute Care

Surg. 2021;91(2S Suppl. 2):S46–55. https://doi.org/10.1097/TA.0000000000003199.

7. Tadlock MD, Carr M, Diaz J, Rhee P, Cannon JW, Eastridge BJ, Morgan MM, Brink E, Shackelford SA, Gurney JM, Johannigman JA, Rizzo AG, Knudson MM, Galante JM. How to maintain the readiness of forward deployed caregivers. J Trauma Acute Care Surg. 2021;90(5):e87–94. https://doi.org/10.1097/TA.0000000000003054.
8. Joseph, B., Tseng, E. S., Zielinski, M. D., Ramirez, C. L., Lynde, J., Galey, K. M., Bhogadi, S. K., El-Qawaqzeh, K., Hosseinpour, H., & EAST Equity, Diversity, and Inclusion in Trauma Surgery Practice Committee (2023). Feeling like an imposter: are surgeons holding themselves back? Trauma Surg Acute care Open, 8(1), e001021. doi: https://doi.org/10.1136/tsaco-2022-001021
9. Jadick R, Hayden T. On call in hell: a doctor's Iraq War story. New York: NAL Caliber; 2007.
10. Marmon LM, Heiss K. Improving surgeon wellness: The second victim syndrome and quality of care. Semin Pediatr Surg. 2015;24(6):315–8. https://doi.org/10.1053/j.sempedsurg.2015.08.011.
11. Bozzay JD, Murphy TP, Baird MD, Dingle ME, Rokayak OA, Renninger C, Boomsma SE, Milam BP, Horrell TJ, Rittenhouse BA, McGlone PJ, Kashtan HW, Buzzelli M, How RA, Lynch BA, Heyda L, Humphries AE, Jessie EM, Patel JA, Hardin R, et al. The last days: the medical response of United States and allied military teams during the Afghanistan Exodus. J Trauma Acute Care Surg. 2023;95(2S Suppl. 1):S13–8. https://doi.org/10.1097/TA.0000000000004062.

28 Leading A Surgical Team into Combat

William Jordan

Introduction

Upon graduation from residency, it's time to get a job. In the military, this typically involves assignment to one of the military medical treatment facilities across the country as a staff surgeon where you'll practice medicine as you would in a normal hospital. (Note, this chapter emphasizes work in the Army, but it is very similar to work in the Navy and Air Force). You'll wake up, go to work, go round, see some clinic, do some cases, and then go home only to do it all over again the next day. It's a great way to establish the routine that up until that point, had been established for you by the mandates of your training. You now get to make that all your own—more or less.

Many physicians join the military for precisely this. It's the same job as a civilian, albeit with considerably less pay. The only difference is that you're wearing clothing that makes it slightly more challenging to see you in the woods, not that you'll ever actually be in the woods. Sure, you'll do the required annual weapons qualification and take the occasional PT test, but is it really The Army?

Some surgeons may catch occasional glimpses and hints of something beyond the hospital parking lot, something spoken

W. Jordan (✉)
Orthopaedic Surgery and Sports Medicine, Woodlands Center for Special Surgery, The Woodlands, TX, USA

A. T. Schlussel et al. (eds.), *The SAGES Manual for Navigating a Successful Military Surgical Career*,
https://doi.org/10.1007/978-3-031-88490-0_28

about only in hushed voices, something dirty, possibly greasy, but definitely with copious amounts of foul language, and then the seeds are planted. Their minds will dwell on these things. They will find themselves wondering; I'm in the Army, but where are all the soldiers? Where's the PT, the lower enlisted, the ancient E-8's living off only caffeine and hatred? What on Earth is a Warrant Officer? I've heard whispers about the E-4 Mafia, but does it really exist? Do people really jump out of airplanes? On purpose?! Inquiring minds want to know!

Well, look no further. Uncle Sugar has a job for you.

Welcome to the everlasting glory of the Forward Surgical Team (FST). 20 Joes. In tents. Usually under rocket attack. Ever wonder what it'd be like to operate wearing a Kevlar and ESAPI plates? For that matter, ever wonder what an ESAPI plate is? Wonder no more! Not every military surgeon will get to command a forward surgical team or a similar-sized element in the Navy or Air Force. For some surgeons this may be the first time that they will interact with the rest of the Army outside of the usual environment of the hospital or clinic.

Echelons of Care

The United States military has developed a system of Levels of Care involved in the treatment and evacuation of wounded in a theater of war or conflict. Each echelon is designed to treat the service member and return them to duty, or if they are beyond the capacity for care at that echelon, to stabilize them for evacuation to a higher level.

Level I

Echelon I care provides immediate life-saving measures, Disease non-battle-related injury (DNBI) prevention, combat stress support, casualty collection, and initial evacuation. Level I care does not require the skills and knowledge of a physician. These healthcare providers at this level consist of the injured soldier, their battle buddy, Combat Lifesavers, and Combat Medics.

Level II

Echelon II care is a Division level asset provided by support battalions, medical battalions, medical companies, and forward surgical teams. The care provided here consists of initial trauma resuscitation, emergency care, dental, lab, x-rays, and very brief holding capacity. This usually involves a Forward Surgical Team (FST), or some variant, co-located with a Battalion Aid Station (BAS). The BAS receives the walking wounded. The FST takes the litters. Surgical care in an FST is provided to those patients who are not stable enough to survive evacuation to Level III. Level II is traditionally located no more than a 30-minute Blackhawk flight away from combat operations (an hour round-trip).

Level III

Echelon III is the highest level of care in the theater of operations and is provided by Combat Support Hospitals. These are usually on or near an airfield to allow for the rapid evacuation of wounded out of theater by fixed wing aircraft. Further surgical stabilization can be performed for patients deemed not stable enough for the flight out of theater to Level IV.

Level IV

For Iraq and Afghanistan, and likely any future Middle Eastern conflict, the Level IV treatment facility is Landstuhl Regional Medical Center. Located at Rammstein Air Base, Germany, this facility receives the wounded from the theater of operations and provides surgical subspecialist care (definitive Ortho, urological, OB/GYN, dental, and oral surgery).

Level V

USA. The soldiers with substantial injuries may be cared for at Brooke Army Medical Center, in San Antonio, TX or Madigan Army Medical Center on Joint Base Lewis McCord. The recovering soldiers can be kept here for continued care until deemed stable and healthy enough for evacuation back to their individual home station and families.

Composition of the Team

Forward Surgical Teams/Forward Resuscitative Surgical Teams (the acronym seems to change every few years) are the core of Level II care. In theater, we live and work on the Forward Operating Bases (FOB) with the combat units and are the first surgeons they see after sustaining injury. We currently operate under the golden hour principle in that the soldiers are no more than one hour away from emergency surgical care. DUSTOFF (the casualty evacuation helicopters) are usually co-located by the FST. This means we are never more than a thirty-minute Blackhawk ride from the area of combat operations, and are quite frequently much closer. This requires the FST to be agile and rapidly deployable. Indeed, the first medical teams into Afghanistan, Iraq, and Syria were all FSTs.

There are four functional areas of the unit:

1. Headquarters—communications and administrative functions.
2. Advanced Trauma Life Support (ATLS)—4 bed emergency resuscitation and triage.
3. The Operating Staff—Room for two patients at a time, Damage Control Surgery.
4. Intensive Care Unit (ICU)—Room for four patients, 24-h hold time max.

The Army team consists of the following personnel: (Navy and Air Force may have slightly different personnel, but it's meant for the same mission and capabilities)

- 1 Commander (MOS varies)
- 1 Executive Officer (70B)
- 1 Orthopedic surgeon (61M)
- 3 General surgeons (61J)
- 2 Certified Nurse Anesthetists (66F)
- 1 Emergency Registered Nurse (66T)
- 1 Critical Care Registered Nurse (66S)
- 1 Operating Room Nurse (66E)
- 3 surgical techs (68D)
- 3 licensed practical nurses (68C)
- 4 combat medics (68W)

Traditionally the Commander is one of the surgeons, though we have tended towards ignoring his doctrinal assignment in the latter years of the OIF/OEF. It's now not unusual to see a PA, CRNA, Nurse, or Medical Service Corps officer in command of these teams.

The team has the capability to split in half with two surgeons in each unit. This allows for rapid flexibility to assist another FST in a different area that has been rendered combat ineffective or to push out forward for major operations that are outside of the Golden Hour radius from the more established location.

Some of the Army's FSTs are airborne, meaning they deploy by parachuting down to the area of operations. They are meant to deploy in a shorter amount of time to the combat zone. The soldiers assigned to these units are all paratroopers and are trained to be dropped into austere environments and establish surgical capacity. From exiting the aircraft to being ready to receive critically wounded patients takes only about 4 hours. As a commander of an Airborne FST you'll be airborne qualified as well and will be on jump status, routinely participating in airborne training operations at home station.

While doctrine has only one surgeon organically assigned to the unit, there are four total surgeons while deployed. These other three surgeons come from medical treatment facilities across the country to be deployed as part of the FST. These surgeons will likely have little contact with the teams prior to the actual deployment and have little understanding of what's expected of them when they are in theater and on mission, other than to provide surgical and trauma care. It's up to you as the commander to help educate them on what the mission is, what the expectations are, keep them focused on the task at hand, and provide anything they need to make that mission happen.

Your mission may be of any duration. OIF and OEF deployments were 9 to 12 months long, but this can be highly variable. For longer missions, your attached surgeons may rotate halfway through. This is to ensure no significant loss of surgical skills (a laparoscopic bariatric surgeon isn't going to be doing any bariatric surgery during a deployment), and to ensure no significant loss of continuity of care of patients at home station. Make sure that your surgeons in both groups are in constant communication with each other throughout the deployment. You are the institutional memory in that you're there for the duration, but the surgeons who're leaving can continue to be a great asset for those replacing them and are just an email away.

A Day in the Life

When not deployed, FST commanders actually have two full-time jobs. You're leading and managing the soldiers of your team, planning their training, and handling all the endless nonsense that is the Army in Garrison, like conducting countless inventories, and dealing with higher command who very rarely have any concept of patient care. The other job is maintaining full operative privileges and a clinical practice at the hospital on post.

On some days, you'll see clinic and do cases at the hospital, and on others you'll do PT with your FST, sit in staff meetings with the Combat Support Hospital Commander and help your soldiers train on and maintain all the equipment of the team. Again, being ready to deploy at a moment's notice.

Much of how you manage this dichotomy will be dependent upon the quality and dependability of the junior officers and non-commission officers under your command. As such, the soldiers assigned to FSTs tend to be among the very best. There is often intense competition among the soldiers assigned to the Combat Support Hospital for selection to the FSTs. My team had some of the most gifted junior NCOs I have ever had the privilege of working with and because of their dependability, professionalism, and expertise, I was able to easily find a stable balance between life in the hospital maintaining my surgical skills and life on the teams keeping my unit combat ready.

The Mission

Put simply: Mitigate death. This is Damage Control Surgery. This is not definitive treatment. This is stabilization. Your task isn't to get the wounded back into the fight. Your task is to get the wounded stable enough to survive the 30-minute Blackhawk flight to the Level III facilities.

For the past 2.5 decades, the main planning focus has been preparing for combat deployment as part of Operative Iraqi Freedom in Iraq or Operation Enduring Freedom in Afghanistan. The units assigned to these missions knew when their deployment was happening, how long they're going to be there, and what to expect while they are there. Many soldiers on the team will have deployed to these theaters numerous times before. This gave them ample time to plan all required training to ensure the soldiers were trained, qualified, and checked out prior to heading downrange.

Now that we have withdrawn from these theaters, we are back to the original doctrine of being "on alert." There will be a rotating roster of units that are on recall status. Some of the teams will need to be rapidly deployable – in the manner of hours. Others will maintain a recall status of days to months. This can prove to be challenging in maintaining an established presence for patient care at the hospital, but the department chiefs and other surgeons in the clinics understand this and will cover down. You are there for the FST, the care you provide at the hospital is a welcome ancillary benefit of your presence, but you are not mission critical to them.

Some missions are combat oriented. At Ft. Bragg, the XVIII Airborne Corps will continually rotate the Brigades and Battalions of the 82nd Airborne Division on varying levels of alert status and the FSTs will rotate on that status with them. When they go, you go. You and your team will be trained to answer that call, get to your team house, pack your gear, and load the aircraft at Pope Army Airfield enroute to destinations unknown on only a moment's notice, only finding out the mission and destination while in the air.

Other missions for which you'll be on alert may not be combat-related at all. One of the FSTs in the army will be on Chemical Biological Radiation Nuclear or high-yield Explosive (CBRNE) attack alert. In the event of a CBRNE attack in the US, this team would be rapidly deployed to set up surgical capacity wherever possible near the area of concern. While on this rotation, you'll receive extra training on what to do and how to care for these types of casualties.

As an orthopedic staff surgeon at Womack Army Medical Center, you'll be doing the same 10 cases that all orthopedic surgeons do: rotator cuff repair, ACL reconstruction, ankle fracture, etc. Fun, but routine. Repetitive. As an FST Commander, you'll do all that as well, and will occasionally jump out of a C-17 at 800 feet altitude into complete darkness at 0200 into a "3 to 5 knot wind" onto Geronimo Drop Zone at the Joint Readiness Training Center and set up surgical capacity in a bunch of tents, treating both actual and "training" patients over the course of 14 days. I can assure you that after a career in military service, you'll remember those 14 days far more fondly than knocking out your 18th ACL of the month at Womack. In over 17 years of military service as both an Infantry Officer and an Orthopedic Surgeon, the 17 months I spent in Afghanistan as part of an FST is what I remember most fondly. Nothing else compares. It's an experience that exceedingly few of your peers in the civilian world can relate to, and it will help separate you from them in the eyes not only of potential employers, but patients as well.

Triage/Evacuation

In theater, you aren't likely to get patients in groups of one or two. They are much more likely to be in groups of eight to ten, and you have only two OR beds. Time spent in the OR must be managed appropriately. Triage is critical. Historically, doctrine has assigned this role to the dentist from the Battalion Aid Station, as they are the most trained/least critically important asset in the setting of a mass casualty scenario. This role is perhaps best served by the most experienced general/trauma surgeon in the unit until critically injured patients become overwhelming at which time the orthopedic surgeon can take over. Secondary to significant advances in modern body armor, most injuries sustained in recent armed conflicts are extremity injuries, but most critical injuries requiring immediate resuscitation and stabilization are axial and truncal. In my opinion, putting ortho in triage puts all three general surgeons in direct patient care for those who might be most emergent. This will be a decision made amongst the four surgeons and will be based off personal experience and comfort with making these critical decisions under periods of duress.

It's important not to let rank have much say here. While we all train in trauma, we don't all practice it on a regular basis. You may have a senior O-6 assigned as one of your surgeons, but the O-4 may be the better trauma surgeon. It's important for each surgeon to check their ego at the door and fill the role that best ensures that your patients are stabilized and evacuated safely and efficiently.

Your patients will have undergone initial evaluation by their battle buddies, combat medics, and the flight medics who've picked them up and brought them to you. There will be bandages, tourniquets, some may have IVs, and occasionally there will be an airway. Some will be CPR-in-progress. The FST is only a stopping point on their way to definitive care. The surgeons in the facility may be capable of much more involved treatment, but it's important not to lose sight of what you're there to do: stabilize them for transport higher.

This can be difficult for some surgeons to deal with. A surgeon in an FST may be more than capable of doing a definitive revascularization procedure for a patient with an arterial injury, but that procedure takes time (which you may not have), resources like blood (which is not easily replaced) and significant protection of the extremity in transport (which you may not get). It's far better to shunt temporarily and let Level III deal with it in a hardened facility further away from the fight with more predictable results. Spending 2 hours revascularizing a brachial artery transection with a saphenous vein graft in a tent in the middle of the night only for that graft to clot off in the back of a blacked-out Blackhawk flying over the mountains of Eastern Afghanistan not only wasted that patient's time but delayed the care of everyone else in line behind him. Shunt it. Move to the next patient.

From an orthopedic standpoint, we don't do any definitive fracture fixation in an FST setting. Wash out the injury, reapproximate the tissue and if it's an unstable fracture, apply an external fixator for the trip to the next level. You operate under the assumption that 100% of your patients are going to get infected, so don't do anything to them that can't be easily un-done when treating the infection. Providing external fixation to an unstable femur or tibia fracture is dramatically more comfortable to the patient and makes transport significantly easier than splinting the extremity alone might do, all while protecting the neurovascular structures which may be only barely intact.

You've got 2 OR beds, but I would caution against routine concurrent use of both unless there are exigent circumstances. Your patient just survived their injury, their battle buddy's care, and a 30-minutes of being tossed around in the back of a helicopter flown by a pilot of questionable sanity (anyone willing to fly a non-sneaky, unarmed helicopter face first, directly into a hot LZ to pick up the wounded deserves their own chapter in the DSM-V). Most of the patients can wait a bit longer for surgery after resuscitation in ATLS. That 2nd OR bed may be best reserved for anyone acutely injured and in extremis that needs definitive surgical stabilization immediately. These patients could come from anywhere, and at any time, but usually arrive during treatment of other casualties. OGA units (Other Governmental Agency – the federal alphabet agencies that are co-located with you) may not use traditional means of CASEVAC and your only warning for arrival of their wounded may be a CH-47 helicopter level screaming across the FOB just barely over the antennas towards your helipad. Or, more likely, the patients sustain injuries directly on the FOB either by enemy action or an accident. The femur fracture washout and ex-fix doesn't need the 2nd OR bed. It needs to wait for the one that's being used, leaving the 2nd bed available in case you get the exsanguinating bowel evisceration from blast trauma, penetrating chest injuries with active poorly controlled bleeding, and any pelvic injury in an unstable patient may require more emergent management than simply waiting their turn for a bed to become available. In my experiences downrange, leaving that 2nd bed available, even though there were casualties that could have used it, allowed for the lifesaving surgery of three patients that otherwise would have expired in ATLS and allowed us to stabilize them for evacuation to Bagram.

You'll fix up the bad guys, too. You'll likely do this more frequently than fixing up the good guys, and you'll nearly always take them back to the OR first, before the good guys. You either come to terms with that concept now or find a new job.

The Law of Land Warfare, the Geneva Conventions, US government policy, military law, and your own Hippocratic oath all boil down to the same thing: Once they hit the front door, all patients are treated in triage order. The bad guys and local national population don't have the training that we do, don't wear ESAPI plates, they don't ride around in MRAPs, and they possess a very poor understanding of the concept of a seatbelt. Their injuries will usually be far more severe than those of coalition forces, and the most severely injured patient gets treated first.

Triaging patients can be somewhat affected by capacity for follow on care. For example, there may be no long-term neurological care available for local national or enemy combatant patients with an entrance/exit cranial wound in country. In a high-volume situation, that patient would more likely be declared expectant than emergent, whereas coalition forces have that long-term care available to them and, capacity permitting, may be treated early and more aggressively for evacuation to Level III and beyond. It is not unusual to have an injured soldier lying in a bed at Landstuhl Regional Medical Center in Germany less than 24 hours after sustaining an injury in Eastern Afghanistan.

With regards to triage, stay flexible. A coalition patient with a catastrophic injury may be triaged into different categories based not necessarily on his own injuries, but the status of the injured patients he arrives with. The concept of "He's not expectant until I need that bed" should be kept in the forefront of your mind. If you can maintain vital body functions without expending critically needed supplies or limiting access to care for other patients, then err on the side of treatment. This may give the opportunity for evacuation to Germany where family may be able to be there to say their goodbyes.

Early in the war, enemy forces were evacuated to Level III. Towards the end, when the host country civilian and military medical care facilities became more established, they were handed off to the local treatment facilities. Your situation will be dependent on the mission at hand, your capacity to treat, and the current political climate. This decision will be made echelons above you by the Medical Brigade and Maneuver Commanders.

Morale

Your mission is to save the wounded. To do that, you need soldiers that can put the needs of the wounded before their own. We as physicians are indoctrinated to this concept over the course of a brutal five-year (and often longer) surgical residency, limited by federal law not to exceed an 80-hour work week. Your E-4 medic might get his first introduction to this when he's standing next to the bullet-ridden guy that just killed a dozen Americans. Your medic may not have slept in 36 hours, certainly hasn't had anything to eat other than Rip-Its and Copenhagen in at least that long, is on his 11th patient, and is angry at a level he's never experienced before. How you maintain the morale of your unit will influence his ability to start that IV and begin treatment of that patient more than any training he's received to that point. Rely on your senior soldiers who've been there before. Keep everyone focused on the mission. As surgeon and commander, you have the wounded you're treating and the service members who are treating the wounded. The care of both of those groups is equally important for a successful mission.

While not entirely inevitable, you and your team may be faced with death. Patients may come in Killed in Action or Died of Wounds enroute. You may have experienced death before, but your soldiers likely haven't, and they will react. Acknowledge their feelings and the raw emotion associated with seeing it right before your eyes and help them through it. Seeing a dead enemy combatant is one thing. Seeing a dead American soldier is harder, and it could be someone you know. Even more challenging, it could be a female American soldier.

In my 17 months down range, I had one female patient die during our treatment from a transthoracic gunshot wound. Both of my deployments to Afghanistan were high-volume trauma situations where death was not unusual, but her death shook everyone. It's difficult to describe how her being female made it different, but there was no doubt that it was. The intensity of our anger was palpable, and it spread throughout the brigade. This situation has traditionally been cited as a reason why mixed-gender combat units were considered less effective than all-male teams. Times have changed. With female soldiers now on the front lines, we must expect female casualties and understand that their loss can feel indescribably different. Worst of all: kids get killed, too. When you see what an IED does to a 6-year-old, they will have to physically restrain you. Now imagine that the guy who placed the bomb that killed the kid is in the very next bed, and he needs an exploratory laparotomy and an ex fix. You'll save that guy's life. You'll save it the same as if he was your own father. But you'll be operating with the fury of a thousand suns while you do it. Your medics may not have the same self-control. Understand this. Have the detachment sergeant watch out for their reactions while you continue with patient care. Remove them from the situation if needed. It's not a sign of weakness to have these emotions. It's only a problem if you act on them.

A deployment overseas or into combat is alternating periods of mind-numbing boredom followed by absolute chaos. With significant amounts of time with nothing to do, it's easy to lose track of where everyone is and keep them on task. Ever so tempting to your soldiers is the time machine of their beds and the sweet release into unconsciousness. Incorporate a daily meeting, even if there is nothing significant to report. Give blocks of instruction or talks on various topics that may be of interest to the group but may not be something they've known to ask about. You'd be surprised at how a 15-minute talk on ballistics highlighting the difference between high velocity vs. low velocity weapons, 5.56mm vs 7.62mm rounds, or JHP vs FMJ will make your medic a better provider. Perhaps more important than giving that talk is assigning that topic to one of your juniors and getting them used to researching, writing, and standing up to teach on a topic. Learning how to react when you get shelled from the cheap seats in a briefing about something you just learned about is a life skill that will take them far. Be creative. It can be about anything: anatomy, exercise physiology, 1990s progressive metal and its influence on the migratory patterns of sub-Saharan wildlife. The topic isn't as important as getting and keeping your soldiers involved in presenting it. Let them pick the topic. Don't make it a chore, make it an opportunity, and reward them for their efforts. The pharmacy technician from the BAS on one of my deployments gave an exhaustive power point presentation on the interconnected relationships between the characters of the Twilight Saga. The team then fought amongst each other for the next 4 weeks about #TeamEdward and #TeamJacob. I put her in for an award.

Incorporate other units. Have the other medics or corpsmen on your FOB ever been in an OR? They will be the most motivated retractor holder you've ever had. The Medical Service Corps platoon leader at the Battalion Aid Station might be considering a career in medicine. I can't think of a better place for her to get an in-your-face hands-on experience than in combat. Get them involved. You remember how amazing it was the very first time you scrubbed into surgery as a student? You can provide hands on training for interested personnel and expand the capacity of your team in a mass casualty scenario just by giving medics training on things to do that might be slightly outside their wheelhouse. The end result is improvement in their skills and a dramatic expansion on the number of people that can help out when things go sideways.

Learn everything you can about your soldier's families. Our surgeon's wife was due to deliver their first child during our deployment. We had a bit of a competition on guessing the date, time, and weight of the baby. The winner, if all three were guessed correctly, was unofficially allowed to name the child. Our ICU nurse pulled the trifecta. I can neither confirm nor deny that there is a young woman named Hurricane Bacon McCollister living somewhere in the eastern US.

It's the little things like this that make it all work. Many times, it will not be fun. You'll live through some of the most terrifying and most heartbreaking events of your life, so take the time to make the fun times fun.

Higher Command

Your boss is unlikely to be anywhere near you in theater. This glorious distance from the flagpole affords you the opportunity to filter and diffuse much of the onerous administrative nonsense that can come from the staff of this commander. Do your very best to ensure that the bureaucracy of unit administration stays as far from your soldiers as possible. You have an executive officer and detachment sergeant assigned to you specifically for this. Let everyone else worry about patient care.

The autonomy that comes from this distance can be a blessing and a curse. You have freedom to employ your unit with little to no influence from the higher command. Do your job well, and they'll leave you alone. The senior ranking officers on the FOB located with you are not in your chain of command. While they may have say in how the units under their command are managed, they have zero direct influence on yours. However, should you struggle with outcomes, or if the surgeons at Level III begin to have concerns that the treatment being provided at your FST isn't what's expected, you can expect an uncomfortable visit from senior surgeons and commanders. The distance can also make you feel very isolated and exposed. That's part of the job.

Wins and Losses

With limited resources and being far forward on the battlefield, you have to play the hand you are dealt. Sometimes, you'll win. Sometimes, you'll lose despite doing everything right. Most of the deaths from combat won't even make it to you. Those who were killed in action or have died of wounds will be intercepted by Mortuary Affairs at the flight line and will only need input from you to make the declaration of death. This can be done by any surgeon on the team or any physician assigned to Charlie Med at the Battalion Aid Station. This is not a task to be assigned to just anyone. Mankind has become exceedingly efficient at delivering violence, and what you see and experience in this role will never leave you. Choose this person accordingly, or do the job yourself.

The wounded are evacuated as a priority and as capacity demands. Those killed in action are evacuated when mission time allows. This is usually at night and is done with a ceremony. The Hero Flight involves a moment of silence across the FOB, with all units standing at attention facing the FST while the deceased are evacuated out to the waiting Blackhawks. The unit will not leave their fallen comrade alone until they are back on home soil. They are loaded, and the flight or aircraft takes off for Level III. In the desolate darkness and silence behind, Taps plays over the loudspeakers. This will change your life. Brings tears. Even today.

You'll have big wins, too. You may get mail from the families and patients who made it across your table once they get back to home station. Some injured soldiers that you'd thought had no chance of making it past Level III might send you a Christmas Card several months later. I met a patient on my second deployment who needed some help adjusting the prosthetic on his left leg. We went to the maintenance shop across the FOB and adjusted the ankle hardware until it worked perfectly. It wasn't until an hour into this that we made the connection that I was the guy who had amputated this Special Forces soldier's leg 2 years earlier at a different FOB on the other side of the country. Special Forces are a whole different breed of soldier.

Is It Worth it?

It's two full-time jobs. It's working for a morale-crushing medical brigade commander who might possibly be some kind of physician but hasn't seen a patient in over a decade and has zero concept of what you might need to accomplish your job as an FST commander, yet gleefully tells you precisely how to do it. You'd be exposing yourself to the enemy, operating in body armor while the FOB gets shelled with 107mm rockets. You'd be keeping yourself ready to deploy anywhere on the face of the planet at a moment's notice. There is truly nothing in all of medicine like it.

Is it all worth it? Without any reservation, yes. You've got your entire career to do cases and see patients in the clinic. It seems a shame not to take advantage of what makes Military Medicine unique. You're in the uniform and obligated to serve for at least four years after residency. Assignment to this role opens an entirely new side of training that's closed off from those assigned to only the medical treatment facilities such as live tissue training, more advanced combat casualty and trauma training, US Army Airborne School, Jumpmaster School, Air Assault School, Expert Field Medical Badge training, land navigation, tactical field operations, weapons training and qualifications, among so many others. But the best part? You get to be the person who coordinates and provides immediate lifesaving care for the 19-year-old rock star who straps himself into a mine-resistant vehicle every single day to do his duty and serve. There is nothing in medicine more professionally rewarding than that.

William Jordan MD, attended college at Houston Baptist University in Houston, TX, on a US Army ROTC scholarship, graduating in 1997. He was commissioned as a Second-Lieutenant in the Infantry and assigned to Fort Benning, Georgia, where he attended the Infantry Officer Basic Course and Bradley Leader's Course. While still a cadet in 1995, he also attended the US Army Airborne School at Fort Benning.

Upon graduation, Dr. Jordan was assigned as the 2nd platoon leader in Charlie Company, 1st Battalion, 26th Infantry Regiment of the 1st Infantry Division in Schweinfurt, Germany. He served as a platoon leader for just over a year, then was promoted to First Lieutenant and assigned as Company Executive Officer to Bravo Company, 1st Battalion, 26th Infantry. In this role, he was deployed to Kosovo during Operation Joint Guardian II from June to December 1999 as part of the initial entry force (KFOR-1A). During this deployment, his unit secured the locations that would become Camp Bondsteel and Camp Monteith in Kosovo. It was during a night patrol in the city of Gnjilane, Kosovo, that he decided to apply to medical school.

After redeploying from Kosovo, Dr. Jordan was assigned to Battalion Staff Operations. Later that year, after a chaotic series of events, he gained acceptance to the University of Texas Health Science Center – Houston Medical School and left active-duty military to begin his studies there in 2001. He graduated in 2005 and attended an Orthopedic Surgery internship and residency at William Beaumont Army Medical Center at Fort Bliss in El Paso, Texas, a combined program with Texas Tech University Health Science Center in El Paso.

After graduation in 2010, Dr. Jordan was assigned to the medical staff at Carl R. Darnall Army Medical Center at Fort Hood, TX (now Fort Cavazos) and immediately deployed in support of Operation Enduring Freedom. He was assigned to the 909th Forward Surgical Team at FOB Shank outside Pol-e Alam, Afghanistan. After six months in theater with the 909th, he extended his deployment for three months to cover at FOB Bostick in northeastern Afghanistan, as the 555th FST there had been operating without an Orthopedic Surgeon.

In March 2011, Dr. Jordan returned to Fort Hood and served as a staff orthopedic surgeon until he was contacted regarding a short-notice requirement for an Airborne Qualified FST commander for a team deploying within a couple of months and was reassigned to the 274th Forward Surgical Team (Airborne) at Fort Bragg and Womack Army Medical Center.

In June 2012, Dr. Jordan deployed his team to FOB Fenty in Jalalabad, Afghanistan, in support of Operation Enduring Freedom. During this deployment, they oversaw the treatment of over 100 combat casualties from coalition forces, enemy combatants, and local nationals, achieving a greater than 97% survival rate to Level III treatment. After nine months, they returned to Home Station, and Dr. Jordan finished his military service as an FST Commander and Staff Surgeon at Womack.

Since 2014, Dr. Jordan has been in private practice in The Woodlands, TX, focusing primarily on shoulder reconstructive surgery.

Military Decorations include: Bronze Star Medal with oak leaf cluster, Meritorious Service Medal, Army Commendation Medal with 2 oak leaf clusters, Army Achievement Medal with 2 oak leaf clusters, National Defense Service Medal, Kosovo Campaign Medal with gold star, Afghanistan Campaign Medal with 2 Campaign Stars, Global War on Terrorism Service Medal, Army Service Ribbon, Overseas Service Ribbon second award, NATO Medal second award, Combat Action Badge, Expert Field Medical Badge, Expert Infantryman Badge, Parachutist Badge, Air Assault Badge.

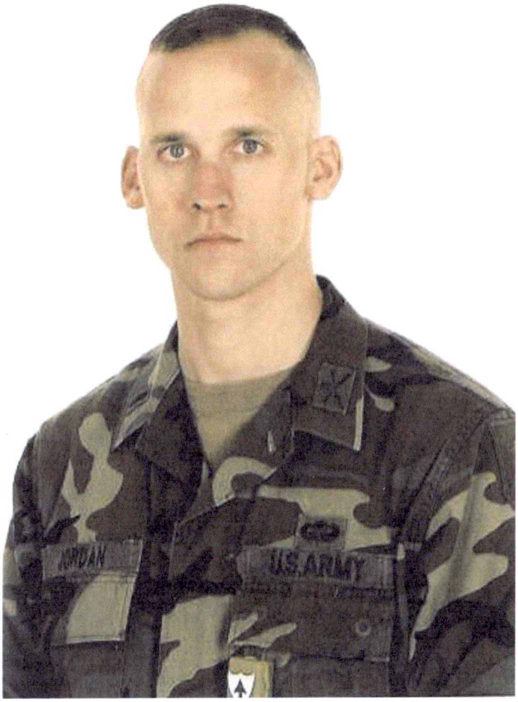

1LT William Jordan: Infantry Officer

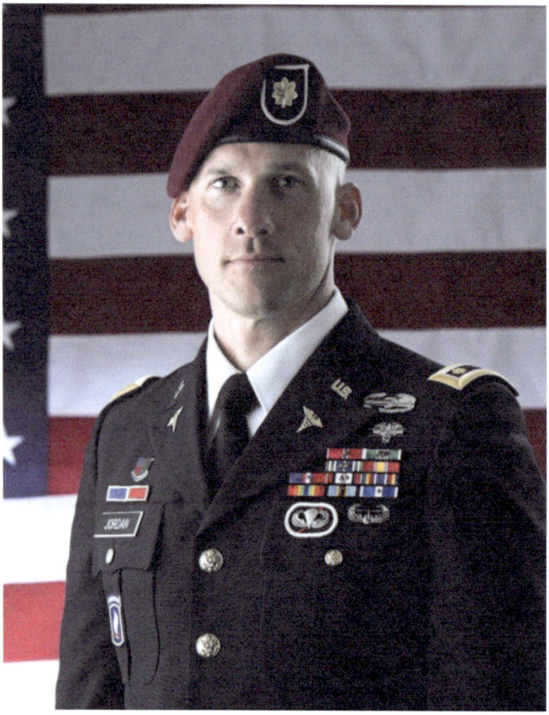

MAJ William Jordan: Orthopedic Surgeon

29 Space Medicine: Role of the Surgeon

Eric Petersen, Kresimira Milas, Kaleigh Stabenau, and Gordon Wisbach

Introduction

Brief History

The early spaceflight era was limited in in-flight medical and surgical need with short missions and highly selected crews. As United States and Russian space station programs increased mission durations, one of the first encounters with possible surgical pathology in space flight occurred when a Salyut 7 cosmonaut developed abdominal pain concerning appendicitis [1]. Though ultimately diagnosed as ureterolithiasis, the event underscored the need for advancing space surgical research.

The US Shuttle program and International Space Station (ISS) programs further increased interest in defining in-flight surgical risk and management. Extensive parabolic flight research per-

E. Petersen · K. Milas · K. Stabenau
University of Arizona College of Medicine—Phoenix, Phoenix, AZ, USA

G. Wisbach (✉)
Department of General Surgery, Navy Medicine Readiness and Training Command—San Diego, San Diego, CA, USA

Department of Surgery, Uniformed Services University, Bethesda, MD, USA

A. T. Schlussel et al. (eds.), *The SAGES Manual for Navigating a Successful Military Surgical Career*,
https://doi.org/10.1007/978-3-031-88490-0_29

formed during the 1990s and early 2000s evaluated restraints, sterility, wound closure techniques, tissue handling, bleeding management, and the feasibility of various emergency procedures [2–14]. Surgery was studied on murine species on the Neurolab STS-90 mission (April 1998), where thoracotomies, laparotomies, craniotomies, laminectomies, and exposure of lower extremity muscles were performed [15]. These studies helped determine that surgery in microgravity was no more difficult than in the standard 1 g environment once adaptation had occurred and appropriate restraints were used.

To this day, no surgeries on humans have been performed in space. Though missions are ongoing, humans have spent <200 person-years in space [16]. The likelihood of a surgical emergency is low, especially in the highly selected government astronaut corps. With the expansion of commercial spaceflight opportunities that include passengers with a greater medical/surgical risk and extended-duration exploration class missions, space surgery is inevitable in the coming decades.

Current State of Healthcare Available

Standards for levels of medical care for NASA programs were initially transcribed in NASA-STD-3001 Volume 1, Revision A (Table 29.1), which served as a foundation for commercial industry [17]:

While subsequent revisions of NASA-STD-3001 have removed this terminology in favor of medical systems based on mission-specific Probabilistic Risk Assessments (PRAs), the underpinning rationales are still applicable [18]. Short-duration missions, such as commercial suborbital flights, fit well into Level of Care One. In the future, Artemis mission profiles and proposed commercial deep-space missions will require more advanced medical systems [19–22]. While surgical capabilities were discussed in the initial standard, the limitations imposed by launch vehicles would determine ultimate inclusion. More research and innovations are required to make surgery in space possible, and mission-specific risks and parameters will determine what surgical capabilities are supported.

Table 29.1 Adapted from NASA-STD-3001, volume 1, revision A

Level of care	Mission profile	Rationale	Provider level	Medical system requirements
Level of care one	Survival training, transfer missions in low earth orbit (LEO), and suborbital flights	Low medical risk, the majority of risk is eliminated with preventative strategies	Any crewmember	Preventive care and first-aid
Level of care two	LEO <30 days	Moderate medical risk, short duration missions and evacuation can limit medical needs	CMO	Level of care one + clinical diagnostics, ambulatory care capabilities, and basic life support
Level of care three	<30 day missions outside of LEO	Moderate-to-high medical risk, short duration mission can limit medical needs but evacuation is more difficult	CMO	Level of care two + limited advanced life support and trauma care, limited dental care
Level of care four	LEO missions >30 days OR lunar/planetary missions >30 days but ≤210 days	Moderate-to-high medical risk, delayed evacuation	CMO	Level of care three + increased level of advanced care, medications, equipment (US, PCBA, AED), and training
Level of care five	Lunar/planetary missions >210 days	High medical risk, evacuation very delayed or impossible	Physician	Level of care four + increased autonomous advanced care, surgical care dependent on up-mass capabilities

Stakeholders

National & International Space Agencies

After NASA's Artemis III mission returns humans to the Moon, a pivot to long-duration lunar missions will occur. Gateway is a planned station in lunar orbit that will be the access point for lunar surface excursions. Research into deep space exploration capabilities will be performed at the Artemis base camp at the lunar south pole, which will provide a test bed for advancing space medical care [23].

With strict health criteria driving crew selection for NASA programs, limited crew numbers per mission, and initial missions lasting <210 days, there will be a low risk of emergent surgery. While the risk will be low, the consequences will be much greater if a surgical emergency were to occur due to a 3-day minimum evacuation to Earth. Lunar surface activities may also heighten the risk of trauma compared to the microgravity ISS environment. Therefore, the Artemis program presents an opportunity to refine space surgery risk models and advance space surgery innovation in preparation for Mars missions.

International space travel involves cooperation and collaboration among different countries. The ISS is perhaps the most prominent example of international collaboration in space [24]. Beyond the ISS, there have been collaborative efforts in space exploration. The ESA has contributed to various Mars missions, and NASA has collaborated with international partners on the Artemis program. International space missions involve scientific collaboration on projects such as telescopes, observatories, and planetary exploration, which often require diplomatic agreements and negotiations, leading to improved international and diplomatic relationships. International cooperation in space is considered essential for addressing the challenges and opportunities of space exploration, including sharing the costs and expertise required for ambitious missions. As technology advances and interest in space exploration grows, international collaboration in space activities will continue to expand.

Department of Defense (DoD)

The DoD has recognized the importance of maintaining a strong space presence for scientific and national security motives as demonstrated by the creation of the US Space Force (USSF; previously the Air Force Space Command) in 2019. The USSF is responsible for a range of space-related activities: satellite operations, missile warning systems, and other space-based defense capabilities [25]. This includes the recognition of future human spaceflight, the potential need for medical capabilities, and increasing national security concerns as other nations become spacefaring [25].

As space missions extend in duration and distance, the need for addressing health concerns, including medical procedures like surgery, becomes more critical. Medical assistance will be relevant for military personnel engaged in future space operations. The USSF collaborates with NASA and other space agencies on various aspects of space exploration and operations. This collaboration extends to sharing expertise and resources related to space medicine and surgical capabilities. While routine surgeries may not be conducted in space on a day-to-day basis, the USSF is interested in emergency medical response capabilities, including invasive medical procedures and telemedicine support and guidance for medical procedures.

Federal Aviation Administration (FAA)

The FAA is tasked with overseeing the safety of those using the National Airspace System as well as the general public. Though the FAA has the authority to issue commercial space licenses, verify that spacecraft with human occupants operate as intended, and provide regulation of flight crew qualifications and training, it does not have the authority to regulate the health and safety of individuals on board spacecraft. While commercial crew will be required to hold a minimum class II FAA medical certificate in the future, a "moratorium" on passenger health regulations has been extended to January 1, 2024 [26]. Currently, the FAA only requires commercial space companies to obtain informed consent from their passengers.

Commercial & Private

Commercial space companies are emerging stakeholders in space surgery. As these space operations depend on paying customers, they will not have restrictive selection criteria. The FAA moratorium on regulating passenger health has allowed a wide diversity of civilians to fly to space, including the youngest and oldest individuals. While the need for space surgery is near zero for experiential suborbital flights, such as those provided by Blue Origins and Virgin Galactic, several companies have plans for space stations and deep space travel that will require surgical capabilities [20–22]. Table 29.2 provides examples of commercial mission profiles. Note the variability in in-transit times (spent in the 0-g environment) and destination time (spent in 0.38 g) in the Mars mission profiles, as well as the total time spent without access to definitive medical care.

Table 29.2 Examples of possible commercial mission profiles, adapted from publicly available information from VAST, SpaceX, and NASA

Destination	In-transit duration	Destination duration	Total mission duration	Mission example
Low earth orbit	4 h to 3 days	Up to 30 days	>30 days	Vast-1 (VAST)
Moon (fly-by)	6–7 days	–	6–7 days	Starship (SpaceX)
Mars (short stay)	360–590 days	30–90 days	400–650 days	Starship (SpaceX)
Mars (extended stay, fast transit)	240–360 days	Up to 600 days	900 days	Starship (SpaceX)
Mars (extended stay, slow transit)	400–500 days	Up to 500 days	900 days	Starship (SpaceX)

Commercial space access is following the path of the aviation industry. Initially, only wealthy passengers could afford flights. Technological advances, deregulation, and commercial competition increased general public access to air travel [27]. Risk profiles for surgical emergencies will differ from healthy professional astronauts, with a tendency toward standard public health risk over time. Companies looking toward long-duration ventures should be active participants in furthering space surgery.

Unique Challenges

Time & Space

Human space travel is currently limited by the capabilities of chemical rockets. While trips to LEO take minutes, lunar trips can take upwards of 3 days. Proposed Mars mission architectures put the one-way transit time between 6 and 9 months. These vast distances and transit times are the largest factors increasing the risk of in-flight medical emergencies. Though several types of new propulsion systems are being developed that could decrease medical risks by reducing transit times, these are not currently being designed into commercial spaceflight operations [28].

Vast distances lead to communication delays. While LEO communications are near real-time, lunar delays average 2–3 s, and Mars delays can reach 4–44 min based on orbital alignment. Mars communications rely upon the Mars Reconnaissance Orbiter which is obstructed from Earth about one-third of the time, and approximately every 26 months, there is a conjunction where Earth and Mars are on opposite sides of the Sun [29]. Real-time telesurgical operations are possible with 0.7–1.2 s delays and sufficient bandwidth, >10–40 Mbps, for visual feedback. Delays from the Moon and Mars exceed this level, and the low 0.5–4 Mbps bandwidth in the Deep Space Network to Mars make Earth-based telesurgery unfeasible [30, 31]. Mission architectures could allow for real-time surgical support from orbital stations above the Moon or Mars to respective bases if surgical robots were prestationed. Surgical telementoring can remain beneficial even with

Table 29.3 Potential surgical support based on approximate mission distance and communication delay

Approximate distance	Mission example	Communication delay	Potential surgical support
<600,000 km	LEO orbit, lunar mission, gateway-to-lunar base communication	<1–2 s	Telesurgery if high bandwidth signal, and telementoring if low bandwidth signal
>600,000 km to 36,000,000 km	Early planetary transit	>2 s and <1–2 min	Voice telementoring possible with low bandwidth and video telementoring possible with high bandwidth
>36,000,000 km	Late planetary transit, Mars missions	>1–2 min	Autonomous surgical care augmented with delayed expert consultation

1-min delays in communication, but this relies upon the operator having some surgical training. Beyond 1–2 min of delay, crew surgical skill augmented with just-in-time training and real-time decision support tools will be the deciding factors during surgical emergencies (Table 29.3).

Mass, Power, Volume, & Cost

Surgical capabilities will be limited by the launch system. The tyranny of the rocket equation and the limitations of chemical rockets often leave only 1–2% of the mass for payloads. SpaceX's Falcon Heavy rocket has a mass of 3,125,735 pounds and can launch 37,040 pounds to Mars, representing a payload percentage of 1.2% [32]. This ratio has historically led to high costs for payloads, on the order of $18,500 per kilogram through the year 2000

[33]. Reusable rockets like Falcon have lowered the costs dramatically, below $3000 per kilogram.

The Orion spacecraft will return NASA astronauts to the moon. The Crew Module (CM) is the habitable component of the spacecraft capable of supporting four astronauts during missions up to 21 days. It has a diameter of 16.5 feet, length of 15.5 feet, and habitable volume of 316 cubic feet, leaving little room for medical systems [34]. The Lunar Gateway station will have two habitable modules, the Habitation and Logistics Outpost (HALO), and the International Habitat (I-HAB) that will provide around 4400 cubic feet of space and support astronauts for at least 30 days [35]. The habitable volume leaves room for a condensed medical system akin to that found on the ISS, which occupies a standard rack (73 cubic feet) [36]. The inclusion of an advanced surgical system would have to demonstrate significant risk reduction to displace valuable volume on such a station.

Lastly, power is a rationed commodity in space flight and is mostly generated from solar panels, the output is inversely proportional to the distance from the sun. For example, the solar irradiance on Mars (586.2 W/m^2) is around half of the irradiance on Earth (1361.0 W/m^2) [37]. Until advanced energy generators are developed, power allocations will be heavily scrutinized in mission design. The Gateway station is being designed to provide 32 W of power when the solar electric propulsion system is inactive, with a peak power to science and utilization of 5.26 kW [35]. Earth-based operating rooms can use more than 2–3 kW in an hour, highlighting a need for innovation to reduce surgical power requirements.

Environment

The launch restrictions placed on modern spacecraft limit the addition of smaller items such as medications, wound supplies, and surgical instruments, while prohibitively larger items such as computed tomography or magnetic resonance imaging systems will not be available. Limited quantity items will require restocking via cargo missions at regular intervals, the ease of which is inversely proportional to the distance from Earth and influenced by terrestrial weather, astrodynamics, and planetary position relative to the destination.

Any extraterrestrial environment that humans visit within the foreseeable future will have a reduction in gravity compared to the 1 g (9.81 m/s^2) force on Earth. Vehicles within LEO and in transit between celestial bodies are essentially at zero gravity. Astronauts on the lunar surface experienced 0.17 g (1.62 m/s^2), and those traversing the Martian landscape can expect to feel 0.38 g (3.73 m/s^2) [37, 38]. The zero gravity environments will be the most challenging in regard to surgery, requiring restraint of the patient, operator, and equipment. There have been several proposed restraint methods, including harnesses, interlocking cleats and floor mats, low-placed horizontal bars for foot restraint, and instrument restraint systems attached to the examination table, patient, or operator [14, 39, 40]. The ISS currently uses a stowable, floor-level examination table with a harness system for patient restraint, designed for medical stabilization [41]. Low gravity also affects bleeding during procedures, where surface tension becomes the prevailing force. Studies in parabolic flight have demonstrated that venous bleeding pools around the source, while arterial bleeding has enough pressure to break surface tension and create a spray [42, 43]. Electrocautery can be used for surgical procedures on spacecraft and requires special consideration of microgravity and spacecraft constraints. Surgeons operating in space will need to use adequate controls, including ventilated operating canopies, to avoid contamination of the cabin environment.

Conversely, the cabin environment could potentially contaminate the surgical field. Barring a closed medical bay with an isolated ventilation system, the surgical suite will be in continuity with the cabin. Previous studies have demonstrated that the microbial count in the cabin atmosphere increases with mission duration, temperature, and humidity [44, 45]. Data from ISS missions have shown a higher atmospheric bacterial burden compared to conventional operating rooms, increasing the risk of wound contamination [46]. Condensation within the cabin can also increase infection risk. Advances in Environmental Control and Life

Support Systems (ECLSS) may reduce this risk by reducing bacterial burden and improving temperature and humidity control.

The ECLSS is responsible for the control of the vehicle atmosphere, including the regulation of gas composition, temperature, humidity, and contaminant removal. A system designed for long-duration spaceflight will need to be capable of regulating the excess gasses that can be introduced into the cabin during surgery, of which oxygen is the most important due to flammability risk. The ECLSS must also be able to remove contaminants introduced into the cabin by the procedure, including blood, vaporized tissue, and potentially infectious organisms.

Physiology

Changes in gravity lead to alterations in human physiology that can impact surgical procedures. An early adaptation to zero gravity involves a decrease in circulating plasma volume accompanied by a proportional reduction in erythrocyte mass. A consistent 10–15% reduction in plasma volume is believed to be secondary to extravasation into extravascular space. This reduction causes increased hematocrit that decreases erythropoietin production, ultimately resulting in a 10–12% decrease in circulating erythrocytes [47, 48] that induces a volume state similar to class I hemorrhage. In combination with cardiovascular deconditioning, this physiologic change results in a decreased ability to respond to volume insults. Blood products and other intravascular volume expanders will be extremely limited to unavailable, compounding the problem. Therefore, surgical techniques that minimize blood loss will be paramount in space. The reduction in hematocrit persists for weeks to months despite a relatively quick increase in plasma volume within 2–3 days upon return to Earth, an important consideration for astronauts arriving to Mars after a journey of several months [48, 49].

As fluid shifts cephalad with gravity unloading, slow or retrograde flow can develop in the large veins of the head and neck. This phenomenon has been demonstrated in ISS astronauts using ultrasound (US) [50]. At least one ISS crewmember has developed an occlusive internal jugular thrombosis in flight, requiring treatment with anticoagulation medication that was treated on board with supplies via a cargo mission, and a potential partial internal jugular thrombosis was identified in another crewmember [50, 51]. It is unknown if spaceflight contributes to a state of relative hypercoagulability, but it will be important for the space surgeon to keep in mind [52].

Wound healing is also negatively impacted in zero-gravity conditions. Wound healing, whether surgically created or traumatic, is a complex cellular process that depends on a functioning immune system. Spaceflight results in a state of immunosuppression. Several studies using animal models in spaceflight have demonstrated changes in wound tensile strength, collagen composition, and bone callus formation [53–56]. Delayed or abnormal wound healing can increase the incidence of postoperative infection, especially when combined with the bacteria-laden cabin atmosphere.

The shifting of internal organs that occurs in 0-g conditions is an important consideration. On Earth, gravity acts upon the organs of the human body, which are kept in place by various attachments. This is evident during laparoscopic abdominal surgery, where operating table positions are utilized to shift the bowel in the surgical field. Fortunately, the mesentery provides an adequate tether for the bowel in zero gravity, making open and laparoscopic abdominal procedures viable [57]. The same is not true for the thorax; gravity unloading interferes with the visualization of the mediastinal structures during a thoracoscopy.

Training & Preparation

Traditionally, astronauts start training for their mission a few years prior to flight. The training tempo is fast, with restricted time for medical training or physician practice maintenance. NASA requires two Crew Medical Officers (CMOs) per mission. Only a fraction of astronauts are physicians, and, therefore, CMOs are often nonphysicians who have received 60–80 h of basic medical training. This education provides in “behavioral health, human physiology, treatment for health events with increased risk, treatment of risks specific to space (space physiology) including but not limited to: kidney stones, SANS, effects of altitude, pressure, CO_2 exposure, medical procedures, and techniques (i.e., ultrasound, cardio equipment, hematology monitoring, toxicology, and countermeasures)" [18]. This training is often sufficient for routine operations on the ISS as CMOs have access to real-time telemedical assistance. Though deep space missions will require Level of Care Five, including autonomous physician CMOs, NASA-STD-3001, Volume 2 states that "medical equipment shall be usable by nonphysician crewmembers if a physician crewmember is not present or is the one who requires medical treatment" [58]. This practical standard limits the types and complexity of surgical operations possible, as nonsurgeon CMOs would not be capable of advanced surgical techniques.

A 2008 Aerospace Medical Association Position Paper concluded that surgical capabilities of the CMO would be the limiting factor for the overall surgical capabilities on any long-duration spaceflight mission [59]. The 2002–2003 NASA Long-Duration Mission Surgical Working Group proposed that 6 months of dedicated surgical training of a physician CMO could make them equivalent to a standard second-year surgical resident, supporting the idea of additional surgical training for deep-space CMOs [60]. Unless changes in astronaut surgical training allotments are made with significant innovations in user-friendly surgical technologies, just-in-time surgical teaching aids, and real-time artificially intelligent surgical support tools, complex surgical operations are unlikely to be performed on NASA missions. Commercial spaceflight companies are actively weighing medical risks in the construction of their own medical systems. Further research into commercial astronaut risks will aid in making informed decisions on the inclusion of surgical subsystems and trained personnel.

Current State of Surgical Care

Prophylaxis

Surgical emergencies cannot be screened for and optimized medically. Trauma risk can be reduced through engineering, administrative, and personal protective strategies, but the reality of spaceflight revolves around significant hazards. Perforated appendicitis or severe cholecystitis can lead to life-threatening sepsis in otherwise healthy individuals. The foundations of space medicine are rooted in preventive care, and previous studies have investigated the utility of prophylactic surgery to reduce mission risk. Weighing the ethical considerations with the postoperative risks, prophylactic appendectomy and cholecystectomy are not currently performed for astronauts [61, 62].

Current Capabilities

The ISS is equipped with the Crew Health Care System (CHeCS), including a Health Maintenance System (HMS) subsystem containing diagnostic and treatment supplies [36]. Medical events on the ISS are categorized into three types: Class I (no mission impact), Class II (require use of the HMS), and Class III (require emergent evacuation). As an ISS crew of 6 members over a 6-month mission adds 3 healthy person-years of risk, each individual mission is unlikely to have a Class III medical event. If one were to occur, the protocol is to stabilize with the supplies in the HMS and then evacuate the affected crewmember to a definitive medical care facility (DMCF) on Earth. The ISS program does not include more than basic surgical capabilities (e.g., laceration repair). Additionally, though there are endotracheal tubes and a portable ventilator for Advanced Cardiac Life Support (ACLS) purposes, there are insufficient supplies to provide regional or intravenous anesthesia for complex operations.

Recent trials have shown that up to 50% of patients may not require surgery for appendicitis over follow-up in terms equivalent to potential Mars missions [63]. How the space flight environment could alter medication stability and efficacy and how these trials' findings apply terrestrial results to deep space missions remain unknown. Small studies suggest most medications remain stable, but some antibiotics decayed prior to set expiration dates [64]. While ISS supplies could support a trial of nonoperative management of diseases such as appendicitis, this is not the current paradigm for treating such Class III events.

Medical Emergencies

In the history of human spaceflight, only three medical evacuations have taken place for prostatitis, dysrhythmias, and severe chronic headaches. This equates to about one medical evacuation per 60 person-years in space.

Trauma management would utilize Advanced Trauma Life Support (ATLS). The patient would be restrained with emergent consultation to ground-based flight surgeons. The airway can be protected with endotracheal intubation or cricothyroidotomy. A portable oximeter, stethoscope, and US could be used to assess oxygenation, ventilation, and the chest and abdomen. Supplemental oxygen can be provided, and a pressure-driven ventilator is also available. The onboard blood pressure monitor can assess perfusion. IV supplies with bubble traps and medications for pain control are also available, but resuscitation fluids are limited. There are no stores of blood on the ISS, with only 4 L of 0.9% normal saline available [36]. Neurologic disability would be assessed clinically. Exposure for missed injuries would be critical. Overall, a similar approach would be used for patients being evaluated for acute surgical emergencies, and the level of the CMO's training would define the potential for the success of such heroic attempts in the austere flight environment.

If the astronauts are able to be stabilized, the pros and cons of evacuation would be weighed by the flight director with input from flight surgeons. Evacuation is not without risk. Pressure suits make ongoing care of the affected crewmember difficult for the patient and CMO. The size of the spacecraft also limits care and the amount of medical supplies able to be transported. There is a risk of advanced shock during the acceleration changes of reentry or when returning to a 1 g environment due to a reduction in plasma volume and baroreceptor deconditioning [48, 60]. Unplanned reentry may be in off-nominal locations and during poor weather conditions. All of these factors will be considered when balancing continued nonoperative management versus evacuation timing for surgical emergencies.

Future Directions

Evolving Role of the Surgeon

Aviation medical standards were initially focused on keeping military aviators operationally ready. The expansion of civilian aviation necessitated the creation of standards for crew and medical recommendations for public passengers. Commercial space travel will diverge from aviation when paying customers travel beyond LEO and rapid evacuation potential. Since 2020, 63 new individuals have flown to space on commercial platforms [65], while 72 individuals have flown on governmental missions. Increasing the number of individuals flying, and changing the diversity of medical risk, creates opportunities for space medicine to build upon its preventive medicine roots. Effectively modeling risk in the changing spacefaring population will require surgical expertise. Risk can then be applied to each mission profile and the surgical capabilities solved. Areas of need will be elucidated based on the balance between risk and launch platform constraints, and innovation in those areas will further reduce mission risk. Those desiring to contribute to the field will benefit from a foundation in preventive medicine fundamentals as well as engineering and biodesign principles to realize the technology needed to make space surgery possible.

Providers trained in trauma and emergency surgical care are well positioned to aid in launch and landing operations. As crewed missions increase, further need in contingency medical response preparedness and response is needed. Knowledge and experience in the areas of disaster preparedness, specific spaceflight hazards, and the physiologic changes of spaceflight are required to successfully provide expert care.

Extended Space Missions

Risk modeling based on in-flight experience from governmental programs that highly select their crew would lead to erroneously low risks for future commercial space missions. Public health data registries for incidence data can be a helpful starting point for commercial mission risk analysis.

From 2016 to 2020, there was an average of 128.44 diagnosis of appendiceal conditions per 100,000 people in the US (0.13% risk per person-year) ([66]; HCUP.NET NEDS reference). This is likely an overestimate for the foreseeable future of commercial spaceflight. For a mission to exceed 1% risk of appendiceal conditions, the mission crew time in space would have to exceed 7.8 person-years. A private space station hosting 30-day visits would need to exceed 95 people to increase the mission risk by 1%. On-orbit surgical capabilities are likely not necessary. Conversely, SpaceX's Starship is designed to hold 100 people while targeting deep space missions. A fully booked Starship mission would need 28.5 days in space to exceed the same metric, and evacuation en route to the Moon or Mars would be delayed if not impossible. Surgical capabilities would decrease mission risk in this scenario.

Future models could take advantage of big data to allow for more accurate analyses by stratifying by specific crew factors. Once mission parameters have been defined and the crew-specific data are collected, surgeries with moderate-to-high rates of anticipated occurrence can be identified. For example, cholecystectomy is the most common inpatient abdominal surgery performed in the US, with an average rate of 100.8 per 100,000 person-years ([67]; HCUP NIP reference). On a 3-year Mars mission with 100 individuals, there would be an approximately 30% risk of someone requiring cholecystectomy. Though preventative medicine principles such as screening for gallstones can reduce in-flight risks, it is still undetermined if it is ethical to require paying customers to undergo prophylactic surgery if stones exist. Thus, the next analysis would identify the amount of risk that could be averted with medical management. Loozen et al. found that up to 87% of patients with acute calculus cholecystitis may be managed conservatively [68]. About 22% of conservatively managed patients recurred, mostly within the first 2 years. These data suggest that the mission risk of cholecystectomy would drop to 3.9%, and operative salvage would more likely be needed early in the mission compared to later, when recurrence could be definitively managed upon return to Earth. The final task would be to determine the resources required for cholecystectomy and to weigh those metrics against the estimated risk.

A single disease and associated operation is only part of the equation. As many of the same tools would be needed in other surgeries that will also present a moderate-to-high risk, a full model of surgical risk is needed to determine what surgeries need to be included in the medical systems.

Training & Preparation

Successful space surgery will rely on building a solid foundation of knowledge, developing a broad surgical skillset, and fostering critical thinking and problem-solving skills to allow the application of the known to the unknown. Basic surgical principles and techniques are shared across surgical specialties, which allows for any surgeon to be trained in the procedures likely to be required. Mentorship is important, and these mentors can take the form of aerospace medical physicians, surgeons across a range of specialties, critical care and medical physicians, and even vehicle and life support system engineers.

Acknowledging that the first surgery in space will likely take place prior to sophisticated technological advancements that allow for a comprehensive operative suite in space, the surgeon will need to be diversely trained and creative. They will need to function as a bedside nurse and be facile with US, the only imaging modality to be flown for the foreseeable future. The surgeon will need to be capable of airway and anesthetic management. Finally, this specialized crewmember will need to be capable of handling a wide variety of emergency procedures, including abdominal and pelvic operations and orthopedic stabilization.

Many opportunities are available for Military medical students, residents, and faculty who are interested in becoming part of the space program, depending on their specific career goals and qualifications. The *NASA Astronaut Selection Program* accepts applications from military personnel with medical training who have relevant professional experience and a high level of physical fitness. *Space Medicine Research & Operations* specializes in collaborating with medical institutions and universities to advance space medicine. *Joint Civil-Military Research and Development* offers Military medical professionals engagement to support joint research and develop projects with NASA or other space agencies. *Educational opportunities* may be offered in military medical schools and residency programs to participate in space medicine electives, rotations, or research projects. This exposure can provide valuable experience and connections within the space medicine community. To pursue these opportunities, military medical professionals should stay informed about space-related initiatives and partnerships, maintain relevant qualifications and experience, and actively seek out collaboration and training opportunities in space medicine and space operations. Networking within professional organizations and attending conferences related to aerospace medicine and space exploration can also be beneficial.

Innovation & Technology

Near-future innovations would focus on the tools needed to bring and sustain terrestrial standards of care to the deep space environment. Reliable, accurate, and reusable point-of-care laboratory tests and US with artificially intelligent image guidance and interpretation support will help with rapid diagnosis. Recyclable needles, syringes, and tubing, in addition to low-profile air-fluid separating pumps, will reduce concern for supply stores. Making previous in-flight crystalloid generation systems more portable and focused on balanced solutions will allow for rehydration on long-duration missions [69]. Once the decision for surgery is indicated, advancements in the areas of virtual reality simulation and artificial intelligence will enhance the surgeon's capabilities. Virtual simulation technologies will allow longitudinal skill maintenance. Carefully crafted just-in-time teaching tools will provide needed insight prior to an operation, and artificially intelligent real-time decision support tools could augment performance. Sterilizable, printable surgical tools, including sutures, will minimize the up-mass required to provide a variety of operations while keeping supplies stocked for the duration of the mission. Minimizing surgical platforms into low-mass/power/volume technologies will be necessary for their inclusion. Wearable or implantable biosensors could help provide perioperative monitoring. With impressive advancements required, investing in space surgical innovation now will give adequate time for technologies to mature in preparation for future deep space missions.

Conclusion

International and commercial cooperation in space travel has been growing significantly, reflecting a shift in the landscape of space exploration and utilization. Conferences, forums, and collaborative initiatives bring together space agencies, industry representatives, and experts from around the world to discuss space-related issues, share knowledge, and explore potential partnerships. These trends signify a shift toward a more inclusive and collaborative approach to space activities, with both international space agencies and commercial entities playing crucial roles. As technology continues to advance and interest in space exploration grows, these trends will continue to evolve, and new forms of international and commercial cooperation in space travel will emerge.

In modern times of Human space exploration, surgical capabilities have not been considered a necessity for space flight. As humans venture further out into the cosmos and spend longer durations in space on exploration class missions, surgical contingencies will be a critical part of mission support. Surgical ability is easily taken for granted to cure and prevent life-threatening complications from common pathologies while on Earth; these same pathologies can lead to loss of life and limb as well as mission failure if surgical capabilities are not available. Reaching level V, or truly autonomous, medical care in space will require the ability to provide surgical and critical care management.

Advancements in space surgical care are crucial for the success of future long-duration space missions and the well-being of astronauts. Improvements in space surgical care benefit astronauts on long-duration space missions and contribute to innovations in terrestrial medicine, especially in remote or resource-limited environments. Ongoing research and collaboration will play a pivotal role in shaping the future of healthcare in space.

References

1. Lebedev V. Diary of a cosmonaut: 211 days in space. Moscow: Nauka I Zhizn; 1983. [English translation c1988 by the G.L.O.S.S. Co.; New York: Bantam Books; September 1990]
2. Campbell MR, Billica RD, Johnston SL. Animal surgery in microgravity. Aviat Space Environ Med. 1993;64:58–62.
3. Campbell MR, Billica RD, Johnston SL. Surgical bleeding in microgravity. Surg Gynecol Obstet. 1993;177:121–5.
4. McCuaig K. Aseptic technique in microgravity. Surg Gynecol Obstet. 1992;175:466–76.
5. McCuaig K. Surgical problems in space: an overview. J Clin Pharmacol. 1994;34:513–7.
6. Pinsolle V, Martin D, de Coninck L, Techoueyres P, Vaida P. Microsurgery in microgravity is possible. Microsurgery. 2005;25:152–4.
7. Kirkpatrick AW, Doarn CR, Campbell MR, Barnes SL, Broderick TJ. Manual suturing quality at acceleration levels equivalent to spaceflight and a lunar base. Aviat Space Environ Med. 2008;79:1065–6.
8. Broderick TJ, Privitera MB, Parazynski SE, Cuttino M. Simulated hand-assisted laparoscopic surgery (HALS) in microgravity. J Laparoendosc Adv Surg Tech A. 2005;15:145–8.
9. Rafiq A, Broderick TJ, Williams DR, Doarn CR, Jones JA, Merrell RC. Assessment of simulated surgical skills in parabolic flight. Aviat Space Environ Med. 2005;76:385–91.
10. Speich JE, Cagle YD, Rafiq A, Merrell RC, Doarn CR, Broderick TJ. Evaluation of surgical skills in microgravity using force sensing. Med Eng Phys. 2005;27(8):687–93.
11. Panait L, Merrell RC, Rafiq A, Dudrick SJ, Broderick TJ. Virtual reality laparoscopic skill assessment in microgravity. J Surg Res. 2006;136(2):198–203.
12. Rafiq A, Hummel R, Lavrentyev V, Derry W, Williams D, Merrell RC. Microgravity effects on fine motor skills: tying surgical knots during parabolic flight. Aviat Space Environ Med. 2006 Aug;77(8):852–6.
13. Panait L, Broderick T, Rafiq A, Speich J, Doarn CR, Merrell RC. Measurement of laparoscopic skills in microgravity anticipates the space surgeon. Am J Surg 2004;188(5):549–552.

14. Campbell MR, Dawson DL, Melton S, et al. Surgical instrument restraint in weightlessness. Aviat Space Environ Med. 2001;72:871–6.
15. Campbell MR, Williams DR, Buckey JC Jr, Kirkpatrick AW. Animal surgery during spaceflight on the Neurolab Shuttle mission. Aviat Space Environ Med. 2005;76(6):589–93.
16. Smith MG, Kelley M, Basner M. A brief history of spaceflight from 1961 to 2020: an analysis of missions and astronaut demographics. Acta Astronaut. 2020;175:290–9. https://doi.org/10.1016/j.actaastro.2020.06.004.
17. NASA-STD-3001, NASA Space Flight Human System Standard, Vol. 1, Revision A: Crew Health. Approved: 07-30-2014.
18. NASA-STD-3001, NASA Space Flight Human System Standard, Vol. 1, Revision B: Crew Health. Approved: 01-05-2022.
19. Artemis. National Aeronautics and Space Administration. Accessed Nov 25, 2023. https://www.nasa.gov/specials/artemis/.
20. The Moon. SpaceX. Accessed Nov 25, 2023. https://www.spacex.com/human-spaceflight/moon/.
21. A Crewed Mission to Mars. National Aeronautics and Space Administration. Updated Nov 16, 2015. Accessed Nov 25, 2023. https://nssdc.gsfc.nasa.gov/planetary/mars/marsprof.html.
22. VAST Announces the Haven-1 and VAST-1 Missions. VAST Space LLC. Updated May 10, 2023. Accessed Nov 25, 2023. https://www.vastspace.com/updates/vast-announces-the-haven-1-and-vast-1-human-spaceflight-mission-launched-by-spacex-on-a-dragon-spacecraft.
23. Artemis Plan, NASA's Lunar Exploration Program Overview. Approved: Sept 2020.
24. International Cooperation. National Aeronautics and Space Administration. Updated Sept 27, 2023. Accessed Nov 28, 2023. https://www.nasa.gov/international-space-station/space-station-international-cooperation/.
25. USSPACECOM Deputy Commander Discusses Deep Space Exploration. US Space Command. Updated Oct 25, 2022. Accessed Nov 25, 2023. https://www.spacecom.mil/Newsroom/News/Article-Display/Article/3198458/usspacecom-deputy-commander-discusses-deep-space-exploration/.
26. Human Space Flight. Federal Aviation Administration. Updated Oct 4, 2023. Accessed Nov 25, 2023. https://www.faa.gov/space/human_space-flight
27. Nilsson JH. Chapter 5: Low-cost aviation. In: Gossling S, Upham P, editors. Climate change and aviation: issues, challenges, and solutions. 1st ed. Earthscan; 2009. p. 113–30.
28. The VASIMR Engine. Ad Astra Rocket Company. Accessed Nov 27, 2023. https://www.adastrarocket.com/our-engine/

29. McBrayer KT, Chai PR, Judd EL. Communication Delays, Disruptions, and Blackouts for Crewed Mars Missions. Presented at: ASCEND; Oct 24-26, 2022; Las Vegas, NV.
30. Communications with Earth. MARS Reconnaissance Orbiter. Accessed Nov 27, 2023. https://mars.nasa.gov/mro/mission/communications/
31. Haidegger T. In-space surgery: impact of robotic technology on future exploration missions. In: Proceedings of iSAIRAS08—9th International Symposium on Artificial Intelligence, Robotics and Automation in Space; 2008.
32. Falcon Heavy. SpaceX. Accessed Nov 27, 2023. https://www.spacex.com/vehicles/falcon-heavy/.
33. Jones HW. The recent large reduction in space launch cost. In: Presented at: 48th International Conference on Environmental Systems; July 8–12, 2018; Albequerque, NM.
34. Orion. National Aeronautics and Space Administration. Accessed Nov 27, 2023. https://www.nasa.gov/specials/orionfirstflight/
35. DSG-RQMT-001, Gateway Systems Requirements. Released: 06-27-2019.
36. International Space Station CHeCS Medical Hardware Catalog: Version 8.2. Released: 11–2008.
37. Mars Fact Sheet. National Aeronautics and Space Administration. Updated Sept 29, 2023. Accessed Nov 27, 2023. https://nssdc.gsfc.nasa.gov/planetary/factsheet/marsfact.html.
38. Moon Fact Sheet. National Aeronautics and Space Administration. Updated Dec 20, 2021. Accessed Nov 27, 2023. https://nssdc.gsfc.nasa.gov/planetary/factsheet/moonfact.html.
39. Houtchens B. Medical care systems for long-duration space missions. Clin Chem 1992;39:13–21.
40. McCuaig K, Houtchens B. Management of trauma and emergency surgery in space. J Trauma. 1992;33:610–25.
41. Taddeo TA, Gilmore S, Armstrong CW. Chapter 6: Spaceflight medical systems. In: Barratt MR, Baker ES, Pool SL, editors. Principles of clinical medicine for space flight. 2nd ed. Springer; 2019. p. 201–32.
42. Stazhadze LL, Goncharov IB, Neumyzakin IP, et al. Anesthesia, surgical aid and resuscitation in manned space missions. Acta Astronaut. 1981;8:1109.
43. Yaroshenko GL, Terentiev VG, Mokrov MN. Characteristics of surgical intervention in conditions of weightlessness. Voenn Med Zh. 1967;10:69–70.
44. James JT. Environmental health monitoring results for STS-40/space life sciences 1 (SLS-1). In: Spacelab life sciences-1 final report, vol. 1. Houston: NASA–Johnson Space Center; 1994. JSC-26786.

45. Pierson DL, Viktorov AN. Microbiological investigations of the Mir space station and flight crew. In: Shuttle-mir science program phase 1A research postflight science report. Unpublished NASA document. NASA–Johnson Space Center: Houston; 1998.
46. Fu Shaw L, Chen IH, Chen CS, et al. Factors influencing microbial colonies in the air of operating rooms. BMC Infect Dis. 2018;18(1):4. Published 2018 Jan 2. https://doi.org/10.1186/s12879-017-2928-1.
47. Alfrey CP, Udden MM, Leach-Huntoon C, Driscoll T, Pickett MH. Control of red blood cell mass in spaceflight. J Appl Physiol. 1996;81(1):98–104.
48. Johnson PC, Driscoll TB, LeBlanc AD. Blood volume changes. In: Johnston R, Dietlein L, editors. Biomedical results of Skylab. Washington: Scientific and Technical Information Office, NASA; 1977. p. 235–41.
49. Kimzey SL. Hematology and immunology studies. In: Johnston RS, Dietlein LF, editors. Biomedical results from Skylab. Washington: Scientific and Technical Information Office, NASA; 1977. p. 249–82.
50. Marshall-Goebel K, Laurie SS, Alferova IV, et al. Assessment of jugular venous blood flow stasis and thrombosis during spaceflight [published correction appears in JAMA Netw Open. 2020 Jan 3;3(1):e1920195]. JAMA Netw Open. 2019;2(11):e1915011. https://doi.org/10.1001/jamanetworkopen.2019.15011.
51. Auñón-Chancellor SM, Pattarini JM, Moll S, Sargsyan A. Venous thrombosis during spaceflight. N Engl J Med. 2020;382(1):89–90. https://doi.org/10.1056/NEJMc1905875.
52. Kim DS, Vaquer S, Mazzolai L, et al. The effect of microgravity on the human venous system and blood coagulation: a systematic review. Exp Physiol. 2021;106(5):1149–58. https://doi.org/10.1113/EP089409.
53. Sears JK, Arzenyi ZE. Cutaneous wound healing in space. Cutis. 1991;48:307–8.
54. Davidson J, Aquino A, Woodward S, et al. Sustained microgravity reduces intrinsic wound healing and growth factor responses in the rat. FASEB J. 1999;13:325–9.
55. Kaplansky A, Durnova G, Burkovskaya T, et al. The effect of microgravity on bone fracture healing in rats flown on Cosmos 2044. Physiologist. 1991;34:S196–9.
56. Kirchen ME, O'Connor KM, Gruber HE, et al. Effects of microgravity on bone healing in a rat fibular osteotomy model. Clin Orthop. 1995;318:231–42.
57. Campbell MR, Billica RD, Jennings R, et al. Laparoscopic surgery in weightlessness. Surg Endosc. 1996;10:111–7.
58. NASA-STD-3001, NASA Space Flight Human System Standard, Volume 2, Revision D: Human Factors, Habitability, and Environmental Health. Approved: 09-15-2023.
59. Ad Hoc Committee of Members of the Space Medicine Association and the Society of NASA Flight Surgeons. Human health and performance for long-duration spaceflight. Aviat Space Environ Med. 2008;79:629–37.

60. Campbell MR, Billica RD. Chapter 7: Surgical capabilities. In: Barratt MR, Baker ES, Pool SL, editors. Principles of clinical medicine for space flight. 2nd ed. Springer; 2019. p. 233–52.
61. Ball CG, Kirkpatrick AW, Williams DR, et al. Prophylactic surgery prior to extended-duration space flight: is the benefit worth the risk? Can J Surg. 2012;55(2):125–31.
62. Reyes DP, Carroll DJ, Walton ME, et al. Probabilistic risk assessment of prophylactic surgery before extended-duration spaceflight. Surg Innov. 2021;28(5):573–81.
63. CODA Collaborative. A randomized trial comparing antibiotics with appendectomy for appendicitis (CODA). N Engl J Med. 2020;383(20):1907–19.
64. Du B, et al. Evaluation of physical and chemical changes in pharmaceuticals flown on space missions. AAPS J. 2011;13:299–308.
65. FAA Commercial Human Space Flight Recognition. Federal Aviation Administration. Updated Oct 26, 2023. Accessed Nov 28, 2023. https://www.faa.gov/space/human_spaceflight/recognition.
66. HCUP Nationwide Emergency Department Sample (NEDS). Healthcare Cost and Utilization Project (HCUP). 2007, 2008, 2009. Rockville, MD: Agency for Healthcare Research and Quality. www.hcup-us.ahrq.gov/nedsoverview.jsp
67. HCUP National Inpatient Sample (NIS). Healthcare cost and utilization project (HCUP). Rockville, MD: Agency for Healthcare Research and Quality; 2012. www.hcup-us.ahrq.gov/nisoverview.jsp
68. Loozen CS, Oor JE, van Ramshorst B, et al. Conservative treatment of acute cholecystitis: a systematic review and pooled analysis. Surg Endosc. 2017;31(2):504–15.
69. IV Fluid Generation. National Aeronautics and Space Administration. Updated Feb 15, 2022. Accessed Nov 28, 2023. https://www1.grc.nasa.gov/space/human-research-program/exploration-medical-technologies/iv-fluid-generation/#the-research.

Part IV

Life Outside of the Operating Room

Maximizing Military Finances

30

Bradley C. Bandera
and Pamela L. Burgess

Start with the End in Mind

Begin with the end in mind. Numerous retirement calculators are available for free on the internet. Utilize several to estimate the required retirement fund. In a study conducted by Qianwen et al., examining outputs from five popular US retirement planning calculators revealed substantial variability due to differing assumptions and inputs. The resulting outputs varied significantly, even for straightforward financial retirement scenarios [1].

Planning for retirement involves considering over 20 factors. Important elements highlighted by nerdwallet.com include annual

Disclaimer: The views expressed in this chapter are those of the authors and do not necessarily reflect the position or policy of the Department of Veterans Affairs or the United States Government.
Disclosure: This article utilized AI for formatting and grammar. The content and thought contained here is purely the work of the authors. It is also not a substitute for individual financial advice.

B. C. Bandera (✉)
University of Nevada School of Medicine, Ioannis A. Lougaris Veterans' Administration Medical Center, Reno, NV, USA
e-mail: Bradley.Bandera@VA.gov

P. L. Burgess
University of Minnesota School of Medicine, Colon and Rectal Surgery Associates, Minneapolis, MN, USA

A. T. Schlussel et al. (eds.), *The SAGES Manual for Navigating a Successful Military Surgical Career*,
https://doi.org/10.1007/978-3-031-88490-0_30

pretax income, current retirement savings, monthly contributions, retirement budget, and additional income sources. It is crucial to adjust for inflation [2]. The Federal Reserve aims for a 2% annual inflation rate, although calculators often vary, with some using 2.5% or 3%. Additionally, factor in the retirement age and required retirement funds. Rates of return pre- and post-retirement typically differ, as many retirees shift savings into less volatile, historically safer investment options.

The objective of investing is to generate sufficient income for later years or when one cannot work. Intentionally avoiding the phrase "save enough money," investing involves allocating a portion of wages into appreciating investments. The individualized goal is often to earn returns surpassing the inflation rate. The extent above inflation depends on an individual's risk tolerance. This leads to discussions on conservative versus risky investing vehicles, which is often a misunderstood concept.

Consider the fallacy of being overly conservative with money, when in fact, inflation erodes the value of stagnant funds. Over 98% of the dollar's purchasing power vanished from 1900 to 2010 [1]. Since 1999, the dollar's value plummeted when compared to gold, losing 80% of that 98%. The loss of purchasing power is only accelerating. To preserve purchasing power, funds must at least match inflation rates. Over the last decade, inflation ranged from below 1% to just above 9%, according to the Consumer Price Index (CPI) [2]. In 2022, the Federal Reserve issued seven consecutive federal funds rate increases to combat inflation. Between March and December, the federal funds rate increased from 0.25% to 4.25%. But banks were slow to raise savings account interest rates. In fact, savings accounts sat at an average national rate of 0.10% or below through July despite a rapidly increasing federal funds rate. National average savings rates hit 0.30% in late December [3]. As Robert Kiyosaki bluntly puts it, "Savers are losers!" Their money's worth diminishes over time due to inflation. Investing entails calculated risks with the money earned put into an investment to outpace inflation and maintain or increase purchasing power.

What Type of Investor Are You?

This is largely broken down into two major categories: passive versus active. This also may change over time. Passive investors know the basics about investing and often use more experienced professionals to invest their money. They frequently invest through a company- or agency-based savings plan like a tax-advantaged retirement plan. This involves a more hands-off approach, where investors aim to replicate the performance of a specific market index or asset class. This strategy often entails investing in index funds or exchange-traded funds (ETFs) that track the market's overall movement. On the other hand, active investing is a more dynamic approach, requiring hands-on management and decision-making. Active investors strive to outperform the market by making strategic choices based on their analysis of individual securities, market trends, and economic indicators.

For military surgeons navigating the demanding landscape of residency, frequent moves, and deployments where communication access is not always reliable, passive investing might be the pragmatic choice. The time constraints inherent in the profession can be the equivalent of two full-time jobs and may make it challenging to conduct the necessary research and monitoring required for active investment strategies. However, as one progresses beyond residency and gains more control over their schedule, the transition to active investing becomes a plausible option. Becoming a proficient active investor demands a deep understanding of the chosen investment vehicles, a significant time commitment, and intellectual honesty about one's capabilities for success in the complex financial landscape. Listening to seasoned investors like Warren Buffet, Howard Marks, Ray Dalio, or Ken Griffin can offer valuable insights and a humbling reminder of the vast knowledge required to navigate macroeconomics, technical analysis, central banking, commodities, currencies, equities, and the bond market effectively. It is crucial for physicians to be candid with themselves about their aptitude, available time, and the potential outcomes of their investment decisions.

Time in the Market and Not Timing the Market

Start Early

Getting started early with investing is fundamental yet often overlooked. The ideal moment to begin never truly arrives as life continually presents expenses and unforeseen costs. But as Robert Kiyosaki, the author of "Rich Dad Poor Dad," emphasizes, "Pay yourself first" [4]. Regardless of bills, allocate at least $100 of your pay now; the objective is to aim for 10% of your pay monthly, but just starting somewhere is crucial. Albert Einstein aptly noted, "Compound interest is the eighth wonder of the world. He who understands it, earns it. He who doesn't understand it, pays it." This concept is vividly illustrated in examples from principal.com [5]. Imagine setting aside $100 a month for 30 years: the saver accumulates only $41,876.65 at a 1% interest rate. Furthermore, with 2% annual inflation, the saver continually loses value over time. In contrast, the investor, with a 6% interest rate, amasses $95,444.17, more than double the amount saved.

Another compelling illustration involves two investors: One starts at 25 and invests $12,000 annually for 15 years, totaling $180,000. By age 67, they enjoy $1,346,939.00. The second investor commences at 35, invests $12,000 annually for 30 years (totaling $360,000), and by age 67 accumulates $948,698.00. The investor beginning 10 years earlier, investing half the amount ($180,000 versus $360,000), gains $398,241.00 more. This vividly demonstrates the significance of time in the market over timing the market. Begin early, even if it is just with $25 in undergraduate or graduate school; the impact of starting early is significant.

Debt Versus No Debt

This is a highly contentious topic, and much like the real world, nothing is simply black or white. Is all debt inherently bad? The answer is found in shades of gray; it depends. Let us consider a few examples to delve into this. Imagine a scenario with a $10,000 credit card balance, subject to a 21.24% annual percentage rate (APR)—the current interest rate listed on my Chase Sapphire Reserve card. In this instance, one pays $2124 in interest. However, if that $2124 was invested at a 6% APR for 12 months instead of accruing interest, it would grow to $2255. Moving on to the car loan, a $50,000 new car acquired with a 10% interest rate incurs an annual interest of $5000. Simultaneously, the vehicle depreciates by 9–11% the moment it leaves the car lot, resulting in an approximate $10,000 loss within a year. Contrasting this with an investment property involving a $10,000 down payment, the property generates a 7% annual return on investment post-expenses. This amounts to a $700 annual profit along with the four significant benefits of property ownership: asset appreciation, tax advantages from depreciation, monthly cash flow, and equity accumulation through mortgage payments. By reinvesting the $700 yearly income, one can significantly expand their investment. Is all debt universally detrimental? The reader holds the ultimate judgment.

At Least Manage Your Debt

Soldiers and Sailors Relief Act Now Called The Servicemembers Civil Relief Act

This is a benefit to those service members on active duty for 30 days or more and is designed with the goal of allowing the member to focus solely on his or her service to the country and to minimize any financial distractions [6]. There are five major benefits. But first, to whom does it apply? It applies to active-duty members of the Army, Marine Corps, Navy, Air Force, and Coast Guard. It also applies to members of the Reserve component when serving on active duty as well as National Guard component mobilized under Federal orders for at least 30 consecutive days. Also included are commissioned officers of the Public Health Service and National Oceanic and Atmospheric Administration.

The benefits include lowering your interest rate to a minimum of 6% on any preservice: home loan, car loan, student debt, or credit debt while on active duty. This does not include debt incurred while on active duty. As an example, if the service member opens a credit card while on active duty, they are subject to the current interest rate. This exists only for preservice debts.

The law also protects against default judgments in any civil cases while on active duty. A court cannot enter a default civil judgment without first filing an affidavit stating whether you are or are not on active duty. If facing a defualt judgement and on active duty for the requisite amount of time but unable to secure an attorney,the court must appoint one to represent the service member.

The third pillar of the act prevents foreclosure without a court order on a home loan obtained prior to active-duty service. This even applies to states that do not require a court order to foreclose. As part of this benefit, a court must also pause or stay a foreclosure if the active-duty service materially affects the ability to pay the loan. The example that comes to mind is a private practice surgeon who is called to active duty with a large pay discrepancy between their private practice and military service, resulting in the inability to make their mortgage payments, resulting in default and foreclosure.

Along those lines, the Service Members Relief Act prevents repossession of any personal property such as a car without a court order. This is as long as the purchase or deposit was made prior to active service. They will eventually be able to repossess the property, but it requires they obtain a court order before doing so.

Finally, the final pillar of protection allows for service members to break any lease entered into prior to active service. This allows them to make any necessary move to accommodate the active-duty service without the hassles and headaches of breaking a lease and the associated fees. Additionally, this applies to any deployment or permanent change of station (PCS) move greater than 90 days.

VA Home Loan

The Veterans Administration (VA) home loan is another potential benefit of military service. The home must be the Service Member's primary residence. This is where the member lives the majority of the year and can prove it. The service member is eligible if they have served for 90 continuous days on active duty [7]. There are some caveats to this rule if the buyer has served less time and numerous caveats if the buyer is a veteran. See the eligibility requirements at VA.gov or follow the references in this chapter.

The benefits are numerous and may be used to purchase or refinance an existing primary residence. The loan requires no money down as long as the home appraises for the sales price or more. If the home does not appraise, the buyer would be responsible for making up the difference. Before paying the difference, ask the seller to lower the price or strongly consider walking away from the property. VA loans typically have a lower interest rate than conventional mortgages and do not require private mortgage insurance (PMI). There is no limit to the amount you can borrow to finance the home. There is no minimum credit score to obtain a VA loan, but lenders do have a minimum credit score, so be sure to check with multiple lenders to get the best terms based on the Service Member's credit. The home may be eligible for additional grants for modifications due to service-connected disabilities. There is no penalty for early loan repayment. The benefit may be used multiple times throughout the Service Member's life. Please see VA.gov for additional details regarding this outstanding benefit.

Let us briefly explain some more about PMI. PMI is a type of mortgage insurance the buyer is usually required to purchase on a conventional loan. The insurance protects the lender if the buyer stops making payments. This is usually required if the purchaser puts less than 20% down due to the perceived increased risk of making the loan or when refinancing and the equity in the home does not meet the 20% threshold. Conversely, if you have a conventional loan and are paying PMI. The owner can ask that it be removed after the equity in the home exceeds 20% of the value [8].

Military Investing

Military finances bring into focus two crucial elements: the Thrift Savings Plan (TSP) and the Blended Retirement System (BRS), tailored to the retirement of military personnel. Much like a 401(k) in the private sector, the TSP/BRS serves as a tax-advantaged vehicle for retirement savings. The Blended Retirement System, introduced in 2018, replaced the conventional 20-year model with a more adaptable structure, offering both defined benefit and defined contribution components. Key features include contributions, government matching, tax advantages, and various investment options, each presenting distinct levels of return and risk. Additionally, a significant facet of the BRS is the implementation of a defined benefit referred to as Continuation Pay. This one-time bonus is extended to service members committing to an additional four years of service after 12 years of completed service. The bonus amount fluctuates based on various factors, including the service member's military occupational specialty and other relevant criteria.

Concerning contributions, three types warrant consideration: elective deferral, catch-up contributions, and employer contributions, also known as employer matching. Contribution limits are subject to change; for 2023, elective contributions are capped at $22,500 annually, sourced from one's paycheck. The catch-up contribution permits an additional $7,500 for individuals aged over 50. These funds are deducted monthly and can be adjusted using MyPay. Notably, deployment to a combat zone impacts TSP contributions, where contributions become tax-exempt, but future earnings are taxable. However, contribution limits remain unchanged even if a service member has worked for another federal agency, as multiple federal employments are regarded as a single employer.

How to Read Your Leave and Earnings Statement (LES)

Start with the basics. Know where your money is coming from and make sure there are no errors. The army is a big organization, and they are known to make mistakes. You can be short money, but also watch for a paycheck that is bigger than anticipated. Or entitlements that you are no longer eligible for (for example, imminent danger pay after returning from deployment), ceasing on time. They will always make things square by paying you back in a taxed lump sum or by garnishing your wages in an amount that is not feasible with your responsibilities.

Check back routinely. Just because you corrected a zip code or marital status, does not mean it stays corrected. Or if things change, such as marriage or dependents, make sure you proceed to the finance office to submit the appropriate updates. Pay attention to the comments on the bottom of the LES. They make announcements, describe corrections made to the pay and identify any debt or wage garnishment and are found in the text at the bottom.

Base Pay: This is your monthly amount of pay based on rank and time in service. This will go up as rates are increased. This is taxed.

BAS (Basic Allowance for Subsistence): This is an allotment for things like groceries and necessities at home. If you are housed on post and have DFAC privileges, you may not be entitled to this. This is nontaxable.

COLA (Cost of Living Allowance): If you live in areas of the USA that have a higher cost of living, you may receive this entitlement. This is taxable. An OCONUS COLA is nontaxable.

BAH (Basic Allowance for Housing): This is an allotment to secure housing. It is based on region and rank, and dependent status. If you are a dual military home, you both get BAH. This is not taxed. If you are assigned post housing, you do not receive this allotment.

Incentive Pay: This is the money you get from the military in its way to try and match the gap between military grade and civilian wages by specialty. This is used as an incentive to keep people with special skills in the service. There is also a bonus once board certification is achieved. This is taxable.

Deployment Specific Pay

HDP (Hardship Duty Pay): $50 per month, when stationed in an area noted to be dangerous, commonly on a combat tour. Nontaxable.

IDP (Imminent danger pay): $225/month for deployment to an area where there is risk of exposure to hostile fire or other ordinance. This is nontaxable.

FSH (Family separation pay): $250/month for deployed soldiers with families, nontaxable.

Kuwait, which can be a common location for deployment of medical personnel, is not considered a combat tour. No IDP or HDP is authorized. FSH is authorized.

TSP and Taxes

The government also contributes to the individual's TSP, notably through matching contributions within the BRS. A standard 1% contribution is automatically made to the TSP for all service members, irrespective of their personal contributions. Moreover, there is a matching contribution for the first 5% of a service member's pay, amplifying the potential for long-term savings. However, it is essential to note that this 5% matching occurs monthly. Therefore, if a service member maxes out their contributions within, say, 10 months, they forfeit the government match for the remaining 2 months. This emphasizes the importance of understanding the monthly match, even if it seemingly contradicts the idea of early market entry for funds invested in the TSP. While the TSP allows investment in chosen funds, it is crucial not to overlook the employer's 5% match.

One of the primary benefits of TSP is that it offers a tax advantage. Contributions to the traditional TSP are made with pretax dollars. This has the advantage of reducing your taxable income in the year the contribution will be made. This is different from a Roth TSP. Contributions to the Roth TSP are done with after-tax dollars. However, withdrawals are tax-free. The paramount consideration between how to contribute being will your retirement tax bracket be higher or lower than your current tax bracket.

Imagine you are a military surgeon with a current annual salary of $100,000, placing you in the 24% tax bracket. You are debating whether to contribute to the traditional or Roth TSP.

Scenario 1: Traditional TSP Contribution

- You decide to contribute $10,000 annually to the traditional TSP.
- As this is a pretax contribution, your taxable income for that year reduces to $90,000 ($100,000–$10,000).
- Given the 24% tax bracket, you will pay 24% in taxes on the remaining taxable income, which amounts to $21,600.
- Your take-home pay after contributing to the traditional TSP is $78,400 ($100,000–$21,600).

Scenario 2: Roth TSP Contribution

- Opting for the Roth TSP, you contribute the same $10,000 annually from your after-tax income.
- Your taxable income remains $100,000 for the year.
- At a 24% tax rate, you will pay $24,000 in taxes on the full $100,000.

In both scenarios, you are investing $10,000 into the TSP. However, the key difference lies in when you pay taxes on that money. With the traditional TSP, you reduce your taxable income immediately, paying taxes later when you withdraw the funds during retirement. Meanwhile, with the Roth TSP, you pay taxes upfront, and all withdrawals in retirement are tax-free.

The choice between traditional and Roth TSP hinges on whether you anticipate being in a higher or lower tax bracket during retirement compared to your current bracket. If you expect your retirement bracket to be lower, the traditional TSP might save you more in taxes. However, if you foresee a higher retirement tax bracket, the Roth TSP's tax-free withdrawals could be more beneficial.

TSP and loans: Within the scope of TSP tax advantages lie the provision of low-interest TSP loans accessible to contributors. Participants in the TSP program can lend money to themselves at a low-interest rate, repayable along with interest through regular monthly payroll deductions. According to the TSP website, the interest rate remains constant throughout the loan's term, aligning with the G Fund's interest rate from the preceding month when the loan request was made. TSP offers two types of loans: a general-purpose loan and a primary residence loan, with a minimum borrowing threshold of $1000. The maximum allowable borrowing stands at 50% of the vested account balance or $50,000, whichever is less, considering both personal contributions, earnings, and any existing loan balances, which diminish the available borrowing limit. So, essentially one can take out a low-interest rate loan from their investment funds and pay themselves back. This serves as an effective means to sidestep the need to sell investments to cover significant planned or unplanned expenses, thereby avoiding short or long-term capital gains taxes based on the investment holding duration.

TSP and investing: Investment options for TSP include several different types of investment funds focusing on different areas. Briefly, there are four broad asset classes: debt (bonds), currencies, commodities (hard like gold and silver versus soft like wheat and sugar) and equities (stocks). TSP offers five core funds meant to cover two of those asset classes: (debt and equity) across various market segments. The funds are managed through Blackrock Capital Advisers. Four of the five funds are index funds which hold securities matching a broad market index. Let us discuss the funds each in a little more detail. For additional details, one can visit www.TSP.gov. Most accounts contain a collection of the funds to offer stability in variety. Decisions which fund to invest in can be made using the investment tool above.

G Fund

The Government Securities Investment Fund (G Fund) invests in treasuries not available to the public. These government treasury certificates are issued specifically for TSP and are the only fund that guarantees the return of the investor's principal.

F Fund

The Fixed Income Fund (F Fund) is another debt instrument. This is an index type fund that invests in a wide range of debt instruments from publicly traded treasury and government securities to corporate and foreign debt/bonds. This fund does pay monthly interest and unlike the G Fund does not guarantee the return of investor's principal.

C Fund

The Common Stock Index Fund (C Fund) is an index fund that invests in the 500 large and mid-cap companies. This is based on the Standard and Poor's (S&P 500) market capitalization weighted index of the 500 leading publicly traded companies in the United States. The index is considered one of the most suitable gauges of large American companies' equity performance.

S Fund

Small Capitalization Stock Index Fund (S Fund) holds securities that is the same as the Dow Jones US Completion Total Market Index. Importantly, this index is composed of 4500 companies outside of the S&P Index. These companies are smaller with historically more potential for growth.

I Fund

The International Stock Index Fund (I Fund) invests in equities mirroring the Europe, Australia, and Far East index as constructed by Morgan Stanley. It is meant to be a broad international index investing in more established companies which are larger. It invests in 20–25 companies in developed countries around the world.

L Fund

The Lifecycle Fund (L Fund) represents a composite fund strategically amalgamating various funds listed within the TSP program. Engineered to suit participants preferring automated portfolio management, the L Fund is meticulously managed by Blackrock. Its primary objective is to cater to contributors who opt out of making personalized allocations. The fund's strategy is structured to emphasize a heavier stock allocation during earlier stages, gradually transitioning toward a more pronounced bond emphasis as the target date nears. An important note about the L Fund is that the designated target date might not precisely align with an individual's retirement age. Instead, it revolves around a specified target date to adjust the fund's risk exposure and asset allocation, which may or may not mirror the retiree's actual retirement age.

Other Investment Opportunities

Deployed service members have access to specialized high-interest savings programs tailored to their circumstances. These programs are specifically designed to provide favorable financial avenues for military personnel in active combat zones. One such initiative is the Savings Deposit Program (SDP), allowing deployed service members to invest up to $10,000 in designated combat zones at a high-interest rate, currently capped at 10% annually. In order to be eligible service members must be deployed in a designated combat zone for at least 30 days or one day in each of the three consecutive months and receiving either Hostile Fire Pay (HFP) or IDP. The program offers a unique opportunity for individuals serving in qualifying areas to grow their savings substantially, well beyond typical savings account interest rates. The SDP's elevated interest rates make it an attractive option for those deployed, enabling them to amass savings at a rate far higher than traditional banking institutions typically offer. This program not only encourages financial prudence but also rewards service members for their dedication and service in challenging deployment environments, providing them with a secure and lucrative means to accumulate savings during their deployment. Not everyone has $10,000 that can sit somewhere untouched for 6 months, but if you had even $5000, you could have an extra few hundred dollars earned during your tour based on the length of your deployment. Money deposited will continue to accrue interest up to 90 days after leaving the combat zone, meaning you can maximize even a 4.5 month tour [9].

Think About Your Home of Record

Throughout one's military career, a service member will live in multiple locations and likely multiple states. The military allows the service member to designate any state they have previously lived in as their home state. The state the service member chooses to designate as their home state directly affects their net take-home pay. Let us examine the 5 states with the highest state income tax rates as of 2022: California, Hawaii, Oregon, Minnesota, and New York. These states will take an additional 1–13% of the service members' income on top of the Federal Government. While Alaska, Florida, Nevada, South Dakota, and Texas are a few of the states that do not have state income tax. Consider choosing one of these states as the service members' home state to minimize their tax burden. Keeping in mind that you should have a connection or intention to return to the state at some point to reside.

Common Pitfalls: Guidelines to Avoid Trouble

As a service member, falling prey to high-interest loans and predatory lenders, as well as individuals seeking access to your finances, is a potential risk. Deployments, despite their tax advantages, can strain one's finances, often leading to granting someone else access to your accounts. While modern internet services facilitate bill payments and income management, unfortunate situations can still arise, leaving you to pick up the pieces. It is crucial to make sound decisions and plan ahead. Obtaining a power of attorney (POA) to enlist family help in addressing home issues is convenient, but ensure it is limited to specific matters. Although it might seem tempting to grant broad POA, there are pitfalls. Such as returning home to discover a boat or new car loan your family member cosigned in your name because of an unrestricted arrangement. Think through who is granted your POA. How long have you known them? What is their financial track record? Are they a temporary or permanent fixture in your life? There are many things to consider when granting a limited or general POA.

Other Low Hanging Fruit

For seasoned military personnel, these aspects might seem familiar, but for newcomers, understanding your expected earnings is crucial. Staying updated on bonus details and their payout schedules is essential. Although the army will eventually square things up, discrepancies are easier to address when they first arise. Familiarize yourself with your entitlements, ensuring timely hazard duty or family separation pay while being cautious not to accept overpayments, as they can be swiftly reclaimed with interest.

Additionally, take advantage of reimbursements offered for various expenses. While paying out of pocket may seem simpler, many support systems are available, covering board expenses, equipment, mileage, travel, and research.

It is impossible to cover all financial management aspects for military surgeons here, but this should prompt self-reflection and encourage further education. The resources provided can guide you toward more comprehensive knowledge on this topic. Each soldier's circumstances differ, involving various income levels and family dynamics. When uncertain, seek help from experienced individuals for personalized advice. Often underutilized military resources include Military One Source [10] and MyPAY [11]—spend time familiarizing yourself with your LES. The SCRA is a valuable benefit, capping preservice loans' interest rates at 6% [6].

Leverage the GI Bill for additional education, ensuring timely enrollment or transfer [12]. Also, the GI Bill can be attained by a servicemember but passed along to relatives. As a surgeon, most are not likely to need the GI Bill, but it can pay for undergraduate education of their children or graduate education for their spouse. Keep a close eye on bonuses, as they fluctuate yearly, often with changing requirements, potentially extending your military service, which might not be unfavorable.

Timing Your Exit from Service: It May or May Not Be Financially Beneficial to Stay the Full 20 [13]

Not everyone has the ability to make the decision on when to leave active service based on finances alone. Family situation often plays a role in deciding to stay on active duty. From purely a monetary position, it may or may not make sense. But if just considering the monetary component, consider the below scenario:

Comparing the military retirement outcomes between an O5 leaving service at 10 years and an O6 retiring after 20 years reveals substantial differences in financial trajectories. Assuming both individuals start their service at age 26 as Captains in the

Army and plan to stop working at age 67 while moving to Nebraska to earn the average general surgeon salary after leaving the military, the disparities are evident. The O5, leaving at 10 years, would enter the civilian workforce at age 36, gaining approximately 31 years of earning potential. Meanwhile, the O6, retiring after 20 years, would start civilian life at age 46, allowing for roughly 21 years of civilian employment. The extended civilian work period for the O5 would likely accumulate higher total earnings over the span of their civilian career, potentially outweighing the retirement benefits gained by the O6 due to the earlier start in the civilian workforce and the additional years of higher civilian income. Ultimately, this comparison underscores the trade-offs between immediate civilian career entry and the benefits of a longer military service in retirement planning for military physicians.

The retirement benefits for an O6 with 20 years of service typically include a pension worth 50% of their base pay, assuming 3 years at that rank and pay. Using the calculated base pay for an O6 retiring after 20 years (around $139,668 annually), the retirement pension would be approximately $69,834 annually.

For the 21 years of civilian work after retirement at age 46, the O6 would accrue retirement benefits totaling around 21 * $69,834 = $1,466,014.

So, considering both civilian earnings and retirement benefits:

- The O5 retiring at 10 years and starting civilian work at age 36 would accumulate around $13,175,000 in civilian earnings over 31 years.

- The O6 retiring at 20 years and starting civilian work at age 46 would earn approximately $8,925,000 in civilian income and accrue retirement benefits of roughly $1,466,014.

These figures showcase the difference in overall earnings between the two scenarios, emphasizing the impact of prolonged civilian employment for the O5 compared to the combined civilian earnings and retirement benefits for the O6.

Another consideration, if time and space allow, would be to extend service via the reserves. For those who participated in the

HPSP program, this would allow you to take advantage of the years of individual ready reserve (IRR) that you participated in during medical school. These years are added to retirement in a one for one fashion. For example, if you left active service at 14 years, and you complete 3 years in the reserves, you earn 3 of your IRR years back which gets you to 20 years of service and consideration for retirement from the reserves. You make it 4 years in the reserves, you get all 4 of your medical school years for 22 years of service for retirement. Not everyone can have extra military service on top of a full-time physician job, but it may be worthwhile to have some discussions on how it could fit into your new lifestyle. The reserve program can be associated with several lump sum annual bonuses that can have an impact on your investment portfolio. This is based on the needs of the Army, but as of the writing of this chapter the general surgery bonus in the Army Reserves was $75,000 annually.

Conclusion

In conclusion, maximizing military finances is not an exercise in futility. Quite the contrary. When done well, one can achieve reasonable wealth and not just be reasonably rich. Start with the end in mind and refine your goals annually as they will most certainly change over time. The goal of investing is to allocate at least 10% of your pay toward investments that will at a minimum keep pace with inflation and hopefully outpace inflation to allow one to retire and maintain the same standard of living. Decide what avenue suits the investor, active versus passive, and start early. Continually re-evaluate the strategy as it is likely to change over time. Start now. It is time in the market, not timing the market. Try to avoid frequent trades as this incurs capital gains tax and take advantage of compounding, the eighth wonder of the world. Minimize high-interest liabilities and maximize high-interest assets. Understand the TSP and BRS to maximize the retirement gains and minimize the service members tax burden. Choose your state of residence wisely to minimize the service members' tax burden. Choose a state where stationed that has no state income tax. Hone your profession and leverage your earnings, and one will realize the potential of being a military physician. Consider using an investment firm or manager to maximize your income, but make sure they are reliable.

References

1. Vollum C. Available from: http://pricedingold.com/us-dollar/#.
2. Consumer Price Index. [10/14/2024]. Available from: https://www.bls.gov/cpi/.
3. Underwood J, Aldrich E. Historical savings account interest rates. In: Forbes; 2022.
4. Kiyosaki RT. Rich dad, poor dad. New York: Warner Books; 1997.
5. 5 reasons why investing young makes a big difference later on. 2023 [10/14/2024]; Available from: https://www.principal.com/individuals/build-your-knowledge/reasons-why-investing-makes-a-big-difference-later-on.
6. The Servicemembers Civil Relief Act (SCRA). [cited 2024 10/14/2024]. Available from: https://www.consumerfinance.gov/consumer-tools/educator-tools/servicemembers/the-servicemembers-civil-relief-act-scra/#1.
7. Eligibility for VA home loan programs. 4/11/2024 [cited 2024 10/15/2024]; Available from: https://www.va.gov/housing-assistance/home-loans/eligibility/).
8. Why might I want a VA-backed purchase loan? 8/15/2024 [cited 2024 10/15/2024]; Available from: https://www.va.gov/housing-assistance/home-loans/loan-types/purchase-loan/#:~:text=No%20down%20payment%20as%20long,a%20manufactured%20home%20or%20lot.
9. Military compensation: savings deposit program. [cited 2024 10/14/2024]; Available from: https://militarypay.defense.gov/Benefits/Savings-Deposit-Program/.
10. Earn, spend, protect, borrow, save and invest. 2023 1/30/2023 [cited 2024 10/14/2024]; Available from: https://www.militaryonesource.mil/financial-legal/personal-finance/military-consumer-protection/.
11. MyPay. 2024; Available from: https://mypay.dfas.mil/#/.
12. How to use your GI bill benefits. 9/23/2024 [cited 2024 10/14/2024]; Available from: https://www.va.gov/education/about-gi-bill-benefits/how-to-use-benefits/.
13. Miltary compensation: high 3 calculator. [cited 2024 10/14/2024]; Available from: https://militarypay.defense.gov/Calculators/High-3-Calculator/.

Suggested Reading

Dahle JM. The white coat investor: a doctor's guide to personal finance and investing. White Coat Investor LLC.; 2014.
Keller G, Papasan J. The millionaire real estate investor. McGraw Hill; 2005.
Kiyosaki RT. Rich dad poor dad. New York: Warner Books; 1997.
Kiyosaki RT. Rich dad's cashflow quadrant. Plata Publishing; 2011.
Sutton G. Start your own corporation. RDA Press; 2013.
Wheelwright T. Tax-free wealth. BZK Press; 2012.

A Historical Perspective on Diversity, Equity, and Inclusivity in the Military

31

Chonna L Kendrick

Introduction

On January 21, 2025, President Donald Trump issued Executive Order 14173, titled "Ending Illegal Discrimination and Restoring Merit-Based Opportunity," which dismantled diversity, equity, and inclusion (DEI) initiatives within the federal government. This order marked a sweeping reversal of decades of DEI efforts, including Executive Order 11246 from 1965, which had mandated affirmative action and prohibited employment discrimination by federal contractors. The shift reflected a broader political and cultural debate over DEI's role in shaping institutions, including the US military, where policies on diversity, equal opportunity, and inclusion have evolved significantly over time.

Historically, through regulations and out of sheer necessity, the military has been able to be at the forefront of pushing diversity throughout its ranks. The history of increasing diversity in military medicine has mirrored the changes throughout the civilian sector.

C. L. Kendrick (✉)
Department of General Surgery, Carl R. Darnall Army Medical Center, Fort Cavazos, TX, USA

1st Cavalry Division Sustainment Brigade, Fort Cavazos, TX, USA
e-mail: chonna.l.kendrick.mil@army.mil

A. T. Schlussel et al. (eds.), *The SAGES Manual for Navigating a Successful Military Surgical Career*,
https://doi.org/10.1007/978-3-031-88490-0_31

The lines of effort toward diversity, equitable treatment, and inclusion are not as evident, however, as physicians rise in rank. There has been a significant amount of progress in the diversification of leadership, but a deficit of diverse leaders continues to exist at higher ranks in the military [1]. The synthesis of diversity, equity, and inclusion contributed to a holistic environment that aimed to optimize the delivery of surgical care and improve the retention of diverse medical providers in the military medical profession. Multiple avenues and lines of effort were put into existence to improve diversity; however, progress is slow, especially in orthopedics and other surgical subspecialties [2]. A deliberate and merit-based approach remains essential to ensuring equal opportunity and broad representation within the military surgical community in alignment with existing policies and legal frameworks.

As the surgical workforce more accurately reflects the community it serves, evidence suggests that surgeons can provide better, more individualized healthcare, ultimately leading to improved patient outcomes and increased patient trust in their surgeon [3]. In this chapter, we will explore the historical evolution of diversity in military medicine, recognizing that understanding the past is essential to shaping the future, as seen through many aspects of military history. We will examine how principles of equal opportunity and representation have influenced military medicine over time, leading to its present state. Lastly, we will look at strategies that have been employed to promote a professional environment rooted in fairness, merit, and operational effectiveness within the military surgical community

For minorities and those Underrepresented in Medicine (URiM), aspiring to pursue surgical roles within the military, the barriers are compounded by both racial and gender discrimination. The military, like the broader medical profession, was predominantly male and white, with deeply entrenched biases against minority and female medical professionals. This discrimination manifested in various forms, including limited recruitment efforts targeting minority and female candidates, biased selection processes, segregation, and unequal access to training and career advancement opportunities [4].

Diversity refers to the recognition and valuation of an individual's unique differences, which may include elements such as ethnicity, gender, socioeconomic background, and religious beliefs [5]. In the military surgical arena, this encompasses a broad spectrum of health professionals, from surgeons to nurses and paramedical staff. A diverse military surgical unit creates a conglomeration of unique skills, experiences, and perspectives that potentially facilitate innovative solutions and improved patient outcomes.

Stereotypes and biases regarding the abilities and aptitude of minority and female medical professionals further hindered their entry into surgical roles within the military. Prevailing attitudes regarding the supposed inferiority of minority and female surgeons contributed to their underrepresentation in surgical teams and leadership positions within military medical units. These biases persisted despite evidence of the competence and qualifications of minority and female surgeons [6]. Historical figures from multiple ethnicities have contributed to the ongoing efforts to advance representation within military surgery and the broader medical fields by breaking barriers, serving with distinction, and advocating for change. Their legacies inspire continued work toward a more inclusive and equitable military medical community.

To truly appreciate the current status of diversity in military surgery, one must consider the history of diversity in the military and medical profession concurrently. Guided by Congress and responding to societal norms over time, African Americans, Hispanic Americans, Asian Americans, women, and members of the LGBTQ community have been banned, limited in number and career opportunities, or prohibited from serving. African Americans were first allowed to serve in the Continental Army in 1775 in small numbers. African Americans were prohibited from enlisting in service until 1862, when they were needed to enhance combat power. Those African Americans who joined in 1862 served in segregated units. After the Emancipation Proclamation was signed in 1863, several states organized African American regiments, and the Army established the Bureau of Colored Troops to supervise the units of federally raised US Colored Troops [7]. The military, like the broader society, enforced racial segregation policies such as the Jim Crow laws and military regulations that limited the opportunities for minorities to serve in various capacities, including medical roles. These policies were not only discriminatory but also detrimental to the overall effectiveness of the military's healthcare system. African American soldiers were typically relegated to segregated units, often with inferior resources and opportunities compared to their white counterparts. This segregation extended to all aspects of military life, including medical care and medical roles within the military [8]. During the American Civil War, African Americans served as surgeons, nurses, and medical assistants, often in segregated units or as civilian volunteers. Dr. Alexander Augusta (1825–1890) was one of the first African American physicians to serve as a surgeon in the Union Army during the Civil War and held the rank of lieutenant colonel, making him one of the highest-ranking African American officers at the time. Augusta's service as a surgeon and officer in the face of discrimination highlighted the capabilities and contributions of African American medical professionals, challenging racial prejudices and opening doors for future African American physicians and surgeons in the military [9]. African American medical professionals were often restricted to providing care within segregated facilities or to segregated units, limiting their ability to contribute fully to the military's healthcare system. This practice of segregation extended to surgical roles, where African American surgeons were often confined to treating African American soldiers or were excluded from surgical teams altogether. Segregation also hindered the career advancement of minority medical professionals within the military. Despite these challenges, pioneering surgeons such as Dr. Charles Drew and Dr. Louis T. Wright made significant contributions to battlefield surgery and blood plasma research. Dr. Drew developed techniques for the storage of blood and plasma, leading to the first blood banks [10]. Dr. Wright introduced the intradermal method of smallpox vaccination, devised a splint for cervical fractures, and a plate for certain types of fractures to the femur [11].

Discriminatory promotion policies and practices meant that even highly skilled and qualified African American surgeons faced barriers to advancement within the military hierarchy. This limited their opportunities for leadership roles and recognition for their contributions to military medicine. The desegregation of the military in the mid-twentieth century after the passage of the Civil Rights Act of 1964 marked a turning point for African American surgeons, opening up new opportunities for training, advancement, and service. This law prohibited discrimination based on race, color, religion, sex, or national origin, which had a significant impact on military policies and practices, including those related to medical roles [8, 12]. Despite resistance and challenges, African American surgeons began to integrate into previously all-white medical units and institutions [12].

Women, like African Americans, began serving in the Revolutionary War as early as 1775, though initially not in uniform. Mary Hays McCauly (also known as Molly Pitcher) was one of the first women on the battlefield, along with Deborah Sampson, who enlisted disguised as a man. Dr. Mary Edwards Walker (1832–1919) was noted as the first female physician on the battlefield, serving as a contract surgeon. She would eventually go on to receive the Medal of Honor for her service during the Civil War, for serving initially as a volunteer surgeon and later as the first female surgeon employed by the US Army. Walker was a steadfast advocate for women's rights and suffrage, breaking gender norms in both the military and medicine [6].

Women were initially hired as contract nurses from 1901 to 1942, and Congress created the Army Nurse Corps in 1901. Although women served as physicians, nurses, administrative staff, spies, and in other positions, women were only attached to the Army in organizations such as the Women's Army Auxiliary Corps [13]. Women were not allowed to officially join the military until June of 1948 when President Harry S. Truman signed the Women's Armed Service Integration Act. This law allowed women to serve as permanent, regular members of the armed forces, opening up opportunities for women to pursue careers in the military [6]. Even after being allowed to join, all positions in the armed forces were not open to women. The process of fully integrating women has also been gradual. It wasn't until 2015 that the Department of Defense officially opened all branches of the military, including combat arms, to women. Despite this, in 2011, Dr. Patricia Horoho became the first female and first nurse to serve as the Surgeon General of the US Army [14]. In 2015, Dr. Nadja West became the first African American Surgeon General of the US Army and the highest-ranking woman to graduate from the US Military Academy at West Point [14]. Both women made significant strides in promoting diversity within the military medical corps.

Since the American Revolution, Hispanic Americans have served and played a crucial role in caring for military personnel and advancing medical practices in the military. They were not tracked separately until 1978, when the Army formed a Standing Committee on Equal Opportunity to review policies regarding treatment and opportunities for minorities. The committee recommended that the services use demographic classifications such as white, black, Hispanic, Asian, and African American. Hispanic Americans did not have to serve in segregated units as African Americans did and generally were integrated into the military services like European immigrants. From Bernardo de Gálvez, who played a key role in the American Revolution, to modern-day Hispanic service members serving in Iraq and Afghanistan, Hispanic Americans have demonstrated bravery, dedication, and sacrifice in defense of the nation. Hispanic American doctors, nurses, medics, and other medical personnel have provided vital medical care on the battlefield, in military hospitals, and in research laboratories. In 1990, Dr. Antonia Novello became the first woman and the first Hispanic to serve as Surgeon General of the United States. Dr. Novello played a key role in promoting public health initiatives and improving healthcare access for underserved populations, including military service members and veterans [15].

Asian Americans have a distinguished military history that dates back to the earliest days of the United States. During the American Civil War, approximately fifty Chinese immigrants served in the Union Army and Navy. In the following decades, Asian Americans continued to enlist and serve in various military conflicts, including World War I, World War II, the Korean War, and the Vietnam War [6].

Despite facing discrimination and challenges, such as the internment of Japanese Americans during World War II, Asian

Americans have proven themselves to be dedicated and capable service members. In the field of military medicine, Asian American healthcare professionals have made significant contributions to the care of wounded soldiers and the advancement of medical practices. Asian American doctors, nurses, medics, and other medical personnel have provided critical care on the battlefield, in military hospitals, and in research laboratories. One notable example is Dr. Margaret Chung, the first known Chinese American female physician in the United States. Dr. Chung served as a contract physician with the US Army during World War I and World War II, treating soldiers and advocating for the inclusion of Asian American women in the military [16].

Japanese-American military medical professionals have also been at the forefront of medical research and innovation. Dr. Richard Kainuma, a Japanese American surgeon, played a key role in developing techniques for treating combat injuries during the Vietnam War. His contributions to military medicine have helped save countless lives on the battlefield [17]. In 2013, Vice Admiral (ret) Raquel Bono, MD, became the first director of the Defense Health Agency, which oversees all of the Department of Defense's medical missions from the battlefield to the outpatient clinic [14]. Asian Americans have demonstrated courage, dedication, and excellence in their roles within the armed forces despite facing discrimination and challenges.

For a long time, members of the lesbian, gay, bisexual, transgender, and queer community served in the shadows, as they were prohibited from openly showing their sexuality under the "Don't Ask, Don't Tell" policy. This policy was repealed in 2010, which allowed these personnel to serve openly in the military. LGBTQ+ doctors, nurses, medics, and other medical personnel have provided essential medical care on the battlefield, in military hospitals, and in research facilities [18]. LGBTQ+ military medical professionals have also been at the forefront of research and innovation in military medicine, but recognition of them for this demographic is limited due to concern for discrimination [18]. Their contributions have helped to improve healthcare outcomes for service members and advance medical practices within the military healthcare system.

In the landscape of military healthcare, equity refers to the provision of healthcare services that do not vary in quality due to personal characteristics such as race, gender, geography, or socioeconomic status. Equity ensures that every service member has an equal opportunity to receive the highest standard of surgical care, a cornerstone principle in military medicine. As surgeons, ensuring equitable practice necessitates the elimination of biases and restrictive norms that could potentially impact surgical outcomes. Ensuring equitable treatment can be achieved through equitable representation of diverse racial, ethnic, gender, and socioeconomic groups in the military surgical profession that mirrors the patient population.

Inclusion fosters a culture where everyone's contributions are valued and integrated into decision-making processes, thus promoting a sense of belonging and mutual respect. In a military surgical context, this means involving every medical team member, irrespective of rank, specialty, or background, in the surgical decision-making and execution process. Inclusion can promote psychological safety, enhance teamwork, and contribute to better surgical outcomes through effective interdisciplinary collaboration [19]. Inclusion is being asked to participate. Belonging is having a voice and influence to become a valued member of the team and even the power to invite others to join the team.

For many years, the military prioritized broad representation, but over the last two decades, it became clear that representation alone was not enough. There needs to be inclusion and a sense of meaningful contribution to truly benefit [20]. In 2003, the Chief of Staff of the Army, General Eric K. Shinseki, ordered the study of the underrepresented women and racial minorities within the ranks. In 2005, the Department of Defense instituted its Diversity Office to focus on the promotion of diversity and assist in the implementation and review of army policies. In February 2008, the Secretary of the Army and Chief of Staff established the Army Diversity Task Force to execute a holistic review and assessment of the Army Diversity Program. In June 2020, the Secretary of the Army and the Chief of Staff of the Army announced "Project Inclusion," an initiative that operationalizes the Army People Strategy Diversity, Equity, and Inclusion Annex. Under this project, the Army has worked to organize and leverage resources across the Army to focus on training, listening sessions, implementation of diversity plans, and policy review. As a result, significant changes have been made to grooming standards and height/weight standards. In addition, there has been an increase in the length of parental leave and more postpartum exemptions in the interest of providing more recovery time for mothers and parents [5].

In prior years, military surgery residency programs and hospitals were able to actively promote inclusion and foster cohesion and teamwork in the surgical ward through various initiatives and practices. Residency programs were able to actively recruit and support underrepresented minority candidates to ensure a diverse cohort of residents. They partnered with organizations that promote diversity in healthcare, attended minority recruitment fairs, and offered scholarships or mentorship programs. Through scholarships such as the Health Professions Scholarship Program, which provides scholarships for medical school in exchange for service, the military aims to remove financial barriers and make medical education more accessible to candidates [21]. The ACGME requires programs to provide cultural competency training for residents and staff to enhance understanding and communication with patients from diverse backgrounds to help reduce bias, improve patient care, and promote inclusivity in the surgical setting. Training is conducted in various formats, including workshops, seminars, online modules, and interactive simulations. The training may cover topics such as communication with diverse patient populations, understanding cultural beliefs and practices, addressing health disparities, and promoting inclusivity in patient care [20].

Military residencies have partnerships with the Association of American Medical Colleges (AAMC), which offers resources, programs, and initiatives focused on promoting diversity and inclusion in medical education and practice [22]. They also provide guidance on recruiting and supporting underrepresented minority students and residents [23]. Another key partnership is with the National Medical Association (NMA). The NMA is dedicated to advancing the health and wellness of underserved communities and promoting diversity in healthcare. They offer mentorship programs, networking opportunities, and advocacy for underrepresented minority healthcare professionals [24]. Each branch of the military, such as the Army, Navy, Air Force, and Coast Guard, may have tailored mentorship programs to support the unique needs and goals of military healthcare providers.

Another way of increasing the diversity of the surgical community that also introduces unique experiences with treating a more diverse population is through initiatives such as Military-Civilian Trauma Training Partnerships. Surgeons enhance readiness and gain experience working with a more diverse faculty and a more diverse, higher acuity patient population. These programs provide exposure to high-volume, complex trauma cases typically seen in civilian Level 1 trauma centers. Some notable partnerships and programs include: The US Army Military-Civilian Trauma Team Training (AMCT3) program at Vanderbilt University Medical Center (VUMC), Cooper and Oregon Health & Science University (OHSU), University of Chicago Medicine Partnership, UNC Health and Army Medicine Collaboration, and VCU Medical Center Military-Civilian partnership [25]. As a result of the partnership, military surgeons are afforded opportunities to be mentors and faculty in pipeline programs. For example, the University of Chicago allows military surgeons to participate in the Medical Careers Exposure and Emergency Preparedness Pipeline Program, which exposes children (ages 13–19) in underserved communities to medical and healthcare-related careers along with guidance on applying to medical professional schools along with ongoing mentorship and training [26]. Exposure to military surgeons in this program and others like this may inspire younger generations to pursue military medicine, thus improving diversity within the military surgical arena [27]. These programs are not only critical for enhancing the clinical competency and preparedness of military medical personnel but also serve as platforms for knowledge exchange between military and civilian healthcare providers, a diverse workplace, and exposure to more diverse patients while inspiring a younger generation [25].

The Challenges of Diversity, Equity, and Inclusion Programs

Enhancing representation and fostering collaboration benefit both surgeons and patients; however, historical factors continue to present challenges to progress. Inexplicably, in 2023, several states eliminated their state funding for DEI initiatives at public education institutions. The American College of Surgeons (ACS), American Society for Metabolic and Bariatric Surgery (ASMBS), Society of Military Orthopedic Surgeons (SOMOS), Society of American Gastrointestinal and Endoscopic Surgeons (SAGES), and Excelsior Surgical Society are just a few surgical societies that have formed committees to promote and address representation within their own membership [28]. Through these societies, surgeons undergoing training and those well beyond residency are challenged to learn about equity and nuances such as microaggressions, implicit biases, and barriers to promotion, retention, and advancement for underrepresented minority surgeons in medicine and in the military [4]. SAGES has created the Fundamentals in Leadership Development Course, which teaches surgeons, residents, and healthcare professionals in leadership or aspiring leadership roles essential skills to promote equity and excellence in academic surgery. It focuses on building and managing diverse teams, enhancing communication, and supporting underrepresented groups. The course aims to develop leadership strategies that foster inclusive, high-performing environments in surgery [29]. In addition, the military surgical residency programs are taking a more holistic approach in selecting trainees with well-rounded life experiences [20].

Within the military surgical community, there continue to be challenges with attrition among female and minority residents. There is a higher, disproportionate rate of attrition among minorities and females in surgical specialties [30]. More specifically, Haruno et al. found that underrepresented minorities and females in orthopedic surgery residency underwent unintended attrition at disproportionately higher rates than their male counterparts [31]. Minorities have previously reported limited access to educational resources, experiences of discrimination and bias, lack of mentorship, and lack of support [24]. They may have challenges related to their ethnicity/race in navigating the hierarchical and competitive culture of surgical training programs, especially those who may feel marginalized or excluded from opportunities for advancement and recognition. These challenges contribute to and hinder the number of underrepresented minorities and women competing for fellowships after residency in some surgical subspecialties. Minority surgical residents have limited access to mentors and support networks who can provide guidance, advocacy, and career development opportunities, making it more challenging to navigate the demands of surgical training [30].

Diversity within surgical teams brings together individuals with different backgrounds, perspectives, and experiences, fostering innovation and creativity in problem-solving, which is important when faced with time constraints, limited resources, and communication barriers in combat or during natural disasters. Diverse teams are more likely to consider a wider range of ideas and approaches, leading to novel solutions and advancements in surgical techniques, technologies, and patient care practices. In combat or humanitarian relief operations, healthcare teams composed of individuals with diverse skill sets, cultural competencies, and language proficiencies can adapt more effectively to dynamic and challenging environments, leading to better coordination of care and operational outcomes [32].

Increased representation of minorities and women within medicine and the military have been shown to improve patient care [28]. Despite widespread access to care in the military, minorities consistently have higher infant mortality rates along with worse health and surgical outcomes compared to white patients. Multiple reasons have been cited for this. There has historically been a lack of representation of minority persons enrolled in medical studies. There is evidence of inherent biases between the providers and the patients. Many patients report a preference for healthcare providers of the same race, feeling more comfortable and involved in decision-making with race-concordant providers [33]. Research also supports that patient outcomes and patient-physician relationships are indirectly improved by sharing cultural, racial, or ethnic backgrounds [33].

Discordance has been associated with diminished trust, decreased adherence to screening protocols, and potentially worse outcomes. When it comes to patient care within the military health system, preventive health screening is improved compared to the civilian patient population due to all service members receiving universal healthcare; however, there are still healthcare disparities present along gender and racial lines when it comes to surgical specialty care [2]. In 2023, data from the Army and Air Force identified that women made up 31% and 33% of surgeons, respectively, between both services. Three percent of Army surgeons identified as African American/Black, and 1% of Air Force Surgeons identified as African American/Black [34]. Hoyt et. Al. published an 18-year analysis of racial and gender diversity of physicians accepted to American military and orthopedic and surgical residencies in 2023. They found that even though the percentage of women enrolled in medical school increased from 32% to over 50%, the percentage of female orthopedic residents only increased by 0.10%. They also found that across all surgical specialties within the military, 31% of the residents selected were women during that entire 18-year period with an increase of 0.94% per year. There was a 1.01% increase in underrepresented minorities per year. Twenty percent of the total number of residents accepted that year (1875) were underrepresented minorities in medicine, and seventy percent of those accepted [35] were white. Their analysis included General Surgery, Obstetrics and Gynecology, Orthopedic Surgery, and Otolaryngology. Based on this study and multiple others, there is progress being made in multiple surgical specialties [2].

As a community, military surgeons are actively taking steps toward improvement, but there is still work to be done to sustain and measure the effort. Overuse or overemphasis on DEI initiatives that are ineffective is not fruitful and may have impacted the policies surrounding DEI today. Efforts to improve equitable healthcare should be effective and easily integrated into daily practice. The goal is to have a medical provider workforce that mirrors the demographics of the patient population that it serves. If resources become available in the future, additional research in DEI could aid in identifying any continued disparities, understanding root causes, and evaluating interventions [36]. Feedback from the patients and surgeons is necessary to help shape education and training around DEI topics. This feedback and research can then be used to create evidence-based, effective policies and guidelines in healthcare and military settings. Policy changes informed by research have the potential to address systemic barriers. Advocacy from strong and competent leaders is of utmost importance to help push the policy and provide lasting, sustainable change [37].

Conclusion

Historically, the military has implemented practices to diversify and increase combat power to achieve victory, but in doing so, it has often mirrored the societal norms of the country. After slavery ended in the 1860s, the military engaged in segregation and limited women's rights and career opportunities. Segregation in the military had far-reaching effects on medical roles, including surgery, by limiting the opportunities for minorities and women to pursue careers in military medicine. The initial barriers to entry for minority and female medical professionals in surgical roles within the military reflected broader patterns of discrimination and exclusion in society. By insisting on serving in a medical capacity, women such as Dr. Mary E. Walker challenged gender barriers in military medicine, paving the way for future generations of women in the field. There continue to be some barriers still apparent today. Overcoming these barriers requires concerted efforts to challenge discriminatory policies and practices and promote diversity, equity, and inclusion within the military healthcare system.

Although the military and federal workforce must navigate within the constructs of current policies and Executive Orders, ensuring that the military is providing well-rounded training in a supportive learning environment to the next generation of surgeons is imperative to enhancing patient care, promoting innovation, and ensuring the readiness of our nation's service members. This also promotes a variety of perspectives and better problem-solving within the multidisciplinary medical team after residency. Ongoing research and education are essential drivers of progress both in healthcare and military settings. By generating knowledge, raising awareness, and informing policy and practice, research and education contribute to creating a more culturally competent environment that supports the well-being and success of all stakeholders. In the end, <1% of the United States' population serves on active duty. For those willing to fight for this country, the United States military should be fostering an environment that embraces and encourages all of its members to overcome the challenges that the military will face.

These executive orders are focused on reshaping the military culture, emphasizing military values, readiness, and lethality over social policies. They emphasize a merit-based system without race—or sex-based preferences, which some may argue is a departure from the previous administration's approach to military policy.

These actions have stirred significant debate, with supporters arguing they restore focus on military readiness and critics claiming they introduce potential discrimination, may reduce diversity, and undermine recruitment and morale. The impact of these orders on military operations, culture, and personnel will likely unfold in the coming months to years.

Acknowledgment The author extends sincere gratitude to Anna Stachura, MD, CPT, MC, USA, for her contribution to providing up-to-date insights on recent executive orders and current policies.

References

1. U.S. Department of Defense. Diversity and Inclusion in the Armed Forces 2020. Accessed December 23, 2023. https://www.defense.gov/Newsroom/Reports/DoD-DEI-2020.
2. Hoyt BW, Anderson AB, Dingle ME, Dickens JF, Eckel TT, Sterbis JR, Potter BK. Racial and gender diversity of physicians accepted to American Military Orthopaedic and Surgical Residencies: an 18-year analysis. JBJS Open Access. 2023;8(1):e22.00091. https://doi.org/10.2106/JBJS.OA.22.00091.

3. Abelson JS, Symer MM, Yeo HL, Butler PD, Dolan PT, Moo TA, Watkins AC. Surgical time out: our counts are still short on racial diversity in academic surgery. Am J Surg. 2017;214(4):712–8. https://doi.org/10.1016/j.amjsurg.2017.07.010.
4. Kim Y, Kassam AF, IE ME, Lee S, Tanious A, Chou EL, Patel SS, Pendleton AA, Dua A. The current status of the diversity pipeline in surgical training. Am J Surg. 2022;224(1, Part B):250–6. https://doi.org/10.1016/j.amjsurg.2021.11.006.
5. Department of the Army. The army people strategy: diversity, equity, and inclusion annex. Washington, D.C.: Department of the Army; 2020.
6. U.S. Army Center of Military History. The army and diversity. U.S. Army Center of Military History. Accessed December 23, 2023. https://history.army.mil/Research/Reference-Topics/Army-and-Diversity/.
7. Dobak WA. U.S. Army Center of Military History. Freedom by the sword: The U.S. Colored Troops, 1862–1867. Washington, D.C.: U.S. Army Center of Military History; 2011.
8. Lee U. U.S. Army Center of Military History. The Employment of Negro Troops [in World War II]. Washington, D.C.: U.S. Army Center of Military History; 1966.
9. Butts HM. Alexander Thomas Augusta—physician, teacher, and human rights activist. J Natl Med Assoc. 2005;97(1):106–9.
10. The Charles R. Drew Papers. U.S. National Library of Medicine. Retrieved August 25, 2012. Accessed December 20, 2023.
11. Fisher WD. African American doctors in world war I. Lincoln, NE: University of Nebraska Press; 2015.
12. MacGregor M Jr. U.S. Army Center of Military History. Integration of the Armed Forces 1940–1965. Washington D.C.: U.S. Army Center of Military History; 1981.
13. Morden BJ. U.S. Army Center of Military History. The Women's Army Corps, 1945–1978. Washington D.C.: U.S. Army Center of Military History; 1990.
14. History of Women in Military Medicine. https://health.mil/About-MHS/Military-Medical-History/Historical-Timelines/Women?type=External+Articles. Accessed December 23, 2023.
15. Changing the Face of Medicine | AntoniaNovello. cfmedicine.nlm.nih.gov. Archived from the original on 2020-07-26. Retrieved 2020-06-15. Accessed December 23, 2023.
16. Walker, M. (2022) Dr. Margaret Chung: First American Born Chinese woman physician | headlines and heroes. Library of Congress Blogs. Retrieved October 27, 2023, from https://blogs.loc.gov/headlinesandheroes/2022/05/dr-margaret-chung/
17. 100th Infantry Battalion Veterans. (2011–2024). Dr. Richard Kainuma: In service of others. Retrieved December 18, 2023, from https://www.100thbattalion.org/history/veterans/medics/richard-kainuma/

18. Aldahondo R, Cole R. The experiences of LGBTQ healthcare professionals within military medical culture. Military Med. 188(11–12):e3606–12. https://doi.org/10.1093/milmed/usad284.
19. Torres MB, Williams-Karnesky RL, Kaulsolh B, Alimi Y, Altieri MS. Increasing membership diversity in surgical societies through intentional inclusion. Bullet Am College Surg. 2021; Accessed December 23, 2023. https://www.facs.org/for-medical-professionals/news-publications/news-and-articles/bulletin/2021/01/increasing-membership-diversity-in-surgical-societies-through-intentional-inclusion/
20. Ononuju UC, Morgan JB, Ode GE. The role of inclusion in increasing diversity and retention across surgical residencies: a literature review. Curr Rev Musculoskel Med. 2023;16(11):557–62. https://doi.org/10.1007/s12178-023-09866-8.
21. Chaurasia AR, Nhliziyo MV, Paul SR, Horton IM, Wright VK, Serjilus A. US Military Physician Workforce Diversity. In: Deville Jr C, editor. Physician workforce diversity. Cham: Springer; 2024. https://doi.org/10.1007/978-3-031-63050-7_27.
22. Wright V, Stepp E, Flemming B, Kandler C, Wait T, Godshall-Bennett L, Robbins R. The impact of racism on health: a health equity training on structural racism for military residents and fellows. MedEdPORTAL. 2024;20:11443. https://doi.org/10.15766/mep_2374-8265.11443.
23. Association of American Medical Colleges. Equity, diversity, and inclusion. Association of American Medical Colleges. Accessed July 20, 2024. https://www.aamc.org/about-us/equity-diversity-inclusion.
24. Suraju MO, McElroy L, Moten A, Obeng-Gyasi S, Alimi Y, Carter D, Foretia DA, Stapleton S, Yilma M, Reid VJ, Tetteh HA, Khabele D, Rodriguez LM, Campbell A, Newman EA. A framework to improve retention of black surgical trainees: a society of black academic surgeons white paper. Am J Surg. 2023;226(4):438–46. https://doi.org/10.1016/j.amjsurg.2023.07.022.
25. Cureton, Gigail. New program teams Army medicine with civilian hospitals. January 2019. Accessed December 23, 2023. https://www.army.mil/article/216704/new_program_teams_army_medicine_with_civilian_hospitals
26. Plackett TP, Jaszczak N, Hampton DA, Prakash P, Cone J, Benjamin A, Rogers SO, Wilson K. Trauma surgical skill sustainment at the University of Chicago AMEDD Military-Civilian Trauma Team Training Site: an observation report. Trauma Surg Acute Care Open. 2024;9(1):e001177.
27. MedCEEP. Our Programs. MedCEEP. Accessed December 23, 2023. https://medceep.com/our-programs.
28. Fisher MWA, Askew M, Baird M, Ozdemir S, Williams S, Ramirez V, Kilcoyne K, Dingle M. Pipeline to military orthopaedic leadership: 20 years of face and gender diversity trends within military orthopaedic surgery fellowship training. JBJS Open Access. 2023;8(4):e23.00019. https://doi.org/10.2106/JBJS.OA.23.00019.

29. Fundamentals of Leadership Development. Course Information: Fundamentals of Leadership Development. Fundamentals of Leadership Development. Accessed October 10, 2024.
30. Williams-Karnesky RL, Kashyap M, Courtney C, Park C, Ritter KA, Hanke R. Shoring up the pipeline: increasing diversity in surgery by enhancing equity and inclusion in the surgical learning environment. Bullet Am College Surg. 2021; Accessed December 23, 2023. https://www.facs.org/for-medical-professionals/news-publications/news-and-articles/bulletin/2021/01/shoring-up-the-pipeline-increasing-diversity-in-surgery-by-enhancing-equity-and-inclusion-in-the-surgical-learning-environment
31. Haruno LS, Chen X, Metzger M, Lin CA, Little MTM, Kanim LEA, Poon SC. Racial and sex disparities in resident attrition in orthopaedic surgery. JBJS Open Access. 2023;8(1):1–8. https://doi.org/10.2106/jbjs.oa.22.00148.
32. Garrett MX. Military diversity: a key American strategic asset. Military Rev. 2021:14.
33. Smedley B, Stith A, Nelson A. Unequal treatment: confronting racial and ethnic disparities in health care. Institute of Medicine; 2003.
34. Kendrick C, Wilson K, Hill E, Worlton T, Kurts R, Alsobrooks S. Diversity state of the union for military surgery and levers to increase diversity. Oral presentation presented at the American College of Surgeons Excelsior Society meeting; 2023.
35. Haruno LS, Chen X, Metzger M, Lin CA, Little MTM, Kanim LEA, Poon SC. Racial and sex disparities in resident attrition among surgical subspecialties. JAMA Surg. 2023;158(4):E1–9.
36. Koehlmoos TP, Korona-Bailey J, Janvrin ML, Madsen C. Racial disparities in the military health system: a framework synthesis. Military Med. 187(9–10):e1114–21. https://doi.org/10.1093/milmed/usab506.
37. Vela AM, Callegari M, Goudy L, Cozzi C, Gibson M, Rooney MJ, Caicedo JC. Analysis of diversity, equity, and inclusion initiatives presented across US Academic Department of Surgery Websites in 2021. J Clin Psychol Med Settings. 2023;30(2):274–80. https://doi.org/10.1007/s10880-022-09932-2.

Mental Health for the Military Surgeon

32

Kelly Beeken

> *We who lived in concentration camps can remember the men who walked through the huts comforting others, giving away their last piece of bread. They may have been few in number but they offer sufficient proof that everything can be taken from a man but one thing: the last of the human freedoms—to choose one's attitude in any set of circumstances, to choose one's own way.*
>
> —Viktor E. Frankl, concentration camp survivor, WWII

For surgeons, the upfront cost of the life years required to learn how to make the correct diagnosis and devise appropriate treatment plans is astronomical. Besides time, the portion of life dedicated to prolonged and intense residency training requires even more of oneself. Surgical training also instills critical knowledge and decision-making capabilities regarding when to take a patient to the operating room. This responsibility admits graduates to a distinct group of physicians with tactile skills and clinical judgment. However, the cost of this education for many is mental, emotional, and spiritual health. This familiar story of struggle and attainment creates incredible physicians but sometimes makes miserable humans and terrible leaders. It is possible to retain the well-being of a whole person while still being a strong physician, but it can only happen with intentionality. While there is no spe-

K. Beeken (✉)
Martin Army Community Hospital, Fort Benning, GA, USA

A. T. Schlussel et al. (eds.), *The SAGES Manual for Navigating a Successful Military Surgical Career*,
https://doi.org/10.1007/978-3-031-88490-0_32

cific published data on military physicians' suicide rates, being a physician [1] and having served in the military [2] are individually independent risk factors for suicide. Moreover, surgeons are even more likely to have suicidal ideation and less likely to seek mental healthcare [3] than the general public.

As a surgeon, some parts of life will be hard; patients will die, academic submissions will be rejected, one will make mistakes and patients will suffer, and like all people, family members will pass away. As a military physician, there is added hardship as friends will have a permanent change of station, people integral to one's support system will drift away, or one may experience the federal tort system's coldness. If you are facing clinical scenarios of anxiety, depression, suicidality, or other mental health diagnoses as a result of such hardships, please seek help. The end of this chapter has a table of options for seeking mental healthcare on active duty. Addressing these issues is beyond this chapter's scope, but both help and recovery exist.

It is essential to create a mindset that helps one grow from these experiences instead of succumbing to them. This is the mindset in which everyone should live. One should strive for an antifragile life, defined by Nassim Taleb as "things [that] benefit from shocks; they thrive and grow when exposed to volatility, randomness, disorder and stressors and love adventure, risk and uncertainty. Antifragility is beyond resilience or robustness. The resilient resists shocks and stays the same; antifragile gets better" [4]. This chapter reviews strategies for achieving peak mental toughness, antifragility, and resiliency, but not treatments for medical conditions.

The Pyramid's Foundation

Sustaining long-term mental toughness without the basics of physical health is fruitless. Sleep is essential to emotional regulation [5], and conversely, emotional regulation is essential to our sleep. When basic physical needs are unmet, the overriding driver of regulation is the sympathetic nervous system. It is the driver most days for many in medicine and can lead to bad decisions. Poor dietary choices are also detrimental to good mental health.

Many physicians opt for simple sugars and processed food because they are shelf-stable, cheap, and easy to access. A 2017 London study showed that simple sugars and sugar-sweetened beverages were associated with depression and mental health challenges [6]. Exercise, on the other hand, has a positive role in emotional regulation, and its benefit cannot be overstated. Exercise releases serotonin, norepinephrine, dopamine, and endorphins. These hormones, associated with releasing brain-derived neurotrophic factors, improve sleep [7] and provide the best foundation for creating an antifragile life. The higher-order work of achieving and sustaining emotional regulation, positivity, and resiliency is virtually impossible without satisfying one's basic physical needs.

To Err Is Human

Surgeons have a unique position in medicine; ultimately, the attending surgeon alone decides if a patient goes to the operating room. The weight of any complications that occur in patient care rests with the surgeon. This is unlike medicine, where the patient's care is frequently spread between the emergency room physician, a hospitalist, an intensivist, and the primary care physician on discharge. The surgeon typically assumes all of these roles. Each day, surgeons walking into the operating room endeavor for perfection, but no one achieves it. Everyone has a complication rate. The only way around this is by self-deception or not operating at all. This also means that the ultimate responsibility of surgical complications can weigh heavily and take a costly emotional toll on the surgeon. This can happen with or without the additional trauma of explaining one's actions in response to a risk management inquiry or a liability claim. Understanding some of the ways to deal with these cases can help transform crippling experiences into opportunities for growth.

Rituals have been used throughout human history to mark significant events and bind the emotional cost of experiences. Practicing rituals is also fundamental in the culture of medicine. A white coat ceremony invites initiates to wear the uniform. Medical school graduates take the Hippocratic oath, spoken for hundreds of years, to welcome a new generation of physicians every July and remind the audience of the honor and great responsibility of practicing medicine. These positive experiences foster a healthy growth mindset.

Adverse events also have their rituals in the form of departmental reviews and Morbidity & Mortality (M&M) conferences. They are the first step in allowing one to process one's complications in a professional environment. In Brown's *Rising Strong*, she establishes a framework for overcoming difficult situations, avoiding chronic shame, and allowing growth [8]. This also provides an excellent framework for working through challenging cases. The first step is to tell the story, what she describes as the reckoning. This means honestly telling the whole story, including fears and insecurities about the case. It can be hard to admit that there wasn't an acceptable maneuver to fix a problem, that a solution had to be invented, or worse yet, that a known solution was not used. All surgeons have moments in the operating room where it seems like the bleeding will never stop, the anatomy doesn't look like anything in the textbook, and their own tachycardia far outpaces the patients.

To successfully reckon with the story, it is vitally important to cultivate relationships with a small group of surgeons who can be called day or night. They do not have to be in the same specialty, hospital, or even in the military, but it must be someone who understands these dark operative moments so the whole story can come out. In the absence of being able to call someone, journaling can be a close second, or there may be a unique nonsurgeon in one's life who can truly understand the experience. Many of the larger medical centers have begun to develop peer support programs where experienced clinicians are available to younger healthcare providers after adverse events or unanticipated patient outcomes occur.

Brown's second stage is the rumble. This is analyzing and dissecting the story with nonjudgmental curiosity to understand which parts are at the core of the emotional struggle. Brown states, "The goal of the rumble is to get honest about the stories we're making up about our struggles, to revisit, challenge, and reality-check these narratives as we dig into topics such as boundaries, shame, blame, resentment, heartbreak, generosity, and forgiveness." [8] For most cases, a bad outcome isn't about every step that happens. It is recognizing the one or two decisions that led to the poor outcome and then one's response to that unexpected outcome. This step requires understanding how the decision was made and determining if those choices were appropriate with the available information.

The rumble often leads to one of two endpoints: either the surgeon made the wrong decision that led to the outcome, or the outcome was inevitable and could happen again without warning. Neither of these outcomes is comforting as the surgeon will likely feel guilty or powerless; it is possible to vacillate between them regarding the same case on different days. The rumble's ritual is the M&M conference. As human beings, it is necessary to have this safe and protected space to tell these stories and explain the rumble in front of colleagues. It allows trusted partners to fill spaces where thinking is still opaque and provide an honest critique. This can quiet the surgeon's doubts about whether they were good enough. Not every hospital or department has an M&M conference, though. The surgeon who does not have one should start their own and carve out a regular time to meet, even if it is done virtually.

The revolution comes last. This is where the things learned from the poor outcome are accepted and applied to practice. It is the moment of owning mistakes, making improvements, and recommitting to living as the surgeon and human one wants to be.

Understanding That Challenges Will Come

Military surgeons, like civilian surgeons, have their identities wrapped up in their work due to spending so many hours to gain the title, causing them to miss birthdays, funerals, and weddings. Military surgeons must also face deployments that cause them to miss even more life milestones. Challenges at work can feel like an attack on identity. But everyone is worthy and matters, even if they never pick up a scalpel again. Living in a way that embraces this includes paying attention to life outside the hospital and pursuing a life that brings joy, happiness, and accomplishment. Sometimes, part of the old identity has to be let go to make room for the new identity that awaits.

Several publications address a proper mindset when facing disappointments or challenges, including *Hunting the Good Stuff* from Master Resiliency Training, Willink's mindset of GOOD [9], Trident Mindset's *Flipping the Script* [10], and even the Christian hymn *It is Well With My Soul* [11]. They all describe moving forward and becoming better because of it. Willink describes that dwelling on the problem will not solve it. One must accept reality and focus on the solution. He emphasizes that one should "take that issue, take that setback, take that problem, and turn it into something good." Similarly, Trident states, "No matter what event life throws at you, you respond with a positive belief (like this is actually a good thing, I'll make the most out of this, I can learn from this, or this doesn't matter in the grand scheme of things), and therefore achieve a beneficial consequence: calmness and happiness."

Life is hard; life as a military surgeon is even more challenging. There will be days when nothing works. The operating room has not pulled the correct preference card, one's first assistant schedules themselves to do something else, a complication occurs, and the emergency room seemingly cannot disposition a single patient without calling for assistance. At the same time, one is harassed by a commander to complete military skills training. There must be a way to deal with these situations that does not deny their existence but allows one to focus on the positive elements. This first requires an accurate view of the situation itself. Pretending that the situation does not exist is not helpful, as this requires more emotional energy to support the cognitive dissonance. Instead, evaluating the situation, being appreciative of where growth is possible, letting go of unrealistic expectations, and practicing mental flexibility create a person who can calmly manage a crisis. A positive outlook fosters creative thinking and novel solutions and allows one to exploit asymmetric situations. Anger leads to a sympathetic response, which has its own consequences for both physical and emotional health and frequently discharges disappointment and frustration on those who cannot change the situation.

In my first month working at a new hospital, I took care of a mother whose baby had died. There is no positive to this. She brought home a coffin instead of a child. It was tragic and terrible. However, I reevaluated the situation and chose to be grateful that I could care for her. Having cared for more than 50 mothers experiencing the same thing over the preceding 15 years, I could offer my expertise even though I was not assigned to the labor and delivery floor on that particular day. I was grateful she was offered all testing options and that I could approach her with compassion and sympathy, not inexperience and awkwardness. I could make her feel cared for.

Showing Up

As a society, we exist around more people than at any other time in human history but have fewer meaningful relationships. It is easy to substitute acquaintance contacts and social media connections for genuine friendship and intimacy. Our minds use television and movies' fictional stories as a substitute for authentic relationships. Humans are social creatures and need social connections. In Ornish's book *Love & Survival: The Scientific Basis or the Healing Power of Intimacy*, he delineates how happy marriages, social circles, spiritual connection, and even owning pets prolong a lifespan [12]. Everyone needs to feel love and express love.

Deep friendships with a small group of people were also evolutionarily protective because they provided a survival advantage in a hunter-gatherer society. It is what we have evolved to need. But, in our highly mobile society and typically in the military, many people do not have a single close friend from a decade ago. This is difficult on several levels. First, long-term friendships tend to be fostered naturally through challenging and vulnerable moments, breeding further trust and intimacy. Second, long-term relationships include people who have already witnessed and proven they can accept failures. It is important to have friends who have already seen stupid decisions, listened to words that didn't come out right, watched romantic relationships fall apart, and proven they care. Everyone has challenges in life and needs support through these challenges.

For many people, these deep friendships also include a romantic relationship. The demands of a surgical career make it easy in medicine to place this relationship on the back burner, imagining that one day there will be time for this. When John Gottman [13] describes what it takes to make marriages work, he describes having partners intentionally study each other's love maps, figuring out what makes them feel loved, cherished, and safe. This is similar to the principles in Gary Chapman's work *The 5 Love Languages: The Secret to Love that Lasts*, where he describes understanding how both parties in the relationship feel the most loved [14]. All relationships take work and time. It takes energy to evaluate a relationship and then effort to improve it regularly if it is going to survive a surgical career. Walt Whitman said, "Be curious, not judgmental." Unfortunately, curiosity is quickly lost in one's most familiar relationships. It takes intentionality to consider: What would make my partner happy? What would most physically satisfy them? How can I help them achieve their goals? What big events are on their calendar? The deliberate, day-to-day work of making and accepting bids for emotional connection and being a part of each other's next steps, decisions, and goals can help mitigate the time sacrificed during a surgical career.

Gottman's book also promotes solving solvable problems [15]. There are many unsolvable problems in relationships. Some examples are a spouse wanting to live close to their parents but orders for a transfer are to a different state or wanting another baby in the setting of infertility. These are problems that have no simple solution. They will require emotional bandwidth to deal with and, ultimately, some level of compromise. So, do not let solvable problems fester. Commit to finding common solutions for solvable problems. Where to go to dinner, which color the dining room should be painted, and whether the kids will play baseball or soccer are solvable problems. Recognize that moving forward with a partner's idea is not losing and that committing to peace and adding to the emotional bank account for the rest of your life are absolutely winning.

Attention: Focusing on the Moment

Most surgeons have no difficulty paying attention in the operating room. As a resident, I distinctly remember the nurse answering my phone in the operating room. The police were at my house because a break-in had occurred. The alarm had gone off, and they had been alerted. The burglars had broken into the garage after being unable to pry open the deadbolt, drank some vodka from my freezer, and dug through the drywall with a garden tool to enter my house. The alarm went off; they grabbed a few things and headed out. All I remember about this is asking my father to go to my house. It never dawned on me that I should go deal with it. I could not leave. I was in the operating room. In any other situation, I would have promptly driven home to address the issue, and if leaving was not an option, I would have been unable to focus and remained preoccupied with the event. As surgeons, most of us have a unique ability to focus in the operating room but cannot turn that same focus on the rest of our lives.

This ability to focus attention is well-described in the book *Peak Mind: Find Your Focus, Own Your Attention, Invest 12 Minutes a Day*; the author says this deep focus is the spotlight of our attention [16]. Despite honing this skill at work for years, being present and focused outside work is still challenging. Mindfulness allows one to train one's attention. Like any other skill, it takes time to build mindfulness, and it atrophies with disuse. Having voluntary control of one's attention, training it to the moments one wants to focus, can be invaluable in being present for those one cares about instead of spending time outside the hospital with a mind still at work. This technique is described in Jon Kabat-Zinn's work *Full Catastrophe Living*, where he describes meditation techniques and the secular practice of mindfulness [17]. In *Peak Mind*, Jha's formula for measurable increases in attention is only 12 minutes a day, five days a week. Just one hour a week is a minimal investment for this substantial ability.

Quality of Thoughts

The happiness of your life depends upon the quality of your thoughts: therefore, guard accordingly, and take care that you entertain no notions unsuitable to virtue and reasonable nature.

—Marcus Aurelius

Everyone has an inner monologue that begins when one wakes up and continues until drifting off to sleep. The aforementioned *Trident Mindset* describes one's inner monologue as both a two-year-old and a chatty drunk friend [18]. Brene Brown, in *The Power of Vulnerability*, describes it as gremlins [19]. For those who have mastered meditation, there may be five to twenty minutes a day when this voice quiets, but that means almost everyone listens to this inner voice for the rest of the day. This means one talks to oneself for more hours a day than to anyone else. Stoic philosophy, recognizing how detrimental a poor inner monologue can be, describes exerting some control because one's thoughts lead to one's emotions and actions. The inner narrative wants to make sense of how the world works. It connects events that are not connected, assumes intentions that are not present, and catastrophizes. So, being aware of one's inner voice is the first step to improving the quality of one's thoughts.

Everyone should be skeptical of one's inner monologue. If one steps back and observes the inner dialogue for even a few hours, it is clear these thoughts are suspect at best and harmful at worst. As described in *Leadership and Self-Deception,* one's inner monologue frequently leads one into the box where one is either the hero or the victim [20]. Others are the enemy, and one recruits allies to one's point of view. However, purity of intent and black-and-white thinking are the stuff of movies and novels. It would be nice if the world worked with the certainty of the characters in a fictional story. They do not grapple with the uncertainty of other people's intentions or the consequences of their actions. The villain always has a clear motive, and the hero has a heart of gold. However, people are complex in real life, yet one's inner monologue often reduces them to a simple common denominator so one can understand events. Thus, the stories one tells oneself affect how one treats others.

Conversely, evolutionary psychology explains that a pessimistic inner dialogue may provide a survival advantage, implying that those more paranoid and skeptical were more prepared for danger. In a world of lion attacks and tribal raids, this led to survival. Today, most people experience this as an inner dialogue that tells them the sky is falling during an average day. One should recognize that this pessimistic inner view likely provided a survival advantage in high school, college, medical school, and residency. Surgeons told themselves that one failing test grade in high school would keep them out of college. Premed students were motivated to work harder when hearing that they would never make it as doctors. Medical students witnessed class members drop out and fretted about any imperfect aspect of themselves. Most residents wrote a resignation letter at some point during training, even though most never submitted it. This continuous dialogue of never being good enough created a cycle of struggle and survival, adding to the formula that eventually developed one into a staff physician. Again, as a staff physician, there are many times when one will compare oneself to one's peers and feel one is, in some way, not worthy. However, this path is one of anxiety, frustration, and never being enough. Overcoming this feeling is a very personal journey. For some, it is a spiritual question of recognizing one's importance as a soul, and for others, counseling is required. However, the first step is identifying what thought patterns reinforce this message and then replacing them.

So, if the quality of life depends on the quality of thoughts, what should we think? Most spiritual traditions and behavioral scientists emphasize practicing gratitude. We all have different cultural and spiritual beliefs, so one should incorporate whatever gratitude practice one finds appealing. It can be significant sweeping events such as physically visiting everyone who significantly impacted you, similar to Walter Green in *This is the Moment* [21], writing a thank you note each month for those one works with, or taking a moment to be internally grateful for the opportunity to care for patients before walking in an exam room. These can leave a positive impact, specifically allowing gratitude to become a habit. Once this happens, showing gratitude for one's loved ones daily is easier. Whether this takes the form of a prayer of thanksgiving, a loving-kindness meditation, a daily gratitude journal, or large-scale gratitude events, they all focus the mind on the type of thoughts that lead to mental resilience, humility, compassion, and antifragility. Additionally, gratitude combats depression and anxiety [22]. To date, I have not met anyone who wishes they had been less grateful.

Do Hard Things

Never give in, never give in, never, never, never, never

—Winston Churchill

Finally, do hard things. Remembering the challenges already conquered when meeting a new crisis can be invaluable. All the stories one tells at the end of life are about hard things. Everyone has a hero's journey and events that forged them into the person they have become. A comfortable life breeds regret. This goes beyond the difficult moments experienced at work because surgeons anticipate hard work. Confronting hard things outside of work allows growth into a complete human being with antifragility in multiple domains. When one's professional identity is threatened by legal claims, injury, one's mental health, or other forces, one should embrace the memory of these challenges and work to overcome current obstacles. In *The Comfort Crisis: Embrace discomfort to reclaim your wild, happy, healthy self,* Easter describes reviving the idea of misogi [23], a ritual performed by Japanese monks who stood in freezing glacial water as a purification method. He repurposes this to physical challenges that represent the opportunity for accomplishment, risking failure, which is the chance to build these intentional trials into modern life. Duckworth describes a similar concept in her book *Grit: The Power of Passion and Perseverance*, in which she discusses how discipline can be forged and how perseverance can serve one in future life challenges [24]. Decide to intentionally go through events that one can recall in times of crisis to remind one of one's strength, character, values, and worth.

Conclusion

Military physicians will face crises and significant stressors in their careers like all humans. Like all physicians, they will routinely deal with life-and-death matters and struggle with the best way to treat patients. The overwhelming majority of military physicians will face location changes that correspond with a change in their daily habits. They will also likely deal with deployment and separation from loved ones, not to mention the stress and danger of combat, which is unique to this profession and makes a career in the military a highly stressful one. Building resiliency should be done and can occur by following a few concepts:

1. Address the importance of physical health
2. Establish rituals to address difficult outcomes
3. Show gratitude
4. Be present and be mindful
5. Understand your inner monologue
6. Choose strategic challenges

With all of this, the ultimate goal is to achieve an antifragile state so that one is not just resilient; one uses challenges to become even better.

Active-duty physicians have access to a wide range of mental health support options. Most primary care clinics have an embedded mental health counselor who can be accessed through one's primary care physician. Alternatively, a referral can be placed to the behavioral health department for therapy or medication management. Both are confidential, but care is recorded in MHS Genesis. There are limits to confidentiality that apply to mental health services in all settings; these include being an imminent threat of harm to oneself or others or abuse of a child or vulnerable adult.

Marriage and family life counselors are master's or Ph.D. level licensed clinical counselors. They work with families, individuals, couples, and children to provide nonmedical problem identification and counseling services. The issues they address include relationships, stress management, grief after loss, occupational and other individual and family issues, and providing crisis intervention when needed. They do not chart in MHS Genesis and do not require a referral.

Most TriCare regions have a telehealth benefit using live audio and video or audio-only services. This can be very beneficial for those with odd or long hours. Active-duty service members often need a referral (family members and retirees usually do not), but the care is charted in the contracted service's medical record. Search your TriCare region's website to find which one is available.

Chaplain services on all posts offer faith-based and confidential family, marriage, and individual counseling to active-duty service members. They do not chart in MHS Genesis and do not require a referral.

Military One Source at www.militaryonesource.mil offers confidential nonmedical counseling, resources, and support. Services are not reported to the command, which means one can receive nonmedical counseling without anyone's knowledge. Nonmedical counseling is short-term (up to 12 sessions per issue). Here are examples of what they can address: relationships, stress/anger management, adjustment issues (to moving, deployment, or a new baby), marital problems, parenting, and loss/grief.

Many civilian counselors offer cash options. If one wants to remain wholly disassociated from the workplace, one can pay out of pocket and have care remain entirely confidential.

Anyone who needs support now or is having thoughts of suicide should call or text 988 to chat with a trained crisis counselor who can help immediately.

Reading List:
Meditation
Wherever You Go, There You Are by Jon Kabat-Zinn Ph.D. (and other works)
Contemplative Prayer: Traditional Christian Meditations for Opening to Divine Union by Thomas Keating
Peak Mind: Find Your Focus, Own Your Attention, Invest 12 Minutes a Day by Amish Jha
Dealing with Challenges
Trident Mindset app www.tridentmindset.com
Rising Strong by Brene Brown, Ph.D. (and other works)

The Comfort Crisis: Embrace Discomfort To Reclaim Your Wild, Happy, Healthy Self by Michael Easter
Communication
How to Know a Person by David Brooks
Talking to Strangers by Malcolm Gladwell
Social Relationships
Eight Dates: Essential Conversations for a Lifetime of Love by John and Julie Gottman
Love & Survival: The Scientific Basis or the Healing Power of Intimacy by Dean Ornish, M.D.

References

1. Kalmoe MC, Chapman MB, Gold JA, Giedinghagen AM. Physician suicide: a call to action. MO Med. 2019;116(3):211–6.
2. Department of Veterans Affairs. In: 2023 National Veteran Suicide Prevention Annual Report. Office of Mental Health and Suicide Prevention; 2023. https://www.mentalhealth.va.gov/docs/data-sheets/2023/2023-National-Veteran-Suicide-Prevention-Annual-Report-FINAL-508.pdf Accessed 06DEC2024.
3. Shanafelt TD, Balch CM, Dyrbye L, et al. Special report: suicidal ideation among American surgeons. Arch Surg. 2011;146(1):54–62. https://doi.org/10.1001/archsurg.2010.292.
4. Taleb N. Antifragile. Harlow: Penguin Books; 2012. p. 3.
5. Vandekerckhove M, Wang YL. Emotion, emotional regulation and sleep: an intimate relationship. AIMS Neurosci. 2017;5(1):1–17. https://doi.org/10.3934/Neuroscience.2018.1.1.
6. Knuppel A, Shipley MJ, Llewellyn CH, Brunner EJ. Sugar intake from sweet food and beverages, common mental disorder and depression: prospective findings from the Whitehall II study. Sci Rep. 2017;7(1):6287. https://doi.org/10.1038/s41598-017-05649-7.
7. Ratey J, Manning R. Go wild: free your body and mind from the afflictions of civilization. 1st ed. Brown and Company, NY: Little; 2014. p. 101–7.
8. Brown B. Rising strong. London: Vermilion; 2015. p. 77.
9. Willink J. Discipline equals freedom: field manual. 1st ed. New York: St. Martin's Press; 2017. p. 58–60.
10. Trident Mindset. Version 4.281.0. Trident Mindset LLC. Updated 02DEC2023. Flipping the script. Lesson 1: We Are Not Disturbed By Things. Tridentmindset.com. Accessed 06DEC2024.

11. Spafford H. (1873–1878) American colony in Jerusalem collection: Part I: Draft manuscript copy of hymn "It is Well With My Soul." The Library of Congress, www.loc.gov/item/mamcol.016/. Accessed 27AUG2024.
12. Ornish D. Love & survival: The scientific basis for the healing power of intimacy. San Francisco: HarperCollins; 1998. p. 23–71.
13. Gottman J, Silver N. The seven principles for making marriage work. London: Orion; 2015. p. 53–66.
14. Chapman D. The 5 love languages: the secret to love that lasts. Chicago: Northfield Publishing; 2015.
15. Gottman JM, Schwartz J, Gottman D, Abrams C, Abrams RC. Eight dates: essential conversations for a lifetime of love. New York: Workman Publishing; 2018. p. 73.
16. Jha A. Peak mind: find your focus, own your attention, invest 12 minutes a day. 1st ed. New York: Harper One, an imprint of Harper Collins Publishers; 2021.
17. Kabat-Zinn J. Full catastrophe living. New York: Bantam Dell Publishing Group; 2013.
18. Trident Mindset. Version 4.281.0. Trident Mindset LLC. Updated 02DEC2023. Self Talk: Lesson 1 Welcome to Self-Talk and Meditation: Lesson 9 Dino Dig. Tridentmindset.com Accessed 06DEC2024.
19. Brown B. The power of vulnerability: teachings on authenticity, connection, and courage. Session 2: Shame triggers. Sounds True; 2012. https://www.soundstrue.com 06DEC2025.
20. The Arbinger Institute. Leadership and self-deception: getting out of the box. San Francisco: Berrett-Koehler; 2000.
21. Green W. This is the moment! Rancho Santa Fe: Walter Green; 2010.
22. Diniz G, et al. The effects of gratitude interventions: a systematic review and meta-analysis. Einstein (San Paulo). 2023;21:eRW0371.
23. Easter M. The comfort crisis: embrace discomfort to reclaim your wild, happy, healthy self. Rodale: Harmony; 2021. p. 31–7.
24. Duckworth A. Grit: the power of passion and perseverance. 1st ed. New York, NY: Scribner; 2016.

LGBTQ+ Surgeon Life on Active Duty

33

Andrew T. Schlussel
and Kayleigh M. Herrick-Reynolds

Introduction: A Message from the Authors

> The ability to serve in the United States Army has been one of the most honorable contributions to our county that I have made. However, this came at a great cost when in 2000 I decided to join ROTC, put on the uniform, and for what I thought at the time, to place my sexual orientation and personal identity into the closet forever. Although my education in surgery and leadership, as well as the multiple relationships I developed with people around the globe, could not be replaced, there remained many challenges both in my professional and personal life by not being able to express my true self. I am delighted and pleased that, two decades later, we can now share a message about LGBTQ+ Life on Active Duty with the greater surgical community.
> —Andrew Schlussel

> Since the attacks of September 11th, I looked forward to the opportunity to serve my country in the military. I always viewed military service as an obligation and distinction that few were privileged to experience. As I grew into myself and fully recognized my queer iden-

A. T. Schlussel
HCA Florida Jacksonville Surgical Specialists, Jacksonville, FL, USA
e-mail: andrew.schlussel@hcahealthcare.com

K. M. Herrick-Reynolds (✉)
Department of Surgery, Walter Reed National Military Medical Center, Bethesda, MD, USA

A. T. Schlussel et al. (eds.), *The SAGES Manual for Navigating a Successful Military Surgical Career*,
https://doi.org/10.1007/978-3-031-88490-0_33

tity, I hesitated to sign up, accepting that my service would take a different form. I remember the repeal of Don't Ask, Don't Tell (DADT) clearly, as it happened while I was preparing to apply for medical school. With this policy change, I felt that a barrier to my service had been lifted and I joined the Army via the Health Professions Scholarship Program (HPSP). I look forward with pride to a career representing both the LGBTQ+ community and the US Army.
—Kayleigh Herrick-Reynolds

LGBTQ+ History

The history of the LGBTQ+ community in the United States military is a story of challenges, resilience, and progress (Fig. 33.1). For much of its history, the military operated under policies that discriminated against individuals based on their sexual orientation, leading to the expulsion of countless service members simply because of their identity. This discrimination persisted through the twentieth century, with LGBTQ+ individuals serving in silence, fearful of the consequences if their true selves were revealed.

Although the country may have viewed the policy of "Don't Ask, Don't Tell" (DADT) in 1993 as progress, it was a compromise reached after President Clinton was unable to keep his promise to completely lift an existing military ban on gay, lesbian, and bisexual individuals serving in the armed forces. This allowed LGBTQ+ individuals to serve in the military as long as they kept their sexual orientation a secret. This policy only recapitulated ongoing discrimination, which ultimately resulted in over 30,000 service men and women to be removed from duty due to their sexual identity and orientation. The repeal of DADT in 2010 marked a significant milestone, allowing gay, lesbian, and bisexual service members to serve openly without the fear of discharge due to their sexual orientation [1] (Table 33.1).

Despite the repeal of DADT, gay, lesbian, and bisexual service members still were unable to receive the same benefits afforded to heterosexual service members as a result of the county's Defense of Marriage Act (DOMA), which prevented same-sex couples from accessing federal benefits given to married opposite sex

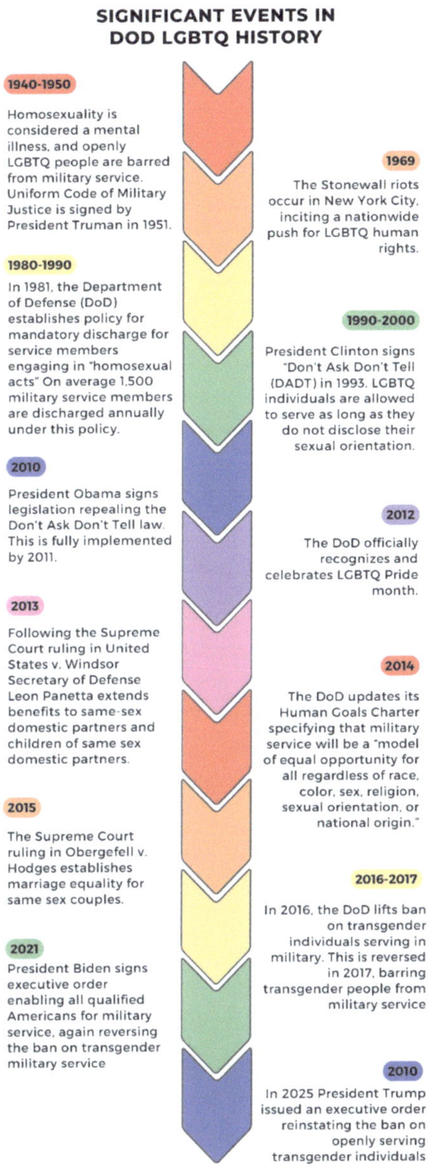

Fig. 33.1 LGBTQ+ Military History. *DOD* Department of Defense

Table 33.1 Resources for programs, policies, societies, and guidelines

Don't Ask, Don't Tell Resources	https://www.defense.gov/Spotlights/Dont-Ask-Dont-Tell-Resources/
Military Service Members' Legal Rights	https://www.justia.com/lgbtq/military-service/
USU SPECTRUM Student Interest Group	https://www.usuhs.edu/campus-life/student-interest-groups#ssg
Army Regulation 600–20 Army Command Policy	https://armypubs.army.mil/epubs/DR_pubs/DR_a/ARN32931-AR_600-20-004-WEB-6.pdf
Excelsior Surgical Society	https://www.facs.org/for-medical-professionals/membership-community/military-health-system-strategic-partnership/ess/
Society of Military Surgeons	https://www.militarysurgeons.org/
Association of Out Surgeons and Allies	https://www.outsurgeons.org/
AMA Advisory Committee on LGBTQ Issues	https://www.ama-assn.org/member-groups-sections/advisory-committee-lgbtq-issues
It's Pronounced Metrosexual	https://www.itspronouncedmetrosexual.com/
Trans student Student Education Resources	https://transstudent.org/
CDC Sexually Transmitted Infections Treatment Guidelines	https://www.cdc.gov/std/treatment-guidelines/
DHA Procedural Instructions: PrEP	https://www.health.mil/Reference-Center/DHA-Publications/2019/12/20/DHA-PI-6025-29
DOD Instruction 1300.28: In-Service Transition for Transgender Service Members (policy rescinded in January 2025)	https://www.esd.whs.mil/Portals/54/Documents/DD/issuances/dodi/130028p.pdf
TRICARE Assisted Reproductive Services	https://www.tricare.mil/CoveredServices/IsItCovered/AssistedReproductiveServices

The Army Military Parental Leave Program	https://www.hrc.army.mil/content/The%20Army%20Military%20Parental%20Leave%20Program%20(MPLP)
USU Faculty Development	https://medschool.usuhs.edu/about/faculty-affairs/faculty-development
ACS: Surgeons as Leaders course	https://www.facs.org/for-medical-professionals/education/programs/acs-surgeons-as-leaders/
SAGES: Fundamentals of Leadership and Development	https://www.sages.org/fld-sign-up/

USU Uniformed Services University, *AMA* American Medical Association, *CDC* Centers for Disease Control, *DHA* Defense Health Agency, *PrEP* pre-exposure prophylaxis, *DOD* Department of Defense, *ACS* American College of Surgeons, *SAGES* Society of American Gastrointestinal and Endoscopic Surgeons

couples. The Supreme Court's landmark 2013 ruling in *United States v. Windsor* struck down the section of DOMA that required the federal government to withhold benefits as unconstitutional, and The Department of Defense (DoD) began to offer spousal and family benefits to those in same-sex marriages on the same terms as it did to those in opposite sex marriages. Presently, these service members have the right to receive military health insurance coverage, a housing allowance, military ID cards, and survivor benefits. Furthermore, these benefits could be requested retroactively from the time of the ruling [2] (Table 33.1).

Further progress was made in 2016 when the DoD lifted the ban on transgender individuals serving openly in the military. This policy change allowed transgender individuals to serve in their preferred gender without fear of discrimination or discharge solely based on their gender identity. Transgender rights in the military have been a topic of significant debate in recent years. In June 2016 under the direction of President Obama, the DoD lifted the ban on transgender people serving openly, allowing them to serve in their self-identified gender. In 2017, President Trump announced that transgender individuals would no longer be allowed to serve in the military in any capacity. This decision faced legal challenges, however, in 2019 the Supreme Court allowed the policy to go into effect temporarily. The policy faced continuous legal disputes. Executive Order 13988, titled Preventing and Combating Discrimination on the Basis of Gender Identity or Sexual Orientation, was the fourth executive order signed by US President Joe Biden on January 20, 2021. However, on January 20, 2025, shortly after taking office, President Donald Trump rescinded the order. Currently, uncertainties remain regarding the provision of gender-affirming care by military physicians, as well as the use of pronouns for service members (Fig. 33.1).

Over the years, the military has evolved to acknowledge the invaluable contributions of LGBTQ+ individuals who serve their country with honor and pride. While the DoD has made great strides over the past 20 years, we continue the collective effort toward achieving equality and inclusion for all members of the armed forces.

Military Medical Education

Medicine and in particular surgery are known to be hierarchical environments and have often been viewed as conservative and resistant to change. There are numerous personal accounts detailing the experience of medical training as a gay person [3]. These accounts emphasize the fear of judgment, the concern that personal identity might impact grades or opportunities, and the constant evaluation of whether a new attending or senior resident will hold an opinion about one's sexual orientation. Survey data has demonstrated an inverse relationship between specialty choice for sexual and gender minorities in medicine and the perceived prestige of that specialty [4]. Combined with the history of the LGBTQ+ community in the military, this climate might contribute to the perception of lack of acceptance, lead to a hesitation to freely express one's sexual orientation when entering a career in military surgery, or even avoid the career (military or medical) altogether. Indeed, a 2023 qualitative study evaluating the experience of 10 LGBTQ+ service members in military medicine identified themes of explicit bias stemming from verbal discrimination, critiques about behavior and affect, and bias in classroom discussions within medical education [5]. Although numerous challenges remain for creation of an inclusive environment for the LGBTQ+ community in military medical education, a number of efforts are also underway.

Prior to January 2025, at the medical student level, the Uniformed Services University of Health Sciences (USUHS) sponsored an LGBTQ+ student interest group, SPECTRUM. Due to a recent shift in federal policy, this interest group, along with many others at USUHS, has been dismantled (Table 33.1). This group was founded in 2017 and strived to advocate for the experiences of LGBTQ+ staff and students on campus. In 2021, to inaugurate Pride month, the group dedicated a brick on campus to the LGBTQ+ students and staff of USUHS, stating, "You are needed. You belong." This token served the purpose of fostering a sense of inclusion and safety for members of the LGBTQ+ community [6].

At the graduate medical education (GME) level, integrating LGBTQ+ identity with the stress of learning to operate and care for patients while also assimilating into a close-knit surgical culture can be a challenge. A 2022 JAMA Surgery paper evaluated self-reported rates of mistreatment among LGBTQ+ general surgery residents compared to their non-LGBTQ+ peers using an anonymous survey of 6381 residents, where 305 respondents (4.8%) identified as LGBTQ+. Using multivariate regression, an association was identified between LGBTQ+ identity and higher rates of bullying (74.8% vs 66.9%; $p = 0.005$), discrimination (59.2% vs. 42.3%, $p < 0.001$), and sexual harassment (47.5% vs. 29.3%; $p < 0.001$). LGBTQ+ residents were also twice as likely to report considering leaving their residency program (OR 2.04, 95% CI 1.52–2.74) or having thoughts of suicide (OR 1.95, 95% CI 1.26–3.04) compared to their non-LGBTQ+ peers. Attending surgeons were cited in this study as the most common source of mistreatment [7].

When applying for general surgery residency in military medicine, applicants will be faced with the decision to disclose their sexual orientation in the interview process. Although sexual orientation is covered under military equal opportunity policies as a protected category [8], and differential treatment based on this identity is considered unlawful discrimination, the fear of implicit bias affecting a career you have dedicated yourself to and sacrificed for, may be difficult to overcome (Table 33.1).

Especially given the limited number of military programs compared to the civilian match, it may feel that you do not have the luxury of "choosing" a program where the culture values inclusion excellence. It may be helpful to use trusted mentors or near-peers with contacts in the places you are rotating to assess the environment before deciding how much to share about your personal life. For residents, faculty, and program directors in leadership positions, basic language changes can go a long way toward creating an inclusive culture and may even aid with recruitment by tangibly demonstrating a welcoming environment for applicants. For example, consider refraining from asking about someone's "wife" or "husband" and rather ask male and female applicants alike about their "spouse" or "partner."

Navigating your Life at Work

Disclosing your sexual identity and orientation to surgical colleagues, department chief, as well as senior and junior service members, is a personal choice that can be challenging for many individuals. Despite the progress that has been made legally, our military and government have many historical roots of bias against the LGBTQ+ community. Whether you are in school, residency or a practicing attending, much of your responsibility as a surgeon requires spending what can seem like countless hours at the hospital. This commitment can often take you away from your family and social community. Having to hide your identity may result in a continued feeling of isolation and mistrust in an already very stressful professional life.

When assigned to a new duty station, the military often assigns you a sponsor. Although this individual may initially be a stranger, they may be able to provide insight into the level of equity in the organization. Developing mentor/mentee relationships is beneficial for multiple reasons for a surgeon in any phase of their career; this is especially important to help navigate the intersection between professional and personal life. This is particularly important for your partner or spouse, as much of the military is centered around family and support for your loved ones when deployed. Most units will also have a Family Readiness Group, which provides a strong support network and means of communications when the servicemember is overseas or deployed. This is especially significant if you find yourself stationed in smaller cities or remote locations further from areas with a robust LGBTQ+ community.

As we move further away from the repeal of DADT, more service members feel at ease being open about their identity. If you are stationed with other openly LGBTQ+ service members, seek their guidance, mentorship, and friendship. You may be surprised to discover many similarities in your career development beyond your sexual orientation. There are private social media groups available for LGBTQ+ military members, stratified by rank and grade, which can be a source of networking when moving to a new station. Being part of surgical societies may also provide an opportunity to meet and network with other LGBTQ+ surgeons outside of your military organization. The American College of Surgeons has Excelsior Surgical Society, and the Society of American Gastrointestinal and Endoscopic Surgeons has the Military Surgical Committee and annual Military Surgical Symposium. Furthermore, many large medical organizations have various diversity committees with a focus on LGBTQ+ physicians such as the American Medical Association. Finally, the Association of Out Surgeons and Allies (AOSA) provides a strong network and community for all surgeons around the world (Table 33.1).

LGBTQ+ Medical Services

Developing a sense of community and trust among your peers not only helps you feel more comfortable and supported at work but also aids you as a provider in establishing a more inclusive practice for LGBTQ+ service members. The long history of denial surrounding LGBTQ+ military medical services has resulted in a significant knowledge gap for military physicians on how to appropriately care for LGBTQ+ patients. Many surgeons and primary care providers remain unfamiliar with how to treat and counsel these patients.

Culturally Competent Medical Care

As healthcare providers and surgeons, it is essential to develop a skill set that enables you to provide culturally competent medical care to all patients. The LGBTQ+ population has numerous biopsychosocial determinants of health that are important to consider, including personal biases from providers and medical personnel. Many patients delay cancer screenings due to possible past discriminatory clinical experiences, and partners of LGBTQ+ service members frequently have less access to insurance and healthcare services compared to the general dependent population. LGBTQ+ patients are more likely to struggle with mental health disorders, reduced quality of life, and increased rates of social isolation, particularly when they are disconnected from their biological family. As surgeon leaders, it is critical to develop a safe place for our patients to seek care.

Healthcare providers treating LGBTQ+ patients may face challenges due to insufficient familiarity with sexual health screening recommendations, awareness of gender-affirming therapies, awareness of higher rates of anxiety, depression, stress, substance use, trauma history or prior negative experience with the healthcare system, and inadvertent use of derogatory terminology. Understanding common terminology used to describe different sexual orientations and gender identities, small physical symbols in the clinic or workspace indicating support for the LGBTQ+ community such as a magazine or poster, and ensuring adequate clinic staff education can help create an inclusive and safe environment for LGBTQ+ patients [9].

Although being knowledgeable and up to date on LGBTQ+ healthcare is essential for all providers, many LGBTQ+ patients often seek out physicians who also identify as LGBTQ+. Many feel they will be heard and understood more effectively, and ultimately receive better surgical care. As with any patient, treat them with respect. Be mindful of pronouns; this can be asked when they check in at the front desk, during their intake with nursing staff, or by simply asking "how would you like to be addressed?" when the consultation begins. For those who have not incorporated this in their practice, it may seem awkward at first, but the patient will feel your sincerity. If you accidentally misgender or use incorrect pronouns for your patient, correct yourself and apologize. Do not belabor the apology as it will make the patient feel that the onus is on them to forgive your mistake.

To gain a deeper comprehension of pronouns, it is essential to grasp key terms and definitions, particularly in relation to a patient's identity, orientation, and expression. Many of the common terms include:

- **Sex assigned at birth**: This is the male, female, or intersex definition assigned at birth based primarily on external anatomy or chromosomal analysis.
- **Gender identity**: An individual's personal and internal understanding or sense of being male, female, neither, both, or another gender. A person's gender identity is self-determined and does not always match their gender expression or their sex

assigned at birth. Gender identities are most often described as male/man, female/woman, or nonbinary

- **Gender expression**: How an individual chooses to express their gender identity in an outward manner. How a patient is treated in society or clinical interactions is often dependent on their gender expression, but it is important to remember a patient's gender expression and identity may not always align.
- **Pronouns** are determined by the individual and are a form of gender expression.
  - Gendered pronouns include she/her/hers and he/him/his.
  - Gender-neutral pronouns include they/them/theirs, used in the singular.
- **Transgender**: A transgender person is a person whose gender identity is not the same as the sex they were assigned at birth. A transgender man is a person whose gender identity is male and their sex is Assigned Female At Birth (AFAB). A transgender woman is a person whose gender identity is female and their sex is Assigned Male At Birth (AMAB). Transgender people do not always identify as male or female, and like anyone else, transgender people may identify anywhere along the spectrum of gender. The term transvestite, is defined as one who dresses in clothes primarily associated with the other sex, is considered offensive and is not appropriate in a clinical setting.
- **Cisgender**: A cisgender person is a person whose gender identity is the same as the sex they were assigned at birth.
- **Sexual orientation**: Sexual orientation describes the type of attraction an individual feels toward other individuals. Sexual orientation also includes individuals who do not feel sexual attraction. Sexual orientation is not the same as gender identity or gender expression.
- **Dead name:** A transgender person's name assigned at birth that they no longer use. **Deadnaming** is the act of referring to a transgender or nonbinary person by their dead name.
- **Misgendering:** Intentionally or unintentionally referring to a person using a pronoun that does not reflect their gender identity.

For a more thorough understanding of gender terminology, valuable resources such as “It’s Pronounced Metrosexual” and “Transstudent Education Resources,” can be explored online [10, 11] (Fig. 33.2 and Table 33.1).

Obtaining an anatomical or organ inventory enables the provider to document the presence or absence of specific organs, facilitating patient-centered care and ensuring appropriate screenings for cervical, breast, and prostate health. Additionally, it addresses sex-specific clinical needs, such as a testicular exam or preoperative pregnancy testing. Furthermore, it is critical to know your patient’s anatomy. Important examples include a transgender woman AMAB with a neovagina and a rectal cancer, or a transgender man AFAB with a new breast mass. For patients who have undergone voice surgery or tracheal cartilage shave, emergency airway planning may differ.

Patients presenting to a surgeon are often seen at very vulnerable times, whether they are in pain, have a new cancer, or another ailment that affects their quality of life. Patients experiencing gender dysphoria may have increased fear of being touched in specific regions or organs. Thoroughly explain how and why you are or will be touching or examining these areas and why it is important to their care. Be an advocate for your patient, if you hear other members of the team misgendering or using the wrong name for the patient, correct the team member to ensure that respect is held for the patient. This is of utmost importance when a patient is sedated or anesthetized as they are unable to advocate for themselves.

In addition, the LGBTQ+ population has higher rates of tobacco use, psychosocial stressors with impact on cardiovascular health, and some reports have higher BMI in sexual minority women [9]. Use of hormonal therapy in gender-affirming care can impact hypercoagulability and risk of deep vein thrombosis, especially in the perioperative setting, as well as general cardiovascular and cerebrovascular health [12].

One area often falling under the purview of the military general surgeon is breast cancer care. For some patients who are transmen AFAB, breast as well as gynecological screening may represent a source of emotional stress. Additionally, transwomen

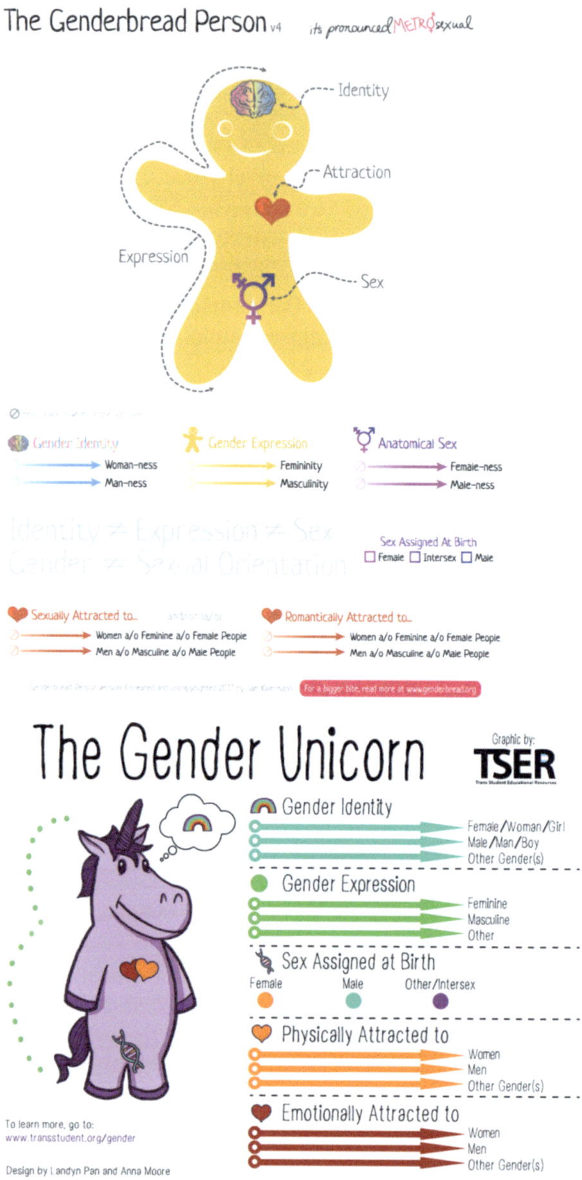

Fig. 33.2 Understanding Gender: The Genderbread Person and The Gender Unicorn [10, 11]. "It's Pronounced Metrosexual" and "Trans Student Education Resources" offer uncopyrighted illustrative material to enhance educational resources for a better understanding of gender expression

AMAB who are receiving hormonal therapy as part of their gender-affirming care have a higher risk of developing breast cancer when compared to cisgender men. The largest study to date evaluating this topic is out of the Netherlands, published in 2019. This was a retrospective national cohort study evaluating 2260 transwomen AMAB and 1229 transmen AFAB with comparison to the adult cisgender population. For transwomen AMAB, there was a 46-fold higher rate of developing breast cancer compared to cisgender men, but still lower than cisgender females. For transmen AFAB, the risk of developing breast cancer was approximately five times lower than expected when compared to cisgender women [13].

Although data is limited, expert consensus guidelines are published by several organizations such as the American College of Radiology (ACR) for breast cancer screening in this patient population [14]. In summary, from the ACR, for transwomen AMAB annual mammography with tomosynthesis is usually appropriate for patients with more than 5 years of hormone use, beginning at age 40 for average risk patients, and beginning at age 25 for those of higher than average risk. For transmen AFAB who have undergone top surgery, different societies have varying recommendations for screening ranging from no screening after surgery to annual MRI. Top surgery differs from a bilateral mastectomy in that some breast tissue is purposefully left behind for contouring of the chest. For AFAB transmen who have undergone only reduction mammoplasty or no surgery, yearly mammography is recommended for average risk patients with consideration for MRI in above average risk patients, similar to the cisgender female population [15].

Sexual Healthcare

Although not specific to the LGBTQ+ population, issues pertaining to sexual healthcare and sexual history are of great importance to the general surgeon. Sexual history should be asked in a non-judgmental forum and include information about number and gender of partners, sex practices including toys and parts of the body involved (anal, oral, vaginal), history of sexually transmitted infections (STI), the use of barrier contraceptives, and pregnancy intention for AFAB patients [16]. Patients should not be deemed at higher or lower risk for STIs solely based on their sexual orientation or gender identity. Careful attention should be paid to an individual's risk factors and practices, especially among men who have sex with men, as some of these patients may not identify as gay or bisexual.

Anorectal pathology is a common surgical referral among our service members. The surgeon should maintain a high index of suspicion for anorectal STIs in patients engaging in anal receptive intercourse. Left untreated, these conditions can lead to numerous systemic complications. Patients determined to be at risk for HPV exposure and subsequent anal dysplasia should be referred to a colorectal surgeon for consideration of treatment options and screening plans. Recent data from the ANCHOR trial, which evaluated individuals living with HIV aged 35 or older with biopsy-proven anal high-grade squamous intraepithelial lesions (HSIL), demonstrated a 57% reduction in the risk of progression to anal cancer in the treatment group compared to the active-monitoring group. This landmark trial stands among the first to provide data-driven support for the treatment of anal dysplasia [17]. Although high-resolution anoscopy should be performed by those appropriately trained, there are few providers other than surgeons who are aware of this intervention. AFAB patients should also be referred to gynecology for cervical cancer screening, especially if an HPV related anal lesion is identified. The Centers for Disease Control and Prevention's (CDC) STI Treatment Guidelines offer easily accessible and streamlined guidance for the treatment and prevention of STIs. Additionally, a mobile application is available for download, enhancing convenience and accessibility [18] (Table 33.1).

Regarding HIV risk, all active duty military members are screened regularly, and this requirement does not change solely based on a service member's sexual orientation or gender identity. Individual high-risk exposures or workplace exposures and the use of post-exposure prophylaxis (PEP) are managed on a case-by-case basis. For patients at high risk wishing to use HIV pre-exposure prophylaxis (PrEP), the DHA has published procedural instructions, established in 2019 [19] (Table 33.1). This instruction follows CDC guidelines, and stipulates that individuals receiving PrEP get HIV testing every 3 months. PrEP is covered for all beneficiaries (military and civilian). Importantly, the use of PrEP does not impact a service member's deployability, as it can be stopped prior to deployment, and the use of PrEP in itself is not an eligibility criteria for re-enlistment or accession into any service branch. With respect to mass casualty situations, although current or past use of PrEP does not preclude participation in walking blood bank programs, blood donation still remains governed by the FDA regulation stipulating that men who have sex with men must defer blood donation for 12 months after the last same-sex sexual encounter. A recent publication assessing active duty gay and bisexual men's interest in PrEP found that although 71% indicated interest in accessing PrEP, gaps in provider knowledge, service member mistrust in the military healthcare system, confidentiality concerns, and a lack of a systemic approach to PrEP remain barriers to access [20].

It is important for military surgeons to be knowledgeable about the medical care needed for LGBTQ+ patients. You may find yourself being the first provider to discuss PrEP, anorectal STI screening and treatment, and HPV vaccination in older men. If you are at a large medical treatment facility, seek out your local infectious disease and mental health providers to partner with them to establish an institution that provides the full spectrum care for this patient population.

Gender-Affirming Care

At the time this chapter was published, Executive Order 13988, which allowed transgender service members to serve openly on active duty, had been rescinded. The information provided below reviews the access to care received by transgender individuals between 2021 and 2025. It is recommended that you remain up to date on current Executive Orders (https://www.whitehouse.gov/presidential-actions/), the Department of Defense, and local command policies.

In-Service Transition for Transgender Service Members was covered under DoD Instruction 1300.28 9 [21]. Army directive 2021–22 (Army Service by Transgender Persons and Persons with Gender Dysphoria) stipulates that military medical providers will diagnose and provide necessary care for transgender Soldiers, and that this care was provided to the Soldier subject to command approval [22]. Following a diagnosis of gender dysphoria, the Soldier was eligible for gender-affirming therapy; once the Soldier was stable in their self-identified gender, as determined by a military medical provider, the Soldier could request command approval for a gender-marker change in Defense Enrollment Eligibility Reporting System (DEERS). Once the gender-marker was changed in DEERS, that Soldier was able to serve in their self-identified gender, including body composition standards, facilities usage, uniform and grooming standards, and physical readiness testing.

Although TRICARE covers gender-affirming hormone therapy for beneficiaries diagnosed with gender dysphoria, it does not cover gender-affirming surgical therapies. Despite this, active duty service members can request a waiver through the Supplemental Health Care Program in cases of "medically necessary, gender-affirming surgery." An array of gender-affirming surgical therapies are available, including vaginoplasty, phalloplasty, masculinizing chest surgery ("top surgery"), voice surgery, facial feminization, augmentation mammoplasty, and in certain instances hysterectomy/oophorectomy or orchiectomy [23]. Availability and access to these procedures were subject to individual surgeon expertise across the military treatment facilities.

Assisted Reproductive Care

Assisted Reproductive Care (ARC) services may be covered by TRICARE in some instances; however, it must be deemed medically necessary and combined with coital conception. Certain Military Treatment Facilities (MTF) with OB/GYN residencies have policies allowing coverage of oral and injectable medications used for in-vitro fertilization (IVF) and intrauterine insemination (IUI) to increase ARC exposure within the residency training program. Even in these locations, the cost of IVF, generally around $8000 per cycle, is paid by the service member. The ARC program at Walter Reed National Military Medical Center (WRNMMC) is one example of such a program. This was established in 1996 and is the largest provider of reproductive health in the military, performing over 600 treatment cycles per year. For females, the age limit is 43, and additional exclusion criteria include BMI >40 and FSH >12. Fertility treatments are considered elective, and for active duty patients, leave for appointments and cycles is at the discretion of the individual's command.

Covered services include hormonal evaluation, semen analysis, semen function testing, chromosomal studies, and diagnostic imaging such as hysterosalpingogram and monitoring ultrasound. TRICARE does not cover costs associated with IVF or IUI, costs related to sperm or egg donors, or surrogacy. Additionally, costs of fertility preservation are not covered (Table 33.1).

Although there are no specific exclusions for same-sex female partners participating in IUI or IVF, the language in the center intake forms and procedures can be stereotypically heteronormative. Given the high demand for these services with a long wait time, there is also no mechanism in place for simultaneous or parallel evaluation of a same-sex female couple when trying to start a family. For example, each person needs to apply and undergo separate evaluation, which can be challenging when choosing donor sperm and needing to undergo genetic testing.

Regarding same-sex male couples, TRICARE does not offer any coverage for gestational carriers, to include being unable to have them be seen within the MTF system. Although donor eggs are used occasionally for heterosexual or same-sex female couples due to age or preference, there is no mechanism for identifying, evaluating, or compensating gestational carriers within the current military health system.

Military parental leave policies have recently been amended and include both the birthing and non-birthing parent as well as adoptive parents and in certain cases foster parents. Parents are granted 12 weeks of parental leave, subject in certain instances to command approval for the timing of when leave can be taken (Table 33.1).

LGBTQ+ Allyship

The Human Rights Campaign defines an Ally as someone who is actively supportive of LGBTQ+ people [24]. Becoming a supportive Ally involves a commitment to understanding and affirming diverse experiences and advocating for LGBTQ+ patients and the community. This includes continued education on terminology and various issues faced by the community, whether this be healthcare needs or policies that impact LGBTQ+ individuals. One should strive to use inclusive language, avoid making assumptions about someone's gender identity or sexual orientation, and be open to feedback. Being an Ally in military surgery cultivates an inclusive environment for your LGBTQ+ colleagues, which ultimately leads to happier, more valued and more productive surgeons.

There are many avenues to support the LGBTQ+ community. The Uniformed Services University (USU) provides the USU Faculty Allyship Curriculum. This program is available to any USU faculty, both billeted and nationally, and aims to support USU students through their time in medical school, promote faculty who recognize the principles of allyship as essential for the success of the USU mission, and foster student-faculty mentoring relationships. They host monthly virtual workshops as well as monthly community conversations designed to increase comfort in communicating across differences and supporting all members of the healthcare team. In addition, The American College of Surgeons offers the ACS Surgeons as Leaders course, which focuses on inclusive excellence, cultivating change, and leading teams. The Society of Gastrointestinal and Endoscopic Surgeons has developed the Fundamentals of Leadership and Development course with online modules followed by in-person small group problem-based didactic discussions, toward a similar end (Table 33.1). Several other nationally recognized non-federal surgical societies, including the Association of Out Surgeons and Allies (AOSA), actively support equitable and inclusive surgical education, and resources are accessible through their membership. As leaders in both surgery and the military, these courses equip you with the knowledge and tools to help cultivate a more inclusive environment within your institution.

Conclusion

The DoD has made significant progress in the care and inclusion of the LGBTQ+ community. However, barriers to care and self-expression still exist that may impact a patient's medical needs or a colleague's professional struggles. There are a number of specific screening and perioperative considerations that the military surgeon should be cognizant of in caring for LGBTQ+ patients. The importance of mentorship, community building, and the essential role of the Ally in fostering a safe, inclusive, and productive environment for LGBTQ+ patients and providers cannot be understated. It remains the individual responsibility of the military surgeon to stay informed and knowledgeable about issues pertaining to LGBTQ+ healthcare in order to fulfill their mission to support a medically ready military force.

Disclaimer The opinions and assertions expressed herein are those of the author(s) and do not reflect the official policy or position of the Uniformed Services University of the Health Sciences or the Department of Defense.

This research was supported (in whole or in part) by HCA Healthcare and/or an HCA Healthcare affiliated entity. The views expressed in this publication represent those of the author(s) and do not necessarily represent the official views of HCA Healthcare or any of its affiliated entities.

References

1. Defense USDo. Don't Ask Don't Tell Resources. 2023. https://www.defense.gov/Spotlights/Dont-Ask-Dont-Tell-Resources/. Accessed 30 Nov 2023.
2. JUSTIA. Military Service members' legal rights. 2023. https://www.justia.com/lgbtq/military-service/.
3. Turban JL. Medical training in the closet. N Engl J Med. 2019;381(14):1305–7. https://doi.org/10.1056/NEJMp1905829.
4. Sitkin NA, Pachankis JE. Specialty choice among sexual and gender minorities in medicine: the role of specialty prestige, perceived inclusion, and medical school climate. LGBT Health. 2016;3(6):451–60. https://doi.org/10.1089/lgbt.2016.0058.
5. Aldahondo R, Cole R. The experiences of LGBTQ healthcare professionals within military medical culture. Mil Med. 2023;188(11–12):e3606–12. https://doi.org/10.1093/milmed/usad284.

6. Neligh I. Student Interest Group brings 'Pride' to USU. 2023. https://news.usuhs.edu/2021/06/student-interest-group-brings-pride-to.html.
7. Heiderscheit EA, Schlick CJR, Ellis RJ, et al. Experiences of LGBTQ+ residents in US general surgery training programs. JAMA Surg. 2022;157(1):23–32. https://doi.org/10.1001/jamasurg.2021.5246.
8. Army Command Policy. Army Regulation 600–20. U.S Government Publishing Office. 2020.
9. Bass B, Nagy H. Cultural competence in the care of LGBTQ patients. StatPearls. 2023.
10. Killerman S. The Genderbread Person v4. It's pronounced metrosexual. 2018. https://www.itspronouncedmetrosexual.com/2018/10/the-genderbread-person-v4/. Accessed 1 Dec 2023.
11. Trans Student Educational Resources. The gender unicorn. 2015. http://www.transstudent.org/gender.
12. Connelly PJ, Marie Freel E, Perry C, Ewan J, Touyz RM, Currie G, Delles C. Gender-affirming hormone therapy, vascular health and cardiovascular disease in transgender adults. Hypertension. 2019;74(6):1266–74. https://doi.org/10.1161/HYPERTENSIONAHA.119.13080. Epub 2019 Oct 28. Erratum in: Hypertension. 2020 Apr;75(4):e10. PMID: 31656099; PMCID: PMC6887638.
13. de Blok CJM, Wiepjes CM, Nota NM, van Engelen K, Adank MA, Dreijerink KMA, et al. Breast cancer risk in transgender people receiving hormone treatment: nationwide cohort study in the Netherlands. BMJ. 2019;365:l1652. https://doi.org/10.1136/bmj.l1652.
14. Expert Panel on Breast Imaging, Brown A, Lourenco AP, Niell BL, Cronin B, Dibble EH, Moy L. ACR appropriateness criteria(R) transgender breast cancer screening. J Am Coll Radiol. 2021;18(11S):S502–15. https://doi.org/10.1016/j.jacr.2021.09.005, PMID: 34794604.
15. Santora T. The confusing world of breast cancer screening for transgender people. Breastcancer.org.
16. Reno H, Park I, Workowski K, Machefsky A, Bachmann L. Sexual history taking. Centers for Disease Control and Prevention (CDC). https://www.cdc.gov/std/treatment/SexualHistory.htm. January 14, 2022. https://www.breastcancer.org/news/screening-transgender-non-binary. October 19, 2023. Accessed 30 Nov 2023.
17. Palefsky JM, Lee JY, Jay N, Goldstone SE, Darragh TM, Dunlevy HA, et al.; ANCHOR Investigators Group. Treatment of anal high-grade squamous intraepithelial lesions to prevent anal cancer. N Engl J Med. 2022;386(24):2273–2282. https://doi.org/10.1056/NEJMoa2201048. PMID: 35704479; PMCID: PMC9717677.
18. Workowski KA, Bachmann LH, Chan PA, Johnston CM, Muzny CA, Park I, Reno H, Zenilman JM, Bolan GA. Sexually transmitted infections treatment guidelines, 2021. MMWR Recomm Rep. 2021;70(4):1–187. https://doi.org/10.15585/mmwr.rr7004a1. PMID: 34292926; PMCID: PMC8344968.

19. Defense Health Agency. Procedural Instruction Number 6025.29. 2019.
20. Beltran RM, Schuyler AC, Blair CS, Goldbach JT, Castro CA, Holloway IW. "That's kind of like the big struggle right now is can we get PrEP?": facilitators and barriers to PrEP uptake among active duty gay and bisexual men. Sex Res Social Policy. 2023;20(2):413–25. https://doi.org/10.1007/s13178-021-00622-6. PMC10212805.
21. Department of Defense. Instruction 1300.28: in-service transition for transgender service members. https://www.esd.whs.mil/Portals/54/Documents/DD/issuances/dodi/130028p.pdf.
22. United States Department of the Army. Army Directive 2021–2022. https://armypubs.army.mil/epubs/DR_pubs/DR_a/ARN32878-ARMY_DIR_2021-22-000-WEB-1.pdf. Accessed 1 Dec 2023.
23. Deutsch MB. Overview of gender-affirming treatments and procedures. UCSF transgender care. 2016. https://transcare.ucsf.edu/guidelines/overview.
24. Human Rights Campaign. Glossary of terms. https://www.hrc.org/resources/glossary-of-terms. Accessed 1 Dec 2023.

Starting a Family in the Military

34

Farah A. Husain and Marissa Beiling

Introduction

The 2022 Department of Defense demographics survey of active-duty soldiers revealed that 17.5% of active-duty military were women, and over 80% were under the age of 35. 47.6% of military members were married. Thirty-seven percent of service members had children, with over 70% of children falling under the age of 11. Looking at female active duty service members, 29% had children, and 45.3% of female service members were in dual-military marriages [1].

Dr. David Bruce Bell once described balancing demands between the military and the family as a battle between "two greedy institutions" [2]. Fortunately, starting a family while serving in the military has become more commonplace with added support structures and is not such a grim prospect. While starting a family is always filled with challenges, the military has explored ways to support families based on service member feedback to

F. A. Husain (✉)
University of Arizona College of Medicine-Phoenix, Obesity and Metabolic Disorders Service Line, Banner University Medical Group, Phoenix, AZ, USA

M. Beiling
Oregon Health and Science University, Portland, OR, USA
e-mail: beiling@ohsu.edu

A. T. Schlussel et al. (eds.), *The SAGES Manual for Navigating a Successful Military Surgical Career*,
https://doi.org/10.1007/978-3-031-88490-0_34

optimize the experience and understanding of the many uncertainties that come with the job.

Military service is said to hasten adulthood. It is, therefore, natural in this process to consider the expansion of the family unit, whether finding a partner or welcoming children. Families face many challenges unique to military service, such as deployments, job changes, and geographic relocations that have been shown to add stress. However, these stressors can allow military members to build strength in their families as a means of emotional support and comfort, as well as stability [3]. The introduction of children is full of surprises, both good and difficult. Children need not only love but also security and stability. Consistency can be difficult to provide with the high operational tempo, leading to frequent deployments and increased dual military families. Dual military service parents are expected to provide a care plan for children as young as 6 months old if both parents are deployed simultaneously. This can cause distress to the parents who feel they are abandoning their child and to the child who feels a great upheaval of their routine. Being a military parent requires an ability to anticipate the uncertainties of the job and operationalize the plan on short notice [4].

Studies have shown that young children in military families mimic their mother's well-being, reinforcing the importance of steadiness and happiness at home. If stressors are added, such as the need to engage in additional parenting roles like managing medical care, advocating for educational/childcare options, and providing specialized therapies, including behavioral interventions, a burden can be added for families. Job-related duties can make it tough to navigate varied service systems and support systems that necessitate a great deal of time, frequent appointments, or in-person follow-up. Sadly, a term coined, "military family syndrome" was developed to describe military families exhibiting mental health issues and challenges at a higher rate than those not affiliated with the military. Research has demonstrated that strong family relationships and positive parent interaction can assist in avoiding such adversity [5].

Families overcoming under stress (FOCUS), a family-centered, evidence-informed resiliency training program started at Harvard and UCLA, is one support structure available. Since Operation

Iraqi Freedom (OIF) and Operation Enduring Freedom (OEF), over two million children have had a parent deployed overseas. Families can adapt well to changes like deployment, but they also can find high levels of stress, trauma, and potential for family discord upon reunion. Creating a strong fighting force can hinge upon providing psychological treatment upon reunion, resiliency training, communication skills, and baseline counseling/support prior to deployments for the entire family. Programs like FOCUS were created to intervene early and help create a positive home environment [6].

Challenges of Starting a Family in the Military

Deployment and Separation

Deployment Support Policies: Military branches have policies in place to support families during deployments. These policies aim to facilitate communication between deployed service members and their families, providing resources such as internet access, video calls, and regular updates. Additionally, family support groups play a crucial role in assisting families during deployment periods.

Coping Mechanisms and Communication Strategies: Military families employ various coping mechanisms during deployment, including maintaining regular communication through emails, letters, and video calls. The importance of open and honest communication between partners is emphasized, and military branches often provide counseling services to help families navigate the emotional challenges of separation.

Frequent Relocations

Permanent Change of Station (PCS) Policies: The Permanent Change of Station policies govern the relocation process for military families. While PCS is a routine part of military life, these policies aim to streamline the moving process and provide resources to assist families in adapting to new locations. This includes financial support, relocation assistance programs, and access to community services.

Creating Stability for Children: To address the impact of frequent moves on children, military schools and education support programs are designed to provide continuity in education. These programs help children transition smoothly between schools and maintain a sense of stability despite changes in location.

Emotional and Mental Strain

Military Family Life Counseling (MFLC) Program: The Military Family Life Counseling Program offers confidential, nonmedical counseling services to military families. This resource is particularly valuable in addressing the emotional strain that can result from the unpredictable nature of military life. MFLC services are available at no cost to service members and their families.

Support Systems and Resources: In addition to counseling services, military families can access various support systems and resources, including chaplain services, family support centers, and peer-to-peer networks. These resources contribute to the emotional well-being of military families by providing outlets for expression and assistance during challenging times. Links to each service's family resources are below:

Army Quality of Life | The United States Army (https://www.army.mil/qualityoflife/)

Family Readiness (navy.mil) (https://ffr.cnic.navy.mil/Family-Readiness/)

Airman and Family (af.mil) (https://www.afpc.af.mil/Airman-and-Family/)

Policies Supporting Military Families

Tricare Coverage

Maternity Care Under Tricare: Tricare offers comprehensive maternity care coverage for military families. This includes prenatal care, labor and delivery, and postpartum care. The coverage extends to both service members and their spouses, ensuring that the entire family receives the necessary medical attention during the crucial phases of pregnancy and childbirth.

Fertility Treatment Coverage: As of 2023, Tricare will cover infertility evaluation. However, per the 2023 website (Infertility Diagnosis and Treatment | TRICARE—https://tricare.mil/CoveredServices/IsItCovered/InfertilityTreatment), Tricare will not cover artificial or intrauterine insemination, any costs related to donors or semen banks, reversal of tubal ligation, reversal of a vasectomy, unless medically necessary, care for erectile dysfunction from psychological causes, noncoital reproductive procedures, services or supplies such as in vitro fertilization (unless you were injured or had a serious illness that resulted in your infertility). Fertility preservation and surrogacy are not covered.

Pediatric Healthcare Coverage: Tricare offers robust pediatric healthcare coverage, ensuring that military children receive high-quality medical care. This coverage encompasses well-child visits, vaccinations, and specialized care, contributing to the overall well-being and health of military dependents. This includes care for children with special needs.

Military Parental Leave Program (MPLP)

The Military Parental Leave Program is a crucial policy introduced to support military families during life-changing events like the birth or adoption of a child. Per Directive-Type Memorandum (DTM) 23-001, parental leave is provided to Active and Reserve component service members (on active duty for 12 months or more) who have given birth, adopted a child, or had a child placed for adoption or long-term foster care with them. Birth parents will be granted 12 weeks of parental leave following a period of convalescent leave, and nonbirth parents will be granted 12 weeks of leave following the birth of their child. Adoptive parents and eligible foster parents will also be granted 12 weeks of parental leave. The MPLP is designed to allow members to care for their children while balancing the needs of their unit.

The leave can be taken by both birth and nonbirth parents and must be administered in accordance with the policies and procedures outlined in the DTM. The expansion of the MPLP, which applies to all eligible Service members as of January 4, 2023, takes precedence over previous DoD issuances and service regulations.

Variations in Leave Duration and Flexibility: While the MPLP establishes a framework for parental leave, variations exist among different branches of the military. The Army, Navy, Air Force, Marine Corps, and Coast Guard may implement the MPLP with some branch-specific nuances. Duration and flexibility can vary, and service members are encouraged to familiarize themselves with their specific branch policies to make informed decisions about their leave options.

Lactation Policies

Military Lactation Support Program: The Military Lactation Support Program is designed to provide comprehensive support for breastfeeding military mothers. It includes the provision of lactation rooms on military installations, ensuring a private and comfortable space for breastfeeding or expressing milk, along with flexible breaks and collaboration with military medical services. This program reflects the military's commitment to creating a supportive family environment.

Resources for Breastfeeding Military Mothers: In addition to physical spaces, military bases offer resources such as lactation consultants and educational materials to assist breastfeeding mothers. The emphasis is on promoting breastfeeding as a healthy choice for military families while providing the necessary support to make it a feasible option for service members.

Adoption and Surrogacy

Military families interested in adoption can benefit from adoption assistance programs offered by the military branches. These programs may include financial assistance, counseling services, and informational resources to guide military families through the adoption process.

Surrogacy Considerations: While surrogacy is a complex and evolving area, military branches are increasingly recognizing the diverse paths to family building. The military healthcare system may provide some coverage for medical aspects of surrogacy, and service members are encouraged to explore available resources and consult with medical professionals for guidance.

Education Benefits and Dependent Care

Military families have access to a range of educational benefits and childcare support designed to ease the challenges of military life. For education, the Post-9/11 GI Bill allows service members to transfer unused educational benefits to their spouses or children, covering tuition, housing, and book costs for college or vocational training. Additionally, the Military Spouse Career Advancement Accounts (MyCAA) program provides financial assistance for spouses pursuing licenses, certifications, or associate degrees in high-demand fields. For childcare, the Department of Defense offers subsidized childcare programs through Child Development Centers (CDCs) on military installations, providing affordable, high-quality care. The Military Child Care in Your Neighborhood (MCCYN) program MCCYN | MCC Central (disa.mil—https://public.militarychildcare.csd.disa.mil/mcc-central/mcchome/mccyn) extends these benefits to off-base childcare providers, ensuring that families have access to reliable childcare options regardless of their location.

Conclusion

As demonstrated by the policies and research, while starting a family during military service has challenges, it is also supported. The military understands that a strong fighting force is created with a strong family behind its members.

While starting a family in the military involves navigating numerous challenges, the support systems in place are designed to help families overcome these obstacles and build strong, supportive relationships. The military's understanding of the critical role that families play in the overall well-being of service members is evident in the comprehensive support structures available, ensuring that military families can face the demands of service with resilience and strength.

References

1. Military community demographics. 2022. https://www.militaryonesource.mil/data-research-and-statistics/military-community-demographics/.
2. Bell D, Schumm W. Balancing work and family demands in the military: what happens when your employer tells you to go to war? In: Halpern D, Murphy S. Work-family balance to work-family interaction: Changing the metaphor. Routledge. 2013. pp. 83–95.
3. Lundquist J, Xu Z. Reinstitutionalizing families: life course policy and marriage in the military. J Marriage Family. 76(5):1063–81.
4. O'Grady AF, Burton ET, Chawla N, Topp D, Wadsworth SM. Evaluation of a multimedia intervention for children and families facing multiple military deployments. J Prim Prev. 2016;37(1):53–70.
5. Classen AI, Horn E, Palmer S. Needs of military families: family and educator perspective. J Early Interv. 2019;41(3):233–55. https://doi.org/10.1177/1053815119847235.
6. Lester P, Mogil C, Saltzman W, et al. Families overcoming under stress: implementing family-centered prevention for military families facing wartime deployments and combat operational stress. Mil Med. 2011;176(1):19–25.

Dual Surgeon Couple/Dual Military Couple Life on Active Duty

35

Kimberly Gerling, John Blickle, Adam M. Pickett, Robert W. Tracey, Ashley E. Humphries, and Michele M. Gage

Introduction

Life as a surgeon is challenging, requiring consistent effort to deliver complex surgical care, develop and maintain skills, progress academically, and teach residents and/or team members, all while maintaining "work-life balance." Life as a ***military*** surgeon compounds these challenges in ways unique from the lives of civilian surgeons, such as deployments to combat zones, extended service in humanitarian missions, or a lack of control over one's current and future

K. Gerling
Johns Hopkins Hospital, Baltimore, MD, USA

J. Blickle
Uniformed Services University, Bethesda, MD, USA

National Capital Consortium, Washington, DC, USA

A. M. Pickett
Anderson Orthopedic Clinic, Arlington, VA, USA

R. W. Tracey · A. E. Humphries
Uniformed Services University, Bethesda, MD, USA

Department of Orthopedic Surgery, Walter Reed National Military Medical Center, Bethesda, MD, USA

A. T. Schlussel et al. (eds.), *The SAGES Manual for Navigating a Successful Military Surgical Career*,
https://doi.org/10.1007/978-3-031-88490-0_35

location of employment. When both spouses are service members, the complexity of these challenges increases even further, and this is a critical topic as there are a significant number of military surgeons who are married to another active-duty service member or "dual-military." According to a US Department of Defense (DOD) demographics survey in 2022, approximately 7% of military couples are dual-military [1]. Of the military branches, the Air Force has consistently had the highest percentage of dual-military couples, but this number has increased in all branches over time [2]. Recognizing the impacts of military life on dual-military families, each branch of service has policies and procedures that influence assignments for dual-military couples. These policies are beneficial to dual-military couples, but when it comes to navigating life and careers as a dual-military surgeon/physician couple, the current most valuable asset is the input from peers and mentors within the dual-military-and-surgical/medical community. Those of us who have experienced the dual-military physician family life firsthand best understand the unique challenges and opportunities facing a dual-military surgeon. In this chapter, we will review the recent demographics of dual-military couples, discuss career progression in graduate medical education, the impact of deployments, resources, and options for dual-military parents, and provide an overview of the policies of each service governing assignments for dual-military couples.

Demographics and Dual-Military Surgeon Survey Results

According to the most recent Department of Defense (DOD) Demographics survey from 2022, 7% of active-duty families consist of dual-military marriages. Based on this survey, approxi-

M. M. Gage (✉)
Uniformed Services University, Bethesda, MD, USA

Division of Surgical Oncology, Walter Reed National Military Medical Center, Bethesda, MD, USA

mately one-third of active duty, dual military households have children (34.7%). Between the services, the Air Force has the highest percentage of dual-military couples (11.2%), followed by the Space Force, Navy, Marine Corps, and Army, respectively [1].

We conducted an informal survey of current and former, retired or separated from the military, dual-military couples with at least one of the spouses being a surgical specialty in order to obtain real-world experiences and opinions on this challenging relationship. We had 23 surgeons respond to our survey, including several who are both dual-military and dual-surgeon (30%). Additionally, approximately one-third of spouses were physicians from nonsurgical specialties, and another one-third had military careers outside of medicine (aviation, logistics, etc.). While the majority of our respondents were general surgeons or general surgery subspecialists (e.g., colorectal, bariatrics, vascular), we also had respondents from other surgical fields such as orthopedic, head and neck, urology, and OB-GYN surgical specialties. All surgeons surveyed had spent significant time away from their spouse either from deployments or temporary duty assignments with the minimum time being 5 months and the longest response time was >65 months, though this was not correlated to career length or stratified based on spouse. Interestingly, one-third of respondents reported both they and their spouse were deployed or on temporary duty (TDY) at the same time—a particularly challenging circumstance, especially in the setting of parenting children.

Graduate Medical Education and Surgical Training

One of the primary concerns of the dual-military couple includes physically staying together through medical training (internship, residency, fellowship, etc.) and beyond. Even at the start of the relationship and career, this can be a daunting first hurdle. For students at the Uniformed Services University of Health Sciences (USUHS), many try to go through the arduous process of branch transfer before their third year of medical school to increase their chances of co-location and career alignment. For those that remain in their respective branches, this can lead to limited options for permanent duty stations and career variability. Unlike civilian dual-physician couples, students must be legally married and enrolled in the service-specific marriage program (see below) to ensure a couple's match when applying to Graduate Medical Education (GME) programs. After enrolling in the branch-specific program, there are few formal avenues to change location once assigned. This requires rebuttals and lengthy reviews by each program. Mentorship and guidance from senior program leaders are key when this situation arises.

For the surgery resident specifically, there are even fewer options for switching residency programs given the smaller program size and inflexibility of the American College of Graduate Medical Education (ACGME). Also unique to surgical trainees is the length of their training pipelines. A 5–7 year surgical training duration (not including subspecialization) is significantly longer than the traditional assignment in the military and other nonsurgery residency training programs. This can limit options for career advancement on the nonsurgeon spouse as the military often looks for traditional "next-assignments" in order to promote.

Following surgical specialty training, deployments and career progression become the primary concerns for dual-military physicians. These challenges often result in one spouse's career taking precedence either by conscious choice or default. More balanced approaches include alternating which person gets the next "best" assignment for their career. While there is no right way for every family, open communication is key. Identifying and correlating early, middle, and late career goals can help identify potential conflicts in career planning. Fellowship training or command opportunities may have to be changed or delayed to accommodate both spouses' goals.

Deployments

Deployments are often the most exciting and daunting aspect of any service member's career. This can be an especially difficult burden when considering the effects on a surgical career and one's family.

Transparency with your military service specialty leader or consultant is paramount. Important issues to discuss include but are not limited to spouse PCS/deployment, pregnancy, and other major life events. Together, you may be able to plan for future deployments to optimize the timing for your family and potentially avoid surprises or scrambling for fellowship match. Transparency with your Chain of Command and colleagues is equally important as they will be able to provide additional support to the nondeployed service member.

Updating your SGLI (life insurance) and your will are also key. Your command administrative and legal departments will be able to assist you with both, and this is something required to be reviewed prior to deployment. To update your SGLI online, take these steps: go to milConnect (https://milconnect.dmdc.osd.mil/milconnect/); sign in; go to Benefits, Life Insurance SOES-SGLI Online Enrollment System; check your coverage and beneficiary information and update accordingly. Your Will needs to be created and executed by your JAG/Legal department.

A Family Care Plan is also necessary as it designates short- and long-term care plans for your children, if applicable for your family. The Family Care Plan outlines designees for the care of your children, and also designates access to funds, a plan for school, and a plan for childcare outside of your spouse. This is important for all service members with children, but especially for dual-military members. The following are the Family Care Plan documents: Navy NAVPERS 1740/6; Army DA Form 5305-R; Air Force Form 357; Marine Corps MCO 1740.113D; Coast Guard does not currently require a Family Care Plan. It is important to have a plan with multiple layers of nonfamily assistance with childcare in the form of Child Development Centers, civilian Day Care, au pair, nanny, or family friends within the community, which makes it necessary to plan well in advance of deployment. Always having a Family Care Plan in place, including the funds to support that plan, even without a looming deployment, is highly recommended.

Childcare

As stated earlier, 2.5% of active-duty service members are dual-military with children [1]. Childcare for the dual-military surgeon couple can be extremely challenging when trying to optimize "work-life balance" in the setting of frequent early/late work hours, overnight call hours, unexpected work-related emergencies, as well as prolonged training exercises or deployments, which can be assigned with little or no advance notice. Furthermore, due to the inability to choose the city/state/country of residence and frequent moves, it is often not possible for locally residing extended family members to assist in childcare, which is not infrequent in the nonmilitary population.

The resources available to families on base are primarily limited to the Child Development Center (CDC). CDCs generally offer care for infant to preschool-age children during standard work hours (6 a.m.–6 p.m.), which does not typically fit a surgeon's work schedule. Some CDCs offer extended hours, though availability is usually challenging. Preference is given to dual-military couples, however, this does not always take into account the long wait times for acceptance and the ever-changing schedules of the surgeon spouse. Additionally, when a child is ill, there is no formal backup when utilizing the CDC (or similar) alone for childcare. While some couples count on extended family for flexible backup childcare support, many dual-military couples require a patchwork of resources. Several military surgeons who were queried for this chapter stated that they required multiple forms of childcare to provide adequate coverage. Consequently, there is a perception that military pay does not adequately account for these financial burdens with dual-military couples.

In addition to the on-base military-operated childcare programs, another resource offered by the military is the Military

Child Care in Your Neighborhood (MCCYN) program. This program allows families to utilize off-base civilian daycares that are enrolled in the program with fee assistance. Even with fee assistance, these facilities are often higher in cost than the CDCs, but can offer advantages such as longer hours and proximity to the family's home. There is also a program for fee assistance for childcare in your home (CCYH). More information regarding these programs can be accessed at www.militarychildcare.com.

Due to the complex schedules and travel of the dual-military surgeon family, daycare alone is not always enough to allow for optimal childcare coverage. Many dual-military families also utilize in-home help with a nanny, babysitter, or au pair. This allows for help with childcare at hours when daycares are typically not open but surgeons are typically working, such as very early in the morning or late in the evening. It is also of great assistance when parenting becomes the responsibility of one spouse, while the other parent is deployed or TDY. Information on nannies and babysitters is best found from other local parents, while information on au pair programs can be found online. We will omit naming specific au pair companies here, as the military does not endorse or promote any specific company, but information is easily searchable on the internet. For local caregivers, local listservs or social media groups can be fruitful resources for identifying potential sitters or nannies. Of course, discretion and safety measures should be taken before hiring any caregiver for a child, and this can add an additional layer of complexity to finding safe and quality childcare. For this reason, additional layers of childcare are best identified as soon as possible when moving to a new location or encountering any other major life change.

Unsurprisingly, almost every response to our survey question regarding the most challenging aspect of a dual-military career revolved around childcare. Many referenced the lack of affordable, flexible care, particularly when one spouse is deployed and the home temporarily functions as a physically single-parenting household. This is especially poignant when the parent remaining at home is expected to continue a busy surgical practice and requires significant financial help to afford flexible childcare. Most of the responses could be simplified into the mantra: "Hire as much help as you can afford." Several couples noted that one spouse changed careers in order to limit the time away from their families and try to minimize the difficulty with child-rearing, particularly during deployments.

Service Policies for Dual-Military Service Members

Each of the major military services has a policy for assignments and joint domicile (JD) for service members married to other service members. The specifics of each of these is beyond the scope of this text but, in general, each service has a formal policy that stipulates that they will try to assign active-duty service members to assignments that are within a reasonable distance of their active-duty spouse. The definition of "reasonable distance" is service specific (e.g., the Navy notes 90 miles, the Army notes 50 miles or 1 h). More importantly, each policy clearly states that the needs of the service outweigh the desires of the dual-military couple and that assigning JD is much more difficult among service members of different branches. Finally, none of these policies apply to nonmilitary spouses.

Despite these stipulations, anecdotal experience and our survey results indicate that the services do usually make an effort to assign dual-military couples to reasonable assignments. Therefore, it is imperative that a dual-military couple completes the requisite steps to enroll in their service-specific programs and keep in close communication with their service specialty leaders or consultants. Failure to do so results in these privileges being waived.

In the Army, this is known as the Married Army Couples Program (MACP) and is governed by Army Regulation 614-200, Enlisted Assignments, and Utilization Management [3]. Navy policy is dictated by their Military Couple and Single Parent Assignment Policy as outlined in MILPERSMAN 1300-1000 [4]. The Airforce policy is known as a "Joint Spouse" assignment and is outlined in a Department of the Air Force Guidance

Memorandum (DAFGM) to their personnel document Total Force Assignments [5, 6].

Additionally, when couples are separated for prolonged periods, there is some financial compensation through the Family Separation Allowance (FSA). This allows for $250 per month to ameliorate the costs incurred with separation. Stipulations include that the separation is "involuntary," more than 30 continuous days, and that they were living together prior to the separation. Voluntary separation is not taken into account. This is more often the case in order to optimize career advancement or family stability when children are involved.

Psychosocial Support

Despite all the challenges that come with being a dual-military couple, there are also significant benefits that can't be overlooked. There is often a better understanding of the career progression and required military commitments that come with having a dual-military partnership. They have a unique evaluation, advancement, and career progression compared to our civilian colleagues. There is a benefit in having an "in-house" mentor or sounding board for various military-related subjects, for example, when writing Officer Evaluation Reports (OERs), Fitness Reports (FitReps), and/or Officer Performance Reports (OPRs). Conversely, survey responses for surgeons married to nonmedical spouses often felt like their busy schedule and personal career demands were not understood, acknowledged, or accounted for by their spouse's command. If not addressed early, this can certainly lead to dissatisfaction and resentment.

The military offers resources for psychosocial support to all servicemembers, including dual-military couples. These include but are not limited to nonmedical counseling, on-base Military and Family Support Centers, chaplains, and more. More information can be found at www.militaryonesource.mil.

Conclusions

Many dual-military surgeon couples, with and without children, have succeeded in reaching the ranks of O-5 and O-6 while maintaining their specialty-specific goals, whether that is to be a busy academic surgeon, high volume surgeon, surgeon-leader, or combination and/or mix of these. Open and frequent communication with your military and medical chain of command is a necessity to optimize life as a dual-military surgeon couple. Similarly, frequent open communication with spouse and family is ideal to ensure career and family goals are in line and optimized for success. Having plans and preparations in place for potential physical separation due to military needs is paramount for success and decreasing stress and hardship during a challenging time. This is exponentially true in the setting of childcare. While the challenges are many, the commitment to service and country is highly honorable and overall supported by the service branches as much as possible.

References

1. U.S. Department of Defense 2022 Demographics Survey. U.S. Department of Defense. 2022. https://www.militaryonesource.mil/data-research-and-statistics/military-community-demographics/2022-demographics-profile/. PDF Download.
2. Parco JE, Levy DA, Air University (U.S.). Press. Attitudes aren't free: thinking deeply about diversity in the US armed forces. Maxwell Air Force Base, Ala.: Air University Press; 2010. xii, 557 p.
3. Army Regulation 614-200. Enlisted assignments and utilization management. 2019.
4. MILPERSMAN 1300-1000. Military Couple and Single Parent Assignment Policy. 2020.
5. Department of the Air Force Guidance Memorandum (DAFGM) to Department of the Air Force Instruction (DAFI) 36-2110, Total Force Assignments. 2023.
6. "Join Spouse assignment consideration keeps mil-to-mil couples together." Kat Bailey. 2017. https://www.afpc.af.mil/News/Article-Display/Article/1200090/join-spouse-assignment-consideration-keeps-mil-to-mil-couples-together/. Accessed 11 Feb 2024.

Retirement, Separations, and Transitioning to Civilian Practice

36

Samuel Douglas

Introduction

The decision to leave the Active Duty military is multifaceted and extends beyond this chapter; however, one should be familiar with the various pathways, their processes, and respective benefits afforded after the service. One may have served 20-plus years and met the full retirement criteria. At the same time, others may have completed their Active Duty Service Obligation (ADSO) and are eligible for separation or Expiration–Term of Service (ETS), which is the date you are released from active duty service. In addition, one may unfortunately experience severe medical conditions or injuries that will result in separation or early retirement, and many of these processes will be similar. Those who joined the Armed Forces, regardless of how long, have provided one of the greatest self-sacrifices one can to this country. Therefore, having a thorough understanding of your earned entitlements and benefits is important, as well as having a framework to successfully embark on the next steps of your surgical career. This chapter will provide a broad overview of some of these key considerations.

S. Douglas (✉)
Department of HPB/Surgical Oncology—Alabama Oncology, Birmingham, AL, USA
e-mail: Samuel.Douglas@AlabamaOncology.com

A. T. Schlussel et al. (eds.), *The SAGES Manual for Navigating a Successful Military Surgical Career*,
https://doi.org/10.1007/978-3-031-88490-0_36

Preparing to Leave

Timeframe/When to Start Planning

As with many things in life, proper prior planning will lead to a more consistent, less surprise-filled journey. With this in mind, it is often helpful to begin planning for your career after your military service at the start of your military career. Some individuals will plan for a full career while others are planning to complete their ADSO and separate immediately, but the reality of the matter is that many individuals are uncertain or change their minds during their military service. For this reason, it is imperative to consider both pathways at various intervals in your career and recognize that the decision to stay in or get out is a personal one that you will need to make after careful consideration. Some major factors that should be considered are the amount of time toward retirement at the end of your ADSO, your career progression, and your personal and family satisfaction. Regardless of whether you decide to retire after 20+ years of service or separate after your initial ADSO is up, it is recommended that you begin preparing for that transition at least 1–2 years in advance.

Retirement vs Separation

A traditional retirement from military service requires 20 years of service, and the exact benefits that you will receive depend on many different factors. Some of the primary factors are: active or reserve component, total amount of time served, grade during the time leading up to and at the time of separation, as well as the type of retirement system which you opted into (High-3 vs Blended Retirement System BRS). Information regarding the Blended Retirement system can be found at https://militarypay.defense.gov/blendedretirement/. All service members since January 1, 2018, have been enrolled in the BRS by default, but those serving before then would have had to opt in during an opt-in period. Regardless of the retirement program, all service members/government employees are eligible to keep any personal money as well as all vested matching government contributions that are invested in the Thrift Savings Program (TSP), which is a military service benefit similar to a 401(k) retirement plan and separate from any retirement pay. This will be discussed in more detail later.

Key Consideration

Under the BRS, even if you do not qualify for a pension (i.e., do not serve a full 20 years), you will be able to keep all of your personal TSP contributions as well as all vested service match (typically 1–5% fully vested after 2 years). This means that even for those who intend to separate immediately upon completion of their ADSO, participation in the BRS is typically financially advantageous. To get an estimate for potential retirement income under various programs, you can utilize several calculators published by the Department of Defense: https://militarypay.defense.gov/calculators/ and additional information regarding military compensation can be found at https://militarypay.defense.gov/.

Reserves

For service members eligible to separate but not to retire, there are potential options to continue military service in the Regular Reserves. There are multiple benefits to service in the Reserves, which include the opportunity to achieve an equivalent 20-year retirement. The timing of the retirement, the financial compensation, and when one would draw that compensation varies based on time spent on active duty, the number of overseas deployments, and how actively you participate with your reserve unit. Each military branch has specific requirements detailed earlier in this book, but the annual time commitment is consistent across all services. Reservists need to earn 50 points per year to qualify for a reserve year that counts toward retirement eligibility. Each 4-h block of time spent with your unit or performing an equivalent duty allocates you 1 point, and every reservist receives 15 membership points automatically at the end of the year. Presently, the

Reserves also provides a 1:1 year credit for Health Profession Scholarship Program students and a $75,000 yearly retention bonus for a 2-, 3-, or 4-year contract. Each military location has a Reserve liaison officer and local Reserve recruiter. If continuing your service interests you, it is recommended that you speak with a local reserve office for the most current details on obligation requirements and benefits. Lastly, it should be noted that most service members will have an Individual Ready Reserve (IRR) obligation of 4 years. While this typically does not count toward retirement, and the main requirement is an annual verification form, there are opportunities to earn points through correspondence courses and other unique opportunities.

Mandatory Programs and Critical Items to Prepare Before Separation

Gathering and organizing all of the required documentation can be daunting. Start preparing a secure file, both electronically and hardcopy, to ensure all necessary documents are available for branch-specific requirements. Despite the mandatory checklist of items required to separate, items can often be missed or overlooked without you or the service recognizing this. This may require you to revise or resubmit documents after separating, and having an organized location will help mitigate any additional delays. Below is a starting point but is by no means a comprehensive list of all the necessary items, and it is highly encouraged to seek assistance from your local facility or a colleague who recently separated from your current duty station.

Transition Assistance Program (TAP)

This is a mandatory program for all service members who have served on active duty for more than 180 days. It offers a wide variety of resources and information. It is required within 12 months of separation but can be taken early. Because it provides so much information, some service members have recommended going through the class twice, with the second time being within the required 12-month period before separation. Because this program is not tailored for specific specialties, it does not provide much assistance with job prospects in the medical field. Still, it can provide much-needed insight into navigating the disability system, VA system, home loans, and many other resources available to veterans.

For job prospects, it is recommended to utilize society job boards, publications, networking, and word of mouth. Surgeons should begin looking for the ideal job 2–3 years in advance and start narrowing down the prospects by state, region, and employment type sought at least 18 months prior to separation. Ideally, a contract should be negotiated and signed 6–12 months before separation or retirement. It should be noted that if plans are for you to go to a fellowship or any other intermediary training, a support stipend can often be negotiated with your ultimate employer to mitigate the pay differential after going from an attending surgeon's payback to a trainee. For more information about the transition assistance program, consult a career counselor from your service and refer to https://www.dodtap.mil/.

Records

Medical

Ideally, all medical records will have been accumulated in an organized fashion throughout your military career, but for most service members, that is not the case. Once the decision is made to separate or retire, the service member should begin requesting and organizing all medical records. This will also aid your provider during the required separation physical exams, disability examinations, and other specialty referrals. This process should start about 12–18 months before the date of separation, and the service member should consider this a major collateral. These examinations are not designed to diagnose and treat new ailments. It is strongly recommended that if you have a new condition or injury that has not been addressed during your time on Active Duty, you should schedule an appointment with your primary care provider as early as possible to ensure any critical imaging, consults, or procedures are completed before you leave active duty. This will ensure you are entitled to appropriate medical benefits through the Veteran Affairs Health Administration and appropriate compensation. This will save you a significant amount of time once you leave active duty and embark on your next stages of life, and it will be financially beneficial to receive this treatment while on active duty.

Service Members who retire can enroll in various TRICARE Plans (https://www.tricare.mil/Plans/Enroll). For those not eligible for TRICARE for life and have separated, you are provided 180 days of the Transitional Assistance Management Program (https://www.tricare.mil/TAMP), which provides health care benefits after regular TRICARE benefits end. This benefit is designed to assist with your transition. After 180 days, TRICARE offers a Continued Health Care Benefit Program, which is similar to a Continuation of Health Coverage (COBRA) and can be purchased in 90-day increments (https://www.tricare.mil/Plans/Enroll/CHCBP_Purchase). Although these programs are through TRICARE, access to care at local military treatment facilities can be challenging due to availability; therefore, it is still important that all medical issues are evaluated while covered by TRICARE Prime.

DD214

This is perhaps one of the single most important documents of your military career. Meticulous attention to detail should be taken to ensure it is 100% accurate by the time of separation. Additionally, multiple physical and electronic copies should be made and kept in separate locations once it is provided. Generally, this will be the primary means of verification of military service for all other entities, including your future employers. The DD214 will be created utilizing your military records, which have been uploaded to your respective branch's website. This will include all documents from when you were a physician and any prior military service. It is critical that you take the time to review all of your online documents, including combat deployment time, overseas service time, awards, schools, and any other important achievements you have accomplished while in military service. If you had prior military service before the multiple online document systems were created or updated, you should bring any hard copies of those documents to your unit's personnel office or to the separation office at your local duty station to ensure these items are entered into your DD214. The number of days spent on active duty, combat deployment time, and certain awards will afford you a greater number of Veteran Affairs benefits for life. Once your draft copy of your DD214 is complete, read this in detail, and do not sign the form until all items are entered to your satisfaction. Although the form can be updated at a later time, it is a challenging process and one that can be mitigated if completed correctly prior to separating.

Performance Appraisal Report (PAR) and Evaluations

These documents should be prepared at regular intervals at all DOD medical facilities. Care should be taken to document any privileges that a surgeon may be eligible for but are not supported by the facility. This is important for future credentialing purposes as some hospitals will require you to have had active credentials for certain procedures before granting them to you at your new job. Most employers and hospital systems are accommodating of military service, understanding the demands of deployments. In some cases, remote locations may not allow surgeons to meet the usual requirements for the number of procedures performed within a specified timeframe. A closing PAR, or evaluation, is typically generated at the end of any tour within a DOD military health system. Care should be taken to organize these and keep them in a safe location, as they may facilitate future credentialing. It is not uncommon for temporary privileges to be granted during times of deployment, Temporary Additional Duty (TAD), or Temporary Duty (TD). Note that some software used by hospital systems to verify your work history may interpret these temporary privileges as ongoing privileges at that hospital. Therefore, close communication with future credentialing personnel is recommended to prevent unintended delays. Different services have different forms of these evaluations, and they should be reviewed prior to leaving the military.

Key Consideration
Before leaving a hospital, it is recommended that you have the OR run a report/pull a record of all your cases that you performed at that hospital. This can be an invaluable resource as you move through the credentialing process. Additionally, although it can be obtained retroactively, it is much more difficult as there are often barriers to accessing the data once you relinquish your hospital privileges. A common example where case volume requirements are commonly inspected is with robotics privileges.

Managing your TSP

As mentioned previously, the TSP is your government employee equivalent of a 401(k) or other retirement account. Any money you invest in it and all government matches is yours to keep after the initial vesting period, even if you do not complete your full retirement. As such, when you leave government employment, you have many of the same options available to you with other employer-sponsored retirement accounts. Specifically, you can leave the funds in the TSP, roll the funds into an individual retirement account (IRA), in certain circumstances, perform an in-service withdrawal (e.g., disability or separate during force reduction), or even convert to an annuity some or all of your funds. One should consider carefully the tax implications of any decision made; TSP funds are notably low-cost and broadly diversified. For more information, you can visit the official TSP website: https://www.tsp.gov/

Managing your VA benefits

One of the first steps to accessing your VA benefits will be to establish an account with https://www.va.gov/. Once completed, this will be the primary access point to all of your veteran's benefits, including disability, education, health care, and many others.

Disability Benefits

Current law assigns different disability ratings for different diagnoses and provides varying levels of benefits based on the assigned rating. Much of the TAP class focuses on how to apply for disability. There are multiple avenues to submit a claim for disability.

Service member initiated claims filed before separation typically allow for the smoothest transition from active duty to disability payments typically with limited delay and payment processing. Claims filed after separation but up to 1 year will have a retroactive date of the date of separation. Claims filed greater than 1 year after separation will have an effective start date of the date of claim. Government (veteran service organizations typically run by a state) and nonprofit organizations (American Legion, Disabled American Veterans, Veterans of Foreign Wars, etc.) provide the opportunity to appoint a power of attorney, and they will submit claims on your behalf. Lastly, there are multiple law firms and legal avenues to file or dispute disability claims.

Common ratings are:

100% Disability: Veterans are eligible for no-cost dental care, a Uniformed Services ID card, and a waiver for Service-Disabled Veterans Insurance (S-DVI) of up to $10,000 if the veteran has been unemployed for at least 6 months. They also qualify for federal student loan forgiveness and access to Space-Available flights (Category 6). Additionally, veterans can receive VA emergency room visits at no cost, along with other benefits below.

50–90% Disability: No-cost self-care and prescription medications with no co-pays, may receive concurrent military retirement pay, and 3 no-cost non-VA urgent care visits.

30–49% Disability: Travel allowance for scheduled appointments for care at the VA Medical Center and VA-authorized healthcare facilities, 10-point veteran preference for federal hiring, and additional compensation for eligible dependents.

10–29% Disability: Waiver of VA funding fee for a home loan, vocational rehabilitation and employment, and burial and plot allowance.

0% Disability: 10-point Veteran preference in federal hiring, no-cost healthcare and prescription drug for service-connected disabilities, small co-pay for all healthcare and mental health care, non-VA urgent care visits $30 per visit, non-VA emergency room for service-connected conditions or nonservice condition conditions if you have no other health insurance, and VA dental insurance program.

It is advisable to consult with your local VA or online for a comprehensive list of entitlements. Different states have different benefits based on the % of disability. Some states waive state taxes on retirement pay, and others exempt disabled veterans from property taxes.

Education Benefits

There are several educational benefits afforded to those who served.

Post-9/11 GI Bill (United States Code [USC] Chapter 33):

Eligibility: For veterans who served on active duty for at least 90 days after September 11, 2001.

Benefits: Can cover tuition and fees, housing allowance, and book stipend.

Benefits can be transferred to a dependent if:

You've completed at least 6 years of service on the date your request is approved, and you agree to add 4 more years of service.

The person getting benefits must be enrolled in the Defense Enrollment Eligibility Reporting System (DEERS)

Montgomery GI Bill (USC Chapter 30):

Eligibility: For veterans who served on active duty for at least 2 years and contributed to the program.

Benefits: Can cover tuition and fees, housing allowance, and book stipend.

Key Consideration

Graduate Medical trainees (residents or fellows) *enrolled in an ACGME accredited residency or fellowship* ***are eligible*** *to receive GI bill education benefits during their GME training*. Trainees enrolled in a *non-ACGME fellowship* ***are not eligible***. Additionally, while the post-9/11 GI bill typically offers a higher overall benefit for most educational opportunities (as it provides a stipend [to you] + tuition [to the school] benefit), only the stipend portion would be paid out to a resident/fellow. As such, the Montgomery GI bill (which pays you a lump sum for each month of benefit) will usually be more advantageous for medical trainees. With that in mind, it should be noted that there is an optional $600.00 one-time buy-in purchase that can be made from your paycheck while on active duty. Utilizing this buy-in will increase your monthly payment by a significant amount over the course of your training. https://www.va.gov/education/benefit-rates/montgomery-600-buy-up-rates/

Reserve Component GI Bill (USC Chapter 1606):

Eligibility: For veterans who served in the National Guard or Reserves for at least 6 years.

Benefits: Can cover tuition and fees, housing allowance, and book stipend.

Vocational Rehabilitation (USC Chapter 31):

Eligibility: For veterans with service-connected disabilities (10% or more).

Benefits: Can cover tuition, fees, books, and supplies, as well as vocational rehabilitation services.

Other VA benefits include access to health care, career and employment resources, housing assistance, life insurance, burials and memorials, records, and other service member or family member benefits—including access to free mental health resources.

Weighing Your Options—Transitioning to Civilian Practice

As you make the decision to either retire or separate, it is extremely important to understand some of the options that are available to you in civilian practice and consider what your "ideal" practice would look like. Additionally, if this is your first non-government contract where you have negotiating power, you should consider obtaining legal counsel. This will help ensure you understand all aspects of your contract and identify key areas important to you to request or negotiate. Understanding what you are signing is of the utmost importance, and sometimes, simply having a lawyer translate the contract into understandable bite-size pieces is worth the cost. Incidentally, retirees have access to JAG services and can utilize them when available.

Practice Location

One of the first differences that you may appreciate during the transition from military to civilian life is that you are now in control of where you go, live, and work. While there are too many unique locations to list here, generally, your potential practice locations can be considered in terms of urban, suburban, or rural. Each of these has its unique benefits and challenges, and the following is a very rough approximation of how the practice of medicine may differ from location to location. It is important to remember that there is a national shortage of surgeons, with an expected worsening of the number of surgeons within the next decade. As such, there may not be availability in your desired location, but there is no shortage of hospitals that need surgeons.

Urban: Densely populated urban medical centers may offer a broader range of demographics and socioeconomic backgrounds. You might see a higher volume of complex cases due to many urban hospitals being referral centers with access to specialists and advanced technology. With more hospitals and specialty clinics, surgeons might need to be part of a larger group or train in a subspecialty to compete. The urban lifestyle can be fast-paced with potentially longer hours, but you may have higher salaries due to a higher cost of living.

Suburban: In suburban practice locations, you might encounter a more balanced mix of common surgeries and more complex cases. There is typically a mixture of hospitals and outpatient surgery centers that may be available. Salaries can be competitive with those in urban areas, but the cost of living is often lower. This may allow for a more balanced lifestyle with potentially more time for family and hobbies.

Rural: Smaller communities will typically have more limited access to specialists, and as such, surgeons may need to be truly a "general" surgeon, handling a wider variety of procedures, including emergency care, trauma, or procedures that might normally be done by other specialties (e.g., C-sections, hysterectomies, tonsillectomies, etc.). It is not uncommon for a rural surgeon to provide both surgical and endoscopic needs to the community, and this may include frequent on-call duties. The workload can be demanding, with long hours on some occasions, but it also offers flexibility during slower periods. Productivity-based compensation might be lower due to lower patient volume; however, some rural practices offer very lucrative incentives to attract surgeons, and the lower cost of living (known as geographic arbitrage) can improve overall financial well-being. Rural life may offer a slower pace and a stronger sense of community.

Academic vs. Community Medicine

Academic: By definition, this will be associated with a university and will require a faculty appointment. Typically, newly appointed faculty will have a lower starting salary, but it increases with promotions and grant funding. The lower salary can be somewhat offset by not paying liability insurance and by having access to trainees, which can help reduce the call burden. Traditionally, advancement in academic medicine followed a research-heavy path. However, there are many different pathways toward promotion, including excellence in clinical care, teaching, and research. Finding a balance between these will be crucial in your early career.

Community: This type of medicine comes in the widest variety, and there is no one-shoe-fits-all description; however, broadly, community practices can be broken down into employed positions or private practice. Most community surgical positions offer higher starting salaries, often with productivity-based bonuses and opportunities for partnership in private practices. Additionally, these roles tend to provide more predictable hours, allowing for better control over work-life balance. Practice in community medicine will often have a heavier focus on patient care, efficient surgeries, and more common procedures. There are a number of community programs that serve as teaching institutions for residents and medical students, but this is not a given and should be discussed with your potential employer/practice.

Practice Types

Solo practice: Solo-owned surgical practices are the ultimate in surgical autonomy. You're the boss, setting your schedule, managing staff, and crafting your patient care approach. The rewards are potentially high, with earnings directly tied to your volume and efficiency. But this freedom comes at a cost. You'll wear many hats—surgeon, business manager, Human Resources (HR)—which can be overwhelming. Work-life balance can suffer as the weight of the practice rests solely on your shoulders. This path is ideal for surgeons who crave independence and the ability to directly impact their patients' lives, but it demands strong business skills and the stamina to handle the pressure of constant responsibility.

Group Practices: Group-owned medical practices are doctor-owned businesses. Many private practice groups offer newly hired surgeons an employed position first and will outline a pathway to partnership in the contract. Partners will share profits and make decisions together, offering more control than employed positions. This model provides greater autonomy than hospital-employed positions while offering the potential for higher earnings through profit sharing. However, smooth operations require strong collaboration and business skills from all the doctors involved.

Key Consideration
When evaluating a private practice group, there are many different pathways to becoming a partner which may range from immediate partnership, gradual partnership (after several years being employed by the group), and/or partnerships that require a "buy-in". To avoid any surprises, it is imperative that you review this carefully before signing the final contract.

Hospital-Employed Physician Practices: Employed surgeon positions offer a trade-off between stability and autonomy. You'll receive a regular salary, benefits, and predictable hours, allowing you to focus on patient care with less administrative burden. However, this comes with less control over your schedule and practice style, potentially lower income, and a focus on productivity or efficiency that might limit time with each patient. This path is ideal for surgeons who prioritize work-life balance, enjoy collaboration, or for new surgeons seeking experience before venturing out on their own.

Key Consideration
As with all practice models, there is a wide variety of hospital-employed physician models that may impact your lifestyle and satisfaction [e.g., call coverage, Paid Time Off (PTO), Advanced Practice Provider (APP) support, clinic staff support, etc.] and it is important to read and understand the details of the contract very carefully as negotiation can be much more difficult with a larger employer.

Locum Tenens: Surgical locum tenens is a high-freedom, high-reward career path. You control your schedule, potentially earn higher pay, and gain experience in various settings. However, the trade-off is instability. Locum tenens jobs are temporary, with no benefits and limited patient connection. You'll also shoulder travel costs and adapt to new environments frequently. This path is ideal for surgeons who crave flexibility, travel, and maximizing income but are comfortable with a less traditional, more independent work style.

Key Consideration

Locums work during your career as a military surgeon can be a great way to experience different locations, practice structures, and hospital systems. It can often serve as a "foot in the door" when looking for a job. Additionally, you should be aware that many locum tenens jobs will pay you as a contractor, meaning you will receive a 1099 and be responsible for paying your own payroll taxes (employer, employee, Social Security, FICA, etc.).

Business of Medicine

Definitions

Fee-for-service (FFS): This is the traditional healthcare payment system in the United States, where providers are paid per service rendered. Providers bill insurance or patients directly for each office visit, test, or procedure.

Capitation: Instead of getting paid per service, providers receive a fixed fee per patient per timeframe, which is intended to cover all anticipated healthcare needs during that period. For example, Health Maintenance Organizations (HMOs) utilize capitation-based contracts with selected providers or hospitals to deliver care to their subscribed patients.

Salary: A guaranteed base pay, like a traditional job. Many contracts are written in a "Salary + Bonus" model where a bonus may be delivered when a surgeon meets certain metrics. There are a number of different bonus models that may be utilized, but for surgeons, compensation is most commonly tied to productivity. Some common bonus structures are:

Productivity Targets: Bonuses for exceeding a set target for wRVUs (work relative value units) or collections.

Patient Experience: Bonuses for high patient satisfaction scores or for exceeding appointment availability targets

Cost Management: Bonuses for keeping costs under control within their patient panel. This is more common for HMO or Accountable Care Organization (ACO) participants.

Specialty-Specific Goals: Bonuses tailored to a specific specialty. For example, a surgeon might receive a bonus for maintaining a low surgical site infection rate, adequate lymph node harvest, low post-bariatric re-admission rate, or any other metric.

Group Performance: Bonuses based on the overall performance of the practice or hospital.

Production-based: Doctors have no set salary floor, but earn based on the volume of services they provide. The most common metric used are the wRVUs (work relative value units) or collections.

Key Consideration

wRVUs are arbitrary units of "value" that are assigned by the Centers for Medicare & Medicaid Services (CMS) for every Current Procedural Terminology (CPT, the procedure done) and are assigned based on perceived complexity and time required. This number is nationwide and does not change based on location. CMS also assigns a "Conversion factor" that dictates how that wRVU translates into real dollars. For example, the current conversion factor is $32.3565 (as of April 2025), so for 1 wRVU, a physician will receive $32.3565 from Medicare payments. NOTE: Private insurers may set their own conversion factors that can vary from physician to physician or hospital to hospital, but in general, will be similar to that set by CMS.

Collections-based: A physician has no set salary floor but is entitled to some or all of the amount actually collected from patients or insurance companies.

Key Consideration

For production-based and collections-based models, many employers will utilize the previous 6 months–1 year and choose a percentage of that to pay out the next 6 months–1 year evenly as a "salary" to ensure consistent cash flow to the surgeon. The employer will typically then distribute any remaining excess on a regular interval. This distribution of monies due is typically known as a "true-up" and is common in a purely production/collections-based practice model. *The surgeon should clearly understand what happens when they under-perform or exceed their employer's production expectations or set salary.*

Reimbursement Landscape

Coding: Current Procedural Terminology (CPT) codes are assigned by CMS to every procedure and are used for billing purposes in the United States. It's a standardized system that ensures everyone—doctors, hospitals, insurance companies—are on the same page regarding what procedures were performed. In civilian medical practice, accurate coding is the lynchpin that ties the surgeon's work to what the insurance or patient pays. CMS also assigns a wRVU to that CPT code and a conversion factor. Taken together, these quantify and then translate the work performed into a dollar amount paid by the insurer.

Coverage: The exact coverage provided under each insurance plan is a balancing act for insurers. They consider medical necessity, cost-effectiveness, and evidence-based practices to decide what gets covered. Imagine a three-legged stool: medical justification, affordability, and proven effectiveness must be present. They rely on medical advisors and their teams to set coverage guidelines, looking at how often a service is used and negotiating rates with providers.

Key Consideration

Until recently, the negotiated rate between an insurer and a hospital system or provider was not routinely disclosed to the public. However, since July 2022, CMS has been enforcing a 2020 transparency law that requires those negotiated rates to be disclosed. Nevertheless, there are currently varying levels of adherence to the law.

Payment: After a healthcare provider submits a bill (claim) to the insurer, the insurer's processing system kicks in. It checks the details like the plan coverage, medical necessity of the service based on the associated diagnosis codes, and if the coding is accurate. They then send an Explanation of Benefits (EOB) to the patient and the provider. This EOB details what the insurer will cover (based on the patient's plan and any cost-sharing requirements) and explains any denied services. Finally, payment is sent to the provider, either directly or after the patient fulfills any patient responsibility, like a deductible or co-pay. Remember, negotiated rates between insurers and providers influence the final payment amount, and these rates are usually confidential. Accurate coding is critical, as errors can delay or deny your claim. The whole process typically takes a few weeks up to a few months to complete.

Key Consideration
It is important to note that because of the length of the billing cycle, it can take several months from the time a service is rendered until payment is received. Combined with the time it takes to build up a large cohort of referring physicians, it can take anywhere from 6 to 12 months for a new provider to reach consistent cash flow.

Payer mix: This term indicates the mixture of payers for a particular practice or hospital and is typically broken down by government (Medicare/Medicaid), private insurers, and self-pay patients. Because there are different negotiated rates, different denial rates, and rates of "non-payment," this is a very important consideration when evaluating a potential practice.

Preparing for Success

Key Contract Considerations

Compensation and Benefits: Although your salary and bonus structure are essential for your contract, they must be understood thoroughly. One should take care to keep this portion of the contract in perspective. Depending on the employment/partnership arrangement, there may or may not be room for substantive negotiations for your gross pay.

Key Consideration
As a general rule, two major ways to increase your net worth are by increasing your take-home pay and reducing your expenses/expenditures. The main ways to improve your take-home pay are earning a higher pay (salary), reaching bonus targets (productivity), and taking advantage of tax-advantaged savings (utilizing traditional

retirement savings accounts [401k, 401a, 403b, etc.] are typically best used during your peak earnings years which will lower your adjusted gross income and subsequent tax bill for that given year.

Work Schedule and Call Duty: Perhaps more important than the raw salary number is your work expectations. These can typically be translated as a productivity expectation and RVUs, cases, admissions, clinic visits, or other metrics. Although they may not be explicitly spelled out in the contract, they should be discussed during negotiations. Call-sharing agreements are sometimes included, but not always. Even if not included in your formal contract, it can be very helpful to have them outlined in writing. Be very wary of verbal agreements.

Early Practice Support, Practice Environment, and Growth Opportunities

Part of the discussion in your negotiations should also be centered around the expectation of growing your practice and building your case volume over the first several years. It is generally noted that it can take 2 or 3 years for a surgeon to reach peak volume, and if not supported during the first 1–2 years, this may not be a viable arrangement. Some things to discuss with your potential employer or partners are what facilities you will use, what support staff you will have, how new consults will be divided up, will your partners have cases prepared for you, or will be expected to garner your own business right out of the gate.

When discussing things such as salary support or guaranteed salary, keep in mind that there is almost always an expectation of production associated with that number. You should discuss how that support will come to you (for example, will it be paid directly to you by a third-party hospital, or paid as part of your salary as part of the practice, will it be paid as 1099 income, etc.). If part of your recruitment package includes loan forgiveness or loan repayment, will this be paid directly to the lender, or will you be paid a 1099 stipend, in which case you will have a tax burden associated? Likewise, for moving expenses, if this is being paid directly to you, there is a high probability that you will also receive a 1099 in which case you will owe some taxes on it.

Key Consideration
It should be noted that Stark law prohibits physicians from referring patients to entities they have a financial relationship with for certain services covered by Medicare or Medicaid. This federal law also prohibits quid pro quo forms of recruitment incentives. However, Medicare *does allow* recruitment incentives for particular regions. Therefore, most hospitals can offer a recruitment package with subsequent obligations attached. The service obligation ("pay-back") cannot restrict your practice to a particular hospital or group. Still, it will restrict your practice to a particular region or geographic location dictated by Medicare. Typically, this is several ZIP Codes around the area to which you are going to work. Most commonly, the requirement is for you to stay in that region for 1–2 years after you have finished receiving benefits from them. For example, suppose you receive a 1-year salary support from a hospital. In that case, you are expected to stay in that region for 2 years after completing that first year of support but it typically does not require you to remain at a particular hospital or group. You should consult with local legal counsel for region-specific rules and regulations.

Finally, your ability to receive referrals will be an integral part of your first 1–2 years in practice. Some of your discussion should focus on what the hospital or practice will do from my publicity and marketing standpoint. This is often a mutually beneficial relationship; hospital systems are generally willing to provide substantial support for this aspect of your early practice.

Continuing education: Hospitals and practices recognize that continuing medical education requires continued Board certification. As such, they will generally be amenable to including or reimbursing the cost of CME and conferences, which is typically $5000–$15,000 annually.

Join professional associations: Being a member of professional societies has numerous benefits; one of the most important is the ability to mentor and be mentored by colleagues and experts in your field. Taking advantage of conference social activities can be both fulfilling and extremely productive. The Society of American Gastrointestinal and Endoscopic Surgeons has supported the military for over a decade through a dedicated Military Committee and the Military Surgical Symposium hosted at its annual meeting. The Excelsior Surgical Society, part of the American College of Surgeons, also offers a day-long forum that brings together military surgeons from the past, present, and future. Both organizations provide excellent resources and networking opportunities from former active duty surgeons.

Network beyond your specialty: One of the first activities as a new surgeon should be meeting all your referring doctors. Generally, this can be the GI doctors and the primary care doctors in your network and region. The hospital physician liaison is typically a great resource to help facilitate this.

Re-engage with past referrers/connections: Many surgeons ultimately ended up settling in an area where they previously lived or trained. Previous acquaintances and social networks can be a tremendous way to (re)establish yourself early in your career.

Establish communication preferences: As you begin building a practice, it is highly advised that you have very clear modes of communication for referring physicians to reach you. Personal cell phone numbers can be a great way for you to communicate directly with your colleagues. Additionally, a well-staffed clinic that answers referrals and promptly schedules patients can be paramount. One of the biggest complaints that referring providers have is that they cannot get their patients seen in a timely manner, and they are lost to follow-up once the patients have not been seen. Whether you are joining a large hospital system or establishing a solo practice, understanding the patient referral pipelines and patient experience is of the utmost importance.

Conclusion

The process of leaving active duty military service can be daunting, but with adequate planning and preparation, it can be made much smoother. Ensuring that all documentation is accurate is crucial, as it directly impacts the pay and benefits you may be eligible for later in life. Understanding the policies and procedures at your local duty station, along with broader Department of Defense guidelines, will set you up for success. Starting early in seeking mentorship and advice from colleagues about your next steps in surgical practice will provide valuable opportunities as you transition to civilian life. Being fully aware of your VA and retirement benefits can help ease the transition process. An O-5 officer (the typical rank at 20 years) can expect to make around $60,000 in retirement, and this can be higher with disability as it adds more pay while decreasing the amount of taxes on the retirement pay. Servicemembers who use TSP can expect to have another large amount of money they can access at age 59.5 years or add to another retirement account, like their new job's retirement benefit. The education bills can be used to pay tuition for the children of servicemembers who qualify, which may make a college or trade school education more affordable. Whether you served 20 years or four, you were part of an elite group of surgeons and leaders, and the country will always be grateful for your selfless service.

37 Becoming a Veterans Affairs Surgeon

Andrew C. Eppstein and Christy Y. Chai

Why I Chose a Career with the VA

> The decision to cultivate a career within VA is ultimately personal. Although I was educated and trained in the civilian sector, I come from a family of veterans. I attribute my choice to my positive experiences as a surgical resident, the supportive staff, wonderful veteran patients, and great mentorship within the Indianapolis VA. As a resident I felt at home with the faculty, staff, and veterans during my rotations at the Richard L. Roudebush VA Medical Center. The supportive training environment was the ideal place to develop my surgical judgment and skills while serving my country as my father and grandfather had. I was fortunate to be recruited back to the same VA and have continued the tradition of striving to improve surgical care for veterans and teach the next generation of surgeons how to manage our complex, inspiring patients.
> —Andrew Eppstein, MD, FACS

A. C. Eppstein (✉)
Section of General Surgery, Surgery Service, Division of General Surgery, Department of Surgery, Richard L. Roudebush Veterans Affairs Medical Center, Indianapolis, IN, USA
e-mail: andrew.eppstein@va.gov

C. Y. Chai
Operative Care Line, Michael E. DeBakey Veteran Affairs Medical Center, Houston, TX, USA

Division of General Surgery and Surgical Oncology, Michael E. DeBakey Department of Surgery, Baylor College of Medicine, Houston, TX, USA

A. T. Schlussel et al. (eds.), *The SAGES Manual for Navigating a Successful Military Surgical Career*,
https://doi.org/10.1007/978-3-031-88490-0_37

I chose to work at the VA to give back to those who have served our country, providing them with the high-quality care they deserve. My nine years as an Air Force surgeon instilled in me a profound respect for the unique challenges and sacrifices of military service members, and I am committed to using my skills and experience to improve the health and well-being of our veterans. Furthermore, working at the very institution where I completed my residency allows me to mentor trainees and give back to those who taught me. It is a rewarding environment where we continually strive to improve and ask, 'How can we make it better?' Every day, I am inspired by the resilience and courage of my patients and motivated by an enthusiastic and hardworking team dedicated to delivering the best care possible. Serving and honoring veterans, while shaping the next generation of physicians, aligns well with my personal values and professional goals, making the VA a deeply fulfilling place to work.
—Christy Chai, MD, FACS, FSSO

Introduction

Whether you are a military surgeon looking to enter the civilian sector, a reservist seeking to extend your federal benefits, or a civilian who wants to practice in an environment different from the traditional academic or community care dichotomy in American health care, a career in the Department of Veterans Affairs as a VA surgeon is worth considering. As VA is a massive, complex bureaucracy, understanding its organization and practices can be daunting and confusing. This chapter seeks to condense and clarify the practice of surgery within the VA system by providing background on the largest healthcare system in the United States and serving as a primer on how you can work in VA.

The Veterans Health Administration [1]

The Department of Veterans Affairs, established as a Cabinet-level entity in 1988, has its origins in the American Revolution. The Continental Congress of 1776 initiated pensions for life for soldiers disabled in duty, setting a precedent for veteran care. In 1811, the US Naval Asylum was approved for disabled Navy veterans, opening in Philadelphia in 1834. Throughout the nineteenth Century, state and federal facilities, including the National Home for Disabled Volunteer Soldiers (established by President Abraham Lincoln in 1865), provided care for veterans. The post-World War I era saw significant consolidation of veterans' services with the creation of the Veterans Bureau. In 1930, President Herbert Hoover's Executive Order 5398 merged the Veterans Bureau, the Bureau of Pensions, and the National Home of Disabled Volunteer Soldiers into the Veterans Administration. This entity underwent significant expansion under General Omar Bradley's leadership after World War II, notably establishing the Department of Medicine and Surgery in 1946, which later became the Veterans Health Services and Research Administration. This period also marked the beginning of collaborations between VA hospitals and academic medical facilities. The Veteran's Administration was elevated to a Department of Veterans Affairs in 1988 by President Ronald Reagan, leading to the current structure where the Veterans Health Services and Research Administration was renamed the Veterans Health Administration in 1991.

The Veterans Health Administration (VHA), a key component of the Department of Veterans Affairs, stands as the largest integrated healthcare system in the United States. It encompasses 144 VA Medical Centers and 1232 Outpatient Sites, strategically distributed across the nation and its territories within 18 Veterans Integrated Service Networks (VISNs). The VISN system, originally numbering from 1 to 23, has undergone reorganization, resulting in the discontinuation of VISNs 3, 11, 13, and 14. This network ensures comprehensive and accessible care for the veteran population. For a detailed and current view, refer to the most recent VISN map provided by the VHA (see Fig. 37.1).

Within each VISN, a range of healthcare facilities operate, including VA Medical Centers (VAMCs), Ambulatory Care Clinics (ACCs), and Community Based Outpatient Clinics (CBOCs). VAMCs are classified into complexity levels, with Level 1 indicating facilities with higher acuity and patient volume, and Level 3 denoting the least complex, as detailed in Table 37.1. Notably, the most complex Intensive Care Units (ICUs) are rated as score 5 in Table 37.1. Additionally, the VA categorizes centers based on operative complexity, as outlined in the VHA Invasive Procedure Complexity for Surgical Programs in Table 37.2. Consequently, the scope of practice and patient acu-

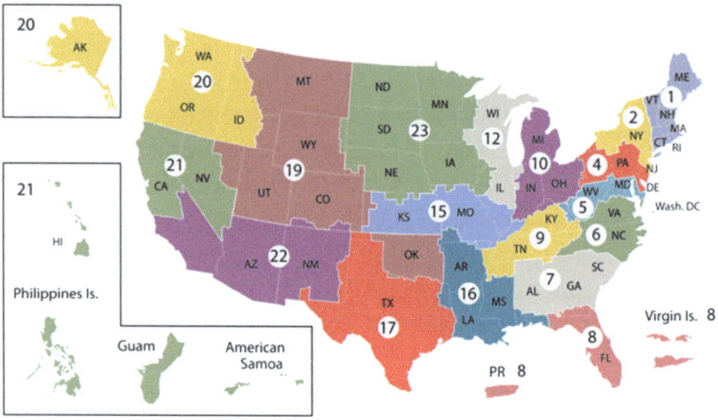

Fig. 37.1 Map of Veterans Integrated Service Networks (VISN) (Source: https://www.va.gov/directory/guide/map.asp?dnum=1)

Table 37.1 Summary of VHA facility complexity model

Level and complexity	Patient volume	Patient risk	Teaching	Research	ICU level[a]
1a—High	Highest	Highest	Highest	Highest	5
1b—High	Very large	Very large	Very large	Very large	4 and 5
1c—High	Large	Large	Large	Large	3 and 4
2—Medium	Medium	Medium	Medium	Medium	3 and 4
3—Low	Lowest	Lowest	Little to none	Little to none	1 and 2

Source: VHA Directive 1220(1), May 13, 2019

[a] The score of 5 presents the most complex ICU level rated 1 in healthcare analysis and information group

ity vary significantly among VAMCs. Acknowledging the distinctiveness of each VA facility is crucial; understanding one does not equate to understanding all. As the adage accurately reflects, "Once you've seen one VA, you've seen one VA," emphasizing that each location provides a singular experience. For those considering an academic career path within the VA system, understanding the complexity level of your specific VA facility is crucial. This knowledge informs the clinical responsibilities and work environment you can expect, as well as the support and resources available for academic endeavors.

Table 37.2 Summary of invasive procedure complexity

Level	Anesthesia	Critical care	OR call	Specialty services	Example procedures
Inpatient complex	General, in-house 24/7	24/7 Intensive Care Team	Readily available 24/7	Comprehensive, 24/7 coverage	CABG, Whipple, craniotomy, transplant
Inpatient intermediate	General	Dedicated Intensivist daily	Available	Comprehensive, immediate thoracic and vascular surgery availability	Shoulder joint reconstruction, bariatric surgery, colectomy, AAA repair
Ambulatory Procedure Center—Advanced	General	n/a	n/a	Inpatient backup within 60 min, cardiology, vascular surgery	Total knee arthroplasty, mastectomy, cholecystectomy, transurethral resection of prostate
Inpatient standard	General	Hemodynamic monitoring, respiratory support	Available	Pharmacy and blood bank during weekdays, emergency department	Appendectomy, tonsillectomy, cholecystectomy
Ambulatory Procedure Center—Basic	General, sedation	n/a	n/a	Backup observation beds, inpatient invasive services, radiology, blood bank, pharmacy	Cataract, inguinal herniorrhaphy, AV fistula

(continued)

Table 37.2 (continued)

Level	Anesthesia	Critical care	OR call	Specialty services	Example procedures
Outpatient intermediate	Moderate sedation	n/a	n/a	n/a	Endoscopy
Outpatient basic	Minimal sedation, local anesthetic	n/a	n/a	n/a	Arthrocentesis, cystoscopy

Source: VHA Directive 1220(1), May 13, 2019

Administrative structures in VA facilities may differ, but typically, a Medical Center Director manages the daily operations of a VAMC and reports to the respective VISN director and leadership team. The Executive Committee, usually comprising Assistant and Associate Directors, oversees various departments such as Engineering, Health Information Management, Police, Supply Chain Management, Environmental Services, and Patient Care Services. The latter encompasses vital non-physician roles, including Nursing, Social Work, and Sterile Processing. Additionally, the Chief of Staff, along with Associate or Deputy Chiefs who report to the Medical Center Director, supervises clinical services. Each service or care line is led by a Service Chief or Care Line Executive and may be further segmented into sections. Section Chiefs are tasked with conducting performance evaluations and ensuring the clinicians in their sections adhere to administrative standards.

Applying to Work at VA

The process of securing employment at the VA offers various pathways, particularly for physicians, who fall under the unique classification of Title 38 employees as per the United States Code. This distinction affords them more flexible hiring options compared to standard federal employment procedures. Federal jobs are generally classified into three categories: Competitive Service, Excepted Service, and Senior Executive Service. Positions within the Competitive Service adhere to stringent hiring and pay scale regulations established by the US Office of Personnel Management (OPM). In contrast, the Excepted Service allows more latitude in recruitment and compensation. The Senior Executive Service typically encompasses leadership roles, including administrative positions within medical centers that do not involve clinical duties. Surgeons, as Title 38 employees, are often placed within the Excepted Service category, which permits higher salary ranges [2] and enhanced benefits (see Appendix 37.1) to attract highly qualified professionals. Furthermore, the VA possesses the autonomy to directly appoint various medical staff such as medical officers, nurses, pharmacists, and radiology technologists, bypassing the extended processes of competitive candidate searches typically required for federal roles. This streamlined approach somewhat speeds up the hiring of essential medical personnel in federal healthcare facilities, yet the process typically extends beyond 3 months.

VA facilities typically list their open positions on USAJOBS.gov [3], where applications and curricula vitae are submitted online. Each facility then coordinates interviews and job offers. In urgent staffing situations, however, a VA facility can bypass the usual posting on USAJOBS under a direct-hire authorization, opting instead for recruitment through traditional methods like word-of-mouth or referrals. When a VA facility collaborates with an academic partner or group practice, unique employment arrangements can arise. For instance, the partnered practice might offer an employment contract with stipulations for part-time VA duties, where the VA compensates the clinician directly for their clinical and/or research efforts. Alternatively, the VA facility might contract with the affiliate, paying a negotiated rate for coverage, with the physician fully employed by the affiliate and not receiving direct payment from the VA. These arrangements can vary based on location and specialty, and often, higher-paying specialties require specific contracts for clinical services.

A prospective VA surgeon should first check USAJOBS.gov [3] for open positions. However, since not all recruitment needs are publicized promptly, or some vacancies might not be listed online, its advisable to directly contact the facilities of interest to inquire about their needs. Furthermore, some facilities may collaborate with recruiters or attend recruitment events beyond USAJOBS[3]. They may also post job announcements on specialized surgical specialty websites and engage with major medical society forums to reach specific groups of candidates. Given that the hiring and onboarding process can be lengthy, early, proactive job searching is more effective than waiting for a vacancy to appear online.

Understanding VA Employment

As civilian federal employees, physicians working within the VA operate under a modified version of the General Schedule (GS) pay system, specifically designated as VM. The GS system correlates with the Military Grade, aligning physicians and surgeons with the upper echelons of the GS scale, primarily at GS-15, equivalent to grade O-6 in the military hierarchy. Title 38 of the United States Code introduces amendments to the GS system specifically tailored for medical personnel, defining three distinct components of physician compensation: Base Pay, Market Pay, and Performance Pay. Base Pay corresponds directly to the assigned GS grade, which features a tiered structure with up to 15 steps, contingent on the duration of federal service. Market Pay is then added to the Base Pay, serving as an adjustment to align overall salaries with specialty and geographic considerations. This component is designed to enhance recruitment and retention efforts, considering factors such as experience, the needs of the hiring facility, and board certification. Finally, Performance Pay constitutes an annual bonus, contingent on the achievement of specific goals and performance measures established by the institution. Currently capped at a maximum of $15,000 or 7.5% of the total Base + Market Pay within a fiscal year, it serves as an incentive for physicians to excel in their roles. Crucially, the direct compensation package is subject to the limitations outlined in Title 3 U.S.C, which prohibits it from exceeding the annual compensation of the President of the United States, currently set at $400,000. Historically, the VA has faced challenges in recruiting and retaining clinicians in highly compensated specialties due to this Federal Pay Cap. To address this limitation, a VA facility may enter contracts with academic medical centers or local practices to hire part-time clinicians for coverage.

Throughout the employment process, salaries are determined based on a combination of Base Pay and Market Pay. These salaries are disbursed bi-weekly and are not contingent on Relative Value Unit (RVU) performance or productivity, although meeting RVU targets may be considered during the end of fiscal year Pay for Performance assessment. Base Pay is subject to an annual Cost-of-Living Adjustment (COLA) provided by the Federal Government, while Market Pay may or may not receive COLA. Additionally, Title 38 physicians' salaries are reviewed every 24 months, or they can request a review sooner if there are changes in qualifications that justify consideration.

The VA operates on a bi-weekly pay period, defining full-time employment as 40 hours per week, totaling 80 hours per pay period. Within the VA, the allocation of work hours is expressed in eighths, with each 1/8th equivalent to 5 hours per week. Consequently, a 1/8th employee contributes 5 hours of work weekly, while a 2/8ths employee dedicates 10 h, and so on, up to 8/8ths for a full-time employee. Employment at the VA involves adhering to regular hours, known as the "Tour of Duty," during which employees must be physically present at their duty stations or actively engaged in their responsibilities. While the standard model consists of 8-h workdays, 5 days a week, meeting the 8/8ths appointment criteria, the VA allows flexibility in structuring the Tour of Duty. For instance, individuals may opt for a schedule of 10-h workdays across 4 days a week while still being recognized as 8/8ths employees. Additionally, telework hours are counted toward the Tour of Duty requirements. Notably, the VA accommodates the allocation of eighths for clinical, administrative and research efforts, enabling the designation of protected administrative and research time within the established work schedule based on your job description and research grant status.

In the context of joint clinical appointments involving a clinician who splits time between the VA and another practice or academic affiliate, compensation is typically structured in eighths. This arrangement covers a scheduled Tour of Duty and the physician is directly remunerated for work within this framework. Alternatively, the VA has the option to enter contracts with group practices, where payment is made to the practice itself, bypassing the pay cap since the physicians are not under direct VA employment. VA facilities also provide the flexibility of intermittent appointments, where clinicians receive a salaried rate solely for the services they perform at the VA. For less frequent procedures, the VA may establish Fee-Basis or Fee-for-Service agreements with part-time surgeons to ensure appropriate compensation. Finally, the VA may extend a WOC (Without Compensation) appointment, granting staff privileges without financial remuneration. This type of appointment is often utilized to accommodate physicians from contracted group practices who occasionally provide patient care, respond to on-call duties, or perform procedures at the VA. Higher complexity inpatient facilities typically require mandatory call coverage, which is included as part of your salary package. Employment or group contract includes call coverage.

"Choose VA" [4]

The VA system is known for being distinct from other healthcare models like academic medicine, community practice, or private practice, particularly in terms of compensation structures, which are limited by federal law. Despite the potential for lower salaries compared to the private sector, there are several reasons why a surgeon might choose to work for the VA.

Service to Veterans

Whether you are a military surgeon looking to continue your service or a civilian surgeon who has become accustomed to the challenges of the current American healthcare system, working within the VA offers you the opportunity to provide care to those who have served our country. The VA's mission echoes President Abraham Lincoln's sentiments in his Second Inaugural Address, pledging to "care for those who have served in our nation's military and for their families, caregivers, and survivors."

While the VA system is not without its flaws and is sometimes burdened by bureaucracy, it makes a genuine effort to deliver timely and equitable healthcare to veterans, irrespective of their socioeconomic status or insurance coverage. Many veterans turn to the VA as a safety net provider when they are ineligible for employment-based insurance or cannot afford private insurance. Some even choose the VA as their preferred healthcare provider, even if they have third-party insurance, due to the respect and fair treatment they receive at VA facilities and the sense of camaraderie they share with their fellow veteran patients and staff. The atmosphere and morale at Veterans Affairs Medical Centers often set them apart from other institutions, contributing to high levels of satisfaction for both patients and employees alike.

Stability

Government jobs, including positions at the VA, often provide greater job stability when compared to the private sector. This stability is especially valuable because private sector jobs can be susceptible to market fluctuations, private enterprise risks, or external factors such as COVID-19. Working within the VA system is often more streamlined than traditional civilian models. The integrated nature of the VA system ensures automatic referrals from clinics to VA Medical Centers, eliminating the need for specialists to establish a referral base, which can take years in a typical setting. Surgeons can start seeing patients and performing procedures shortly after beginning clinical duties, usually within a week or two of employment. Civilian surgeons will find a turn-key practice free from the headaches of establishing a referral base, negotiating with insurance companies, and enduring poor work/life balance and expensive insurance coverage, while benefiting from superior retirement options.

Benefits Package (See Appendix 37.1)

While the salary might be capped, the overall benefits package, including a comprehensive range of insurance programs through national and regional carriers, including health, dental, vision, and life insurance, along with health care flexible spending accounts, retirement plans, and paid time off, can be competitive. The Federal Employee Health Benefits (FEHB) program [5] offers various health insurance plans, while dental and vision insurances are available through the Federal Employees Dental and Vision Insurance Program (FEDVIP), with enrollment managed separately at BENEFEDS.com [6]. Additionally, employees can allocate pre-tax dollars for health care expenses not covered by insurance via a Health Care Flexible Spending Account (HCFSA) managed at FSAFEDS.com, with automatic reimbursement and no receipt submission required. There is also a Dependent Care Flexible Spending Account (DCFSA) for childcare and care of incapable dependents. Basic life insurance coverage is automatically provided through the Federal Employee's Group Life Insurance (FEGLI), with options for additional coverage.

In addition, VA employees enjoy 11 paid Federal holidays annually, during which there are no scheduled clinical activities. VA-employed clinicians also accumulate a significant amount of leave for vacation or sick time. In a 2-week pay period, they accrue 8 h (equivalent to 1 day) of Annual Leave and 4 h of Sick Leave. This translates to 26 days of vacation and 13 sick days that can carry over to subsequent years and accumulate. When scheduling leave, weekends and federal holidays are not counted against this leave balance. For instance, a 1-week vacation would only use 5 days of annual leave, or 4 if it falls during a federal holiday. Additionally, new parents can claim up to 12 weeks of paid parental leave, and active reservists and National Guard members receive up to 15 days of leave. These generous leave benefits are not commonly offered by most hospital systems.

Certainly, one of the most enticing reasons to remain in federal service is the comprehensive retirement program, which includes a pension for dedicated long-term service. For healthcare professionals who have previously served in the military, the VA provides an opportunity to extend their federal career in a civilian capacity while enhancing their long-term retirement benefits. The VA's retirement program aligns in certain aspects with the Blended Retirement System offered by the Department of Defense and is referred to as the Federal Employee Retirement System (FERS) [7]. FERS encompasses three distinct components that provide financial support to retirees: Social Security, the Thrift Savings Plan (TSP) [8], and the Basic Benefit Plan [7]. As Social Security is not exclusive to federal employment, as it is available to all eligible Americans based on work history and disability status, we will focus on discussing the unique features of the TSP and the Basic Benefit Plan, which are specific to federal service.

The Thrift Savings Program (TSP) [9] is a federal retirement savings plan, like private sector 401(k) or 403(b) programs. Employees can make pre-tax contributions to a Traditional TSP, reducing taxable income but deferring taxes until withdrawal, or opt for a Roth TSP, with after-tax contributions and tax-free withdrawals upon retirement. Contributions can vary, within IRS limits, and can be managed through DFAS MyPay [10] and the TSP website. Federal employees can supplement their military retirement with TSP and, if hired after October 1, 2020, are enrolled automatically with 5% salary contributions. Existing 401(k), 403(b), or traditional IRAs can be rolled into TSP, except for Roth IRAs. Additionally, employees benefit from automatic agency contributions exceeding IRS limits, starting with an automatic 1% of pay, and up to 4% additional matching on a 5% employee contribution, providing substantial retirement funds at no extra cost.

The Federal Employee Retirement System (FERS) offers a pension known as the Basic Benefit Plan upon qualified retirement from federal service. This annuity is determined by factors including age, salary, length of service, and hiring date. Employees contribute a percentage of their Adjusted Basic Pay to the pension, with rates varying based on hiring date. For those hired between January 1, 1987, and December 31, 2012, the contribution is 0.8%, labeled as FERS on pay stubs. For employees hired in 2013, it is 3.1%, and for those hired after January 1, 2014, it is 4.4%. The annuity calculation considers the length of service and the High-3 Average Salary, which is the highest average pay earned during any three consecutive years of service. Notably, it excludes military pay, overtime, holiday pay, or bonuses. The formula for employees under 62 at retirement or older than 62 with less than 20 years of service is (0.01 × High-3 Average) × years of service = annuity. For those over 62 with 20 or more years of service, it is (0.011 × High-3 Average) × years of service = annuity. Monthly pension amounts are obtained by dividing this annuity by 12. To be eligible for the pension, a vesting period of 5 years of creditable federal service is required. Military service can be included in the calculation if it ended honorably and was performed before retirement from civilian service. To incorporate military service, Military Retired Pay must be waived, and a deposit of 3% of military basic pay earned during military service, plus interest, must be paid. Exceptions apply for service-connected disability or retirement under specific provisions of Chapter 1223, Title 10, U.S.C., related to reserve component retirement.

Education Support and Loan Repayment Program

As a physician, dentist, or podiatrist you may be eligible to apply for Education Debt Reduction Program (EDRP) [11]. If approved, you may be eligible to receive reimbursement for your student loan payments up to $40,000/year up to 5 years. Additionally, the VA offers opportunities for ongoing education and professional growth, making it an attractive option for individuals committed to lifelong learning and seeking to enhance their expertise. Furthermore, there is a provision for Continuing Medical Education (CME) expense reimbursement, with a cap of $1000, subject to certain restrictions. Within the VA, you will encounter appreciative patients, complex medical and surgical cases, and abundant opportunities to both teach and acquire new skills.

Reduced Overhead and Community of Support

In private practice, surgeons must manage or contribute to the management of a business, whereas in the VA, the focus can be solely on patient care. Because the VA is the sole payor for most patients, a surgeon seeing someone in clinic can schedule them for surgery immediately without insurance preapproval or filling out administrative paperwork for coverage. VA facilities do accept patients with third-party insurance, so occasionally a veteran may need insurance paperwork completed or even a peer-to-peer call, but this is exceptionally rare.

At the VA, the surgical practice operates on a salaried model rather than being driven by the number of procedures performed. This means there is no financial incentive to recommend unnecessary surgeries, and there is no competition among practice partners for cases. In fact, given the often-complex medical conditions seen in the veteran population, the emphasis is placed on conducting thorough patient evaluations and optimizing their medical status before considering surgery in collaboration with a team of clinical experts. While productivity remains a factor, it is not the sole focus. Administrative monitoring ensures that work effort and Relative Value Units (RVUs) are in line with those at comparable VA facilities. Whether you serve full- or part-time, your employment at VA is without employment contracts, noncompete clauses, restrictive covenants, or other significant restrictions on outside work. Working within the VA can provide a sense of community and support among healthcare professionals who share a common goal of serving veterans in a diverse, inclusive working environment.

Work-Life Balance

VA positions often offer more reasonable working hours in comparison to the on-call demands and long hours commonly found in private practice or hospital settings. Unlike private hospitals driven by the need for increased operative throughput to maximize profitability, VA surgeons are not pressured to work excessively long hours. While emergency cases are promptly accommodated and call teams are mobilized when necessary, there are limits placed on elective cases running after hours to ensure adequate nursing and surgical staff coverage the following day. Therefore, surgeons can anticipate adhering to the Tour of Duty schedule established at the time of their hire, as mentioned earlier, to ensure compatibility with their home and family life, unless scheduled for evening or weekend calls. The specific call schedules are determined by each VAMC based on their practice needs.

Research Opportunities

The VA health system offers an extensive research program for those with an inclination toward medical research, especially in areas concerning veteran-specific health issues. As the nation's largest integrated health system, the VA encourages and supports healthcare professionals who are eager to drive innovation, lead transformative projects, and develop new programs. This support is provided through an array of training opportunities and grant offerings. With its vast repository of electronic medical records, some of which span several decades, the VA presents a unique and rich environment for research, presenting an invaluable asset for medical investigations. The VA's dedicated Office of Research and Development [12], a separate entity from other federal research bodies, underscores its deep commitment to advancing medical science. The VA health system has a history of pioneering research, with many prominent academic surgeons having leveraged the VA's resources to bring forth substantial innovations and improvements in medical care. Many of these renowned surgeons are or were members of the Association of VA Surgeons [13], which is an excellent starting point for networking with other dedicated VA surgeons.

Malpractice Coverage

Working as a VA surgeon offers significant malpractice coverage benefits. Physicians are automatically insured against malpractice without any personal cost. Complications are internally reviewed for educational, non-punitive purposes, adhering to Just Culture principles. Regular monitoring of clinicians through Ongoing Professional Practice Evaluation (OPPE) ensures compliance with VA standards, with supervisors auditing patient charts. Failing to meet these standards triggers a Focused Professional Practice Evaluation (FPPE) to address deficiencies. Persistent non-compliance can lead to loss of privileges, termination, or state medical board reporting. Malpractice claims are governed by the Federal Tort Claims Act [14]. Veterans or their families file claims with the VA, not against individual providers. The VA, or its Office of General Counsel, handles the suits, informs providers, and may seek third-party VA opinions to assess standard of care breaches. The outcome, whether dismissal or settlement, is managed by the VA without cost to the providers. However, serious care standard violations could lead to National Practitioner Data Bank reporting and further monitoring through FPPE.

Perspectives from Inside the VA

Numerous compelling reasons make working for the VA an attractive choice for surgeons, particularly in today's challenging healthcare landscape in the United States. This environment is marked by shrinking reimbursements, challenging malpractice conditions, interference from insurance entities and hospital administrations, and often, an imbalanced work-life equation. With such appealing advantages, one might wonder: Is there a downside?

It is essential to provide a clear assessment of both the advantages and disadvantages of the VA healthcare system. While the VA appears to be a unified health system, it comprises diverse facilities with varying cultures, efficiencies, inefficiencies, strengths, and weaknesses. Even within the same VISN, facilities often operate independently, leading to differences in practice patterns influenced by local culture, academic affiliations, and the presence of learners. The level of facility complexity significantly impacts the resources available, affecting the range of surgical procedures and patient treatments possible. A surgeon specializing in complex laparoscopic or robotic procedures or surgical oncology would find a better fit at a level 1 facility, as level 2 or 3 facilities may lack the necessary support. Paradoxically, despite the increased workload and complexity at level 1 facilities, which are often located in major metropolitan areas and affiliated with academic medical centers, the compensation may be lower compared to surgeons in lower complexity facilities in less desirable geographic areas. The discrepancy in compensation within the VA, where more demanding work in complex facilities offers less pay than standard facilities, exacerbates the struggle to retain talented medical professionals.

The Veterans Affairs (VA) system is grappling with the limitations of its aging electronic medical record (EMR) system, VistA. Once at the forefront of EMR technology, VistA now struggles to meet contemporary standards, particularly with its Computerized Patient Record System (CPRS) interface, which frustrates users who are accustomed to more current commercial software. The system's widespread use across VA facilities is marred by inconsistent EMR builds and varied software packages, which hinder seamless operation. Often, the integration of additional software is necessary to retrieve remote patient data and records from community health providers, resulting in a fragmented and user-unfriendly interface. In response, the VA launched the Electronic Health Record Modernization Program in 2018, aiming to overhaul and enhance the EMR system. While the modernization efforts are ongoing, the anticipation for transformative changes in the VA health care system's EMR continues to grow.

Working within the Veterans Affairs (VA) system presents a unique opportunity for medical professionals to engage in education, as the VA is a cornerstone of medical training in the United States. With 60–70% of US physicians gaining experience in the VA, surgeons are expected to embrace the educator role. The presence of medical and physician associate students, residents, and nursing and surgical technologist students is commonplace. Surgeons provide valuable mentorship, contributing to the proficiency of the future medical workforce and benefiting from a dynamic work environment and collaborative service management. However, this educational focus means accommodating learners with varying skill levels and reliability, which can affect workflow efficiency due to the VA's emphasis on comprehensive training over rapid case turnover. Surgeons must be adept in supervision and patient with trainees. Those who perceive learners as a hindrance may find high-complexity VA facilities challenging, but for those who are passionate about teaching, the VA offers a deeply gratifying career path.

The comparatively measured pace at the VA, when contrasted with community medical practices, is an important consideration for practitioners. Surgeons in the VA system must possess a blend of adaptability and advocacy skills, prepared to navigate, and address systemic delays while championing patient care. While these delays are typically more inconvenient than dangerous, urgent patient needs necessitate a proactive stance from surgeons to ensure expedited and appropriate care. Fortuitously, most VA staff are committed to exceptional service, often exceeding their responsibilities to support veterans. A surgeon who approaches their role with patience, understanding, and effective communication is likely to foster positive interactions, achieve greater job satisfaction, and cultivate strong working relationships.

The VA is dedicated to improving quality and patient safety through its VA Surgical Quality Improvement Program (VASQIP), akin to the National Surgical Quality Improvement Program (NSQIP) implemented by the American College of Surgeons and initially developed by VA. Quality is maintained through physician involvement in peer review, overseen by a non-punitive Peer Review Committee. Additionally, services can independently host Morbidity and Mortality conferences separate from their academic affiliates. Supervisors are responsible for monitoring their services and sections through Ongoing Professional Practice Evaluations (OPPE) and audits of documentation by subordinates and physician extenders. However, this commitment to quality often results in substantial administrative paperwork. While these programs are becoming more commonplace in civilian programs, they are standard in the VA setting. The Talent Management System (TMS) administers online teaching modules, many of which are mandatory but may seem unrelated to one's specialty. The VA also employs a time-consuming program called ePerformance to assess employee effectiveness, although it may not be well-suited for physicians and could be viewed as an administrative burden. Unfortunately, non-clinical workload may not decrease with time, as new organizational requirements are regularly introduced.

Summary

Working as a VA surgeon presents a unique opportunity for professional growth as a surgeon, leader, and educator. The VA system offers a range of ongoing prospects for continuous learning and professional development, spanning from clinical expertise to administrative leadership. It fosters a stable work environment that encourages program development, innovation, and diversity, complemented by comprehensive benefits [15] (see Appendix 37.1) such as a wide range of insurance, retirement plans, and the potential for education loan repayment programs. However, the VA experience comes with its own set of challenges. Navigating through bureaucratic processes and managing significant administrative tasks can be demanding. Surgeons may encounter limitations in earning potential, variations in patient caseload, and emotional challenges when treating aging individuals with complex medical problems. The decision to make a lifelong career within the VA or to view it as a stepping stone to other opportunities hinges on individual professional goals and personal values.

Disclaimer The views expressed in this chapter are those of the authors and do not necessarily reflect the position or policy of the Department of Veterans Affairs or the United States Government.

Appendix 37.1. Compensation and Benefits [16]

- **Social Security paid by VA** = 6.2% of taxable wages on behalf of the employee. If an individual has taxable wages over the taxable maximum of $147,000, VA will contribute $9114
- **Employee Assistance Program (EAP)** = free legal and medical services
- **Medicare paid by VA** = 1.45% on behalf of the employee
- **Flexible Spending Account (FSA)** = you may contribute up to $3200 a year to your health care FSA with a $640 max carry over (as of 2024) and save up to 30% on dependent care expenses
- **Life Insurance** = VA pays 1/3 of insurance cost for basic life insurance
- **Thrift Savings Plan (TSP) Federal 401(K)** = VA provides up to 5% employer contributions (1% automatic contribution and up to 4% employer matching contributions)
- **Federal Employee Retirement System (FERS)** = for employees hired after 1/1/2014, VA contributes 16.6% annually to FERS-FRAE basic/defined benefit traditional pension
- **Competitive Salaries** = At VA, you receive a salary (base pay + market pay) based on your years of VHA service, local labor market salaries, duty location, and other factors. However,

by law, VA physicians' direct annual compensation cannot exceed the US President's, which is $400,000 per year.

- **Regular Salary Increases** = Receive annual increases when signed into federal law (as of 2022, the 5-year average was 1.72%), and receive longevity step increase every 2 years based on years of VHA service and increases to market pay when appropriate (market pay is reviewed every 2 years)
- **Performance Pay** = Your compensation includes additional annual performance pay up to 7.5% of annual salary up to a max of $15,000
- **Employment Without Strings** = Whether you serve full- or part-time, your employment at VA is without employment contracts, noncompete clauses, restrictive covenants, or other significant restrictions on outside work
- **Liability protection** = VA health care providers are covered under federal tort laws and may be defended by the United States against allegations of malpractice or negligence (38 U.S.C. §7316)
- **Transit Benefit Program** = You may qualify for transit subsidy monthly benefits of a max of $280/month; check with your local VA Medical Center (conditions apply)
- **Education Debt Reduction Program (EDRP)** [11] = As a physician, dentist, or podiatrist you may be eligible to apply for EDRP. If approved, you may be eligible to receive reimbursement for your student loan payments up to $40,000/year up to 5 years.
- Depending on the conditions and competitiveness of the hiring process, recruitment, retention, or relocation incentives may be negotiated on a case-by-case basis prior to employment.

References

1. United States Department of Veterans Affairs. History overview. https://department.va.gov/history/history-overview/. Accessed 1 Dec 2023.
2. Office of the Chief Human Capital Officer. Title 38 pay schedules. VA. https://www.va.gov/ohrm/pay/. Accessed 30 Nov 2023.

3. United States Office of Personnel Management. USAJOBS. U.S. Government. https://www.usajobs.gov/. Accessed 30 Nov 2023.
4. United States Department of Veterans Affairs. Choose VA. https://choose.va.gov/. Accessed 20 Nov 2023.
5. United States Office of Personnel Management. The Federal Employees Health Benefits (FEHB) Program. https://www.opm.gov/healthcare-insurance/healthcare/. Accessed 30 Nov 2023.
6. United States Office of Personnel Management. BENEFEDS. FEDPOINT. https://www.benefeds.com/. Accessed 30 Nov 2023.
7. United States Office of Personnel Management. FERS information. https://www.opm.gov/retirement-center/fers-information/. Accessed 30 Nov 2023.
8. Thrift Savings Plan. U. S. Government. https://www.tsp.gov/. Accessed 30 Nov 2023.
9. Thrift Savings Plan. About the Thrift Savings Plan (TSP). https://www.tsp.gov/about-the-thrift-savings-plan-tsp/. Accessed 30 Nov 2023.
10. United States Department of Defense. Defense Finance and Accounting Service. https://www.dfas.mil/. Accessed 30 Nov 2023.
11. United States Department of Veterans Affairs. Education support. https://vacareers.va.gov/employment-benefits/education-support/#repay. Accessed 30 Nov 2023.
12. United States Department of Veterans Affairs. Office of Research & Development. https://www.research.va.gov/funding/. Accessed 30 Nov 2023.
13. Association of VA Surgeons. https://www.vasurgeons.org/. Accessed 30 Nov 2023.
14. United States House of Representatives. Federal Tort Claims Act. https://www.house.gov/doing-business-with-the-house/leases/federal-tort-claims-act. Accessed 30 Nov 2023.
15. United States Department of Veterans Affairs. Total Reward$. U. S. Department of Veterans Affairs. https://vacareers.va.gov/employment-benefits/total-rewards/. Accessed 30 Nov 2023.
16. United States Office of Personnel Management. Federal Employee Compensation Package. https://www.opm.gov/policy-data-oversight/pay-leave/pay-administration/fact-sheets/federal-employee-compensation-package/. Accessed 30 Nov 2023.

38 Joining the Military as a Mid-Career Surgeon

Kirby R. Gross

Several factors are important to ensure a rewarding experience for mid-career surgeons who join the military. The most critical of these factors is the alignment of the goals and objectives of the surgeon to the goals and objectives of the military health system in the Department of Defense. While the alignment of goals of the employee and the organization is true of any professional in any employment situation, this is particularly true for healthcare professionals who join an organization whose primary mission is quite different than healthcare delivery.

The overarching mission of the Department of Defense is to ensure the security of the nation. The Department of Defense is an expansive organization that has many implied tasks. The military health system, nestled within the Department of Defense, has a vast range of missions and tasks. These include maintaining the health readiness of the force, directly delivering care in military treatment facilities, advancing knowledge relevant to the military mission, and training and educating military health system members, among others. The military health system mission extends to deployments, both during active conflict and in peace.

K. R. Gross (✉)
Cooper Medical School of Rowan University, Camden, NJ, USA
e-mail: gross-kirby@cooperhealth.edu

A. T. Schlussel et al. (eds.), *The SAGES Manual for Navigating a Successful Military Surgical Career*,
https://doi.org/10.1007/978-3-031-88490-0_38

Aligning a surgeon's goals and objectives within the military health system, which has such a vast array of tasks, in concept, would seem to be an easy task. However, assigning the specific surgeon to the specific assignment may not occur for the surgeon's first duty station. For example, a thoracic surgeon with an interest in surgical education may wish to be assigned to a military treatment facility with robust clinical practice and graduate medical education. However, several other thoracic surgeons may also have similar wishes. Newly onboarded surgeons must maintain patience as they amass some seniority.

As mid-career surgeons are considering joining the military, it is imperative that frank discussions be carried out with the surgical specialty leader of the branch (Army, Navy, or Air Force) to which they are considering joining. Mid-career surgeons joining the military are described as "Direct Accessions," or "Direct Commissions." These terms are in contradistinction to other routes to a military career, such as through the Service Academies (United States Military Academy, United States Air Force Academy or United States Naval Academy), Reserve Officer Training Corps or Officer Candidate School. Of course, officers who joined the military through a service academy, ROTC, or the Officer Candidate School join well before becoming a surgeon, and they typically receive most (if not all) of their medical training while in the military. A separate chapter addresses considerations when deciding to join the military. The mid-career surgeon who is considering joining the military will initially meet military healthcare recruiters. Military healthcare recruiters are not clinicians. Military healthcare recruiters are familiar with the administrative processes to bring a potential military surgeon on board. They are familiar with compensation issues and military life in general. However, they will not be able to provide specifics as to the practice of surgical care within the Department of Defense. The surgical specialty leader (consultant) will present a realistic picture of what the newly onboarded surgeon may expect. In conversations with the consultant, the prospective military surgeon can assess whether their goals and objectives may also be met by service in the reserves or national guard. Reserve and National Guard surgeons deploy as well as active surgeons. The surgeon who wishes to maintain a busy clinical practice yet desires to gain experience in the austere and operational environment may better meet their goals and objectives in the Reserves or Guard.

A surgeon's goals and objectives may be to satisfy a sense of patriotism, service, or family tradition. These are all very laudable. These emotions may be accentuated by threats upon our nation or active conflict. During times of conflict, the mid-career civilian surgeon may consider joining the military. If these circumstances apply as a mid-career surgeon is considering joining the military, a frank conversation with the service specialty consultant is still in order. The specialty consultant would provide some perspective as to the role the newly onboarded surgeon may have during times of conflict. For the surgeon who is looking for experience in a theater of operations, an assignment to a state-side billet would be disappointing.

With success in the military requiring an alignment of goals of the surgeon within the military health system, the direct accession surgeon is joining the military with a sense of service. Specifically, no individual of any occupation should join the military "just for a change" or to flee personal or professional circumstances. The challenges that preexist will continue. In fact, the challenges that preexisted may be accentuated in the relatively more regimented professional environment of the military.

The characteristics of the ideal candidate to join the military as a mid-career surgeon are three: (1) The surgeon has goals that align with the DoD mission, (2) patience, and (3) flexibility.

Implied in the concept that a surgeon's goals and objectives align with the DoD mission is the acceptance that the surgeon has a specific role in a much larger effort. By accepting this concept, the mid-career surgeon recognizes that their significance in their new employment situation will be different than their role in their previous civilian practice. After recognizing the critical importance of aligning goals and objectives with the direction of the military health system, acknowledging the need for patience is needed. In civilian practice, a surgeon has a great influence on clinic schedules and operating room schedules and can readily influence changes within their practice. In general, military surgeons will have less ability to impact their day-to-day clinical practice than their civilian counterparts.

Patience is a particular necessity of the mid-career surgeon joining the military. A mid-career surgeon who joins the military will notice a distinctly different pace between their civilian practice and a military treatment facility. In civilian practice, clinical productivity while providing optimal care is very important. Productivity is important in civilian practice to ensure that hospitals and surgical practices remain financially viable. Such pressures do not exist in military practice. Funding for healthcare is provided from a budget. The efficiency of a military treatment facility or clinic is not necessarily positively rewarded as in civilian practice. Good reasons exist for the difference in pace between civilian practice and military practice. Service members assigned to military treatment facilities, including surgeons, have time away from clinical practice for physical training, field training, and military training. The mid-career surgeon will receive military-specific training upon joining their service. The length of this training may vary from service to service and the urgency for onboarding medical providers. Generally, the length of this training can be expected to be 2–3 months. The training consists of a general introduction to the military, such as rank structure, service organization, and policies/procedures. In addition, weapons qualification, land navigation, and other basic field skills will be taught. The need for the military treatment facility staff to be off-site periodically increases inefficiency. In addition, the junior military members who serve as support staff are typically relatively inexperienced compared to civilian institutions. In addition, junior military members change duty stations at least every 2 years. Civilian practices have turnover as well. However, it is much less frequent and generally at a more experienced employee level than military treatment facilities. Government employees who are nonmilitary members make up part of the employee pool in military treatment facilities. However, they are not incentivized to enhance clinical efficiency.

Patience is also necessary for mid-career surgeons, as they join the military as the newly onboarded surgeon seeks to effect change in their new practice environment. The surgeon new to the military may feel obliged to suggest ways to enhance efficiency and increase productivity. After all, no one advocates for inefficiency and a lack of productivity. However, their recommendations may not be incorporated because the pressures in civilian and military practices are different. W. Edwards Deming, an American engineer, statistician, and management consultant, is credited with the quote, "Every system is perfectly designed to get the result that it does" [1, 2]. Civilian practice systems and the military health system are different. A challenge the experienced military surgeon and a newly onboarded surgeon both face routinely is "how much effort to invest to improve the system." A surgeon will bring scrutiny to themselves and may not be effective in bringing change. Patience in this circumstance is a virtue for the newly onboarded surgeon. Taking guidance and counsel from well-respected and senior surgeons is wise. The experienced colleague will assist by providing perspective on what issues can be improved and at how much effort. In a civilian practice, a surgeon will advocate to a decision-maker who may also be a clinician with similar objectives. Not so in the military environment. Decision-makers may be administrators who have variable inclinations to accept the input of clinicians, particularly a surgeon new to the military.

Even though the mid-career surgeon may have specific goals and objectives upon joining the military, flexibility is a quality that may provide greater opportunity for reward during years of military service. A surgeon who seeks to focus on the delivery of high-quality clinical care may realize that the military provides excellent opportunities for leadership training. Adjusting one's goals and objectives while still aligning with the military health system frequently occurs. Such an adjustment provides a military medical career to be very rewarding.

Aligning one's goals with the military, being patient, and maintaining flexibility permit a surgeon to have a satisfying career. These attributes suggest that the military health system is arbitrary and unyielding, with the surgeon being forced to adapt to the military. Compared to a civilian health system, the military health system changes more slowly. However, change does occur. When a mid-career surgeon positively impacts the military health system, the impact can be immense. As an example, the development and implementation of a Department of Defense deployed trauma system had an immeasurable impact on combat casualty outcomes during the United States' response to the attack on September 11, 2001. The development of the deployed trauma system was impacted by both active, Reserve, seasoned military surgeons and newly onboarded military surgeons. During active combat operations, aligning the goals/objectives of surgeons with the entire Department of Defense is readily accomplished. The effort still needed patience and flexibility by the surgeons involved in the process.

The military health system has a more formal structure and more standardized processes than civilian health systems. Newly onboarded military surgeons will find that some techniques to effect change in civilian practice will be effective in the military. John B. Kotter outlined eight steps to effect change [3]. Even without a formal leadership position, these steps will help guide the informal military medical leader to have a positive impact. As the direct accession surgeon gains seniority and assumes formal leadership positions, these techniques can be particularly powerful after the surgeon becomes familiar with military processes and culture. With time and greater tenure, the direct accession surgeon may have an advantage in implementing change due to exposure to techniques from the civilian environment that may not be utilized in the military environment.

Challenges and Advantages of Joining the Military as a Mid-Career Surgeon

A surgeon can have a very rewarding experience in the military while joining mid-career. Typically, a military surgeon begins their military career during their years of education as an undergraduate, medical student, or resident. After years of service, the military surgeon migrates to the civilian sector. The more traditional path provides an introduction to military culture, processes, and colleagues gradually. The mid-career surgeon new to the military will quickly adapt to the culture and language. Some of the processes and practices will seem foreign and frustrating. Successful mid-career surgeons have become efficient with the use of time. Successful mid-career surgeons have also had a degree of autonomy that does not exist in military medicine. The mid-career surgeon coming into the military must keep in mind the overall mission of the military health system. The attributes mentioned earlier (1) ensuring an individual's goals align with the military health system mission, (2) patience, and (3) flexibility must be kept in mind. The mid-career surgeon must not become passive and docile as opportunities to improve military healthcare present themselves. They must use leadership skills and experience gained during their years of practice to make a positive impact.

Deployments may present challenges to the mid-career surgeon. Physical durability and fitness are a must while deployed. Separation from family and friends may be a hardship. However, provided the mid-career surgeon joined the military understanding the physical challenges and risk of family separation, deployments will be understood as part of being a military surgeon. In fact, while deployed, much of the administrative burden is lifted. Also, surgeons will find their input and skills are relatively more valued than in garrison.

In many respects, the mid-career surgeon has an advantage over their colleagues whose education and training have been isolated to the military. The mid-career surgeon will have had a wealth of clinical and leadership experience. The newly onboarded surgeon may serve as a clinical mentor for junior colleagues. Mid-career surgeons will likely identify opportunities to positively impact the military health system. After gaining knowledge of the military health system, the direct accession surgeon can be an agent of change. Even before assuming formal leadership positions, the newly onboarded surgeon can be an informal leader by using leadership techniques that have proven successful in their civilian careers. After gaining tenure and formal leadership positions, the direct accession surgeon can be a powerful influence to enhance the military health system.

In summary, several key points will facilitate the success of mid-career surgeons as they join the military. First, they have assured themselves that they can align their goals and objectives with the goals and objectives of the military health system.

Second, the direct accession surgeon maintains patience as they are incorporated into the military health system, which moves at a different pace and has different pressures. Third, the mid-career surgeon remains flexible. The military health system will provide opportunities that may not be immediately apparent to mid-career surgeons as they take their oath of office.

References

1. https://www.goodreads.com/quotes/7224415-every-system-is-perfectly designed-to-get-the-result-that.
2. Schulman J. Every system is perfectly designed to get the results it gets. In: Schulman J, editor. The problem of practice variation in newborn medicine. Cham: Springer; 2022. https://doi.org/10.1007/978-3-030-94655-5_19.
3. https://hbr.org/2021/11/how-to-become-morecomfortable-with-change.

Kirby R. Gross M.D. F.A.C.S., Colonel (Retired), Medical Corps, U.S. Army COL (Retired) Gross has insight on joining the military as a mid-career surgeon. He had been in practice in northern Indiana for 17 years when he approached a US Army Healthcare Recruiting Office after September 11, 2001. After Officer Basic Course at Fort Sam Houston, TX, from July 2002 to September 2002, he was assigned to Blanchfield Army Community Hospital. In January 2003, he deployed with the 86th Combat Support Hospital from Ft. Campbell, Kentucky. While deployed, he served as Deputy Commander of Clinical Services even though he had been in the Army less than 1 year.

Upon redeployment, he took command of the 801st Forward Surgical Team (subsequently re-flagged as the 772nd FST). The FST was deployed from September 2005 to August 2006. By the time of his retirement in July 2023, COL (Retired) Gross had been deployed ten times for a total of 62 months. Several deployments were in direct support of Tier 1 assets. He deployed as Director of the Joint Theater Trauma System on three occasions.

COL (Retired) Gross credits his first several years in the Army as shaping his career. His early deployments occurred during the early phases of the war. Not only were clinical skills required, but the ability to interface and shape the deployed trauma system. Being thrust into leadership positions early, an ongoing interest was sparked in deployed trauma system development. In addition to serving as the Joint Theater Trauma System Director three times, he also served as the Joint Trauma System Director in 2015 and 2016.

COL (Retired) Gross's last two garrison assignments were at military civilian partnerships. He was the Director of the Army Trauma Training Detachment at Ryder Trauma Center at Jackson Memorial Hospital in Miami from 2016 to 2020. COL (Retired) Gross's final garrison assignment was with the AMEDD Military Civilian Trauma Team Training Program at Cooper University Hospital in Camden, New Jersey. After retirement in July 2023, COL (Retired) Gross remained on as attending surgeon at Cooper University Hospital.

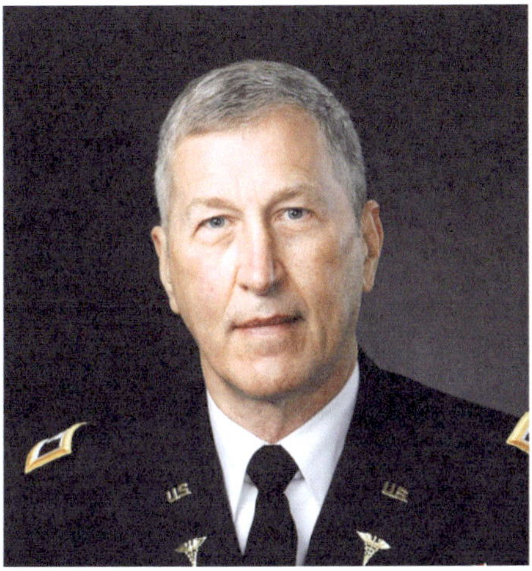

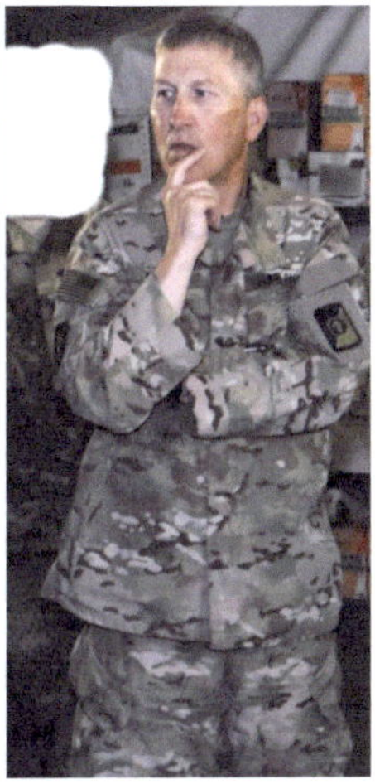

Index

A. T. Schlussel et al. (eds.), *The SAGES Manual for Navigating a Successful Military Surgical Career*,
https://doi.org/10.1007/978-3-031-88490-0

E

F

J

MIX
Papier aus verantwortungsvollen Quellen
Paper from responsible sources
FSC® C105338

If you have any concerns about our products,
you can contact us on
ProductSafety@springernature.com

In case Publisher is established outside the EU,
the EU authorized representative is:
Springer Nature Customer Service Center GmbH
Europaplatz 3, 69115 Heidelberg, Germany

Printed by Libri Plureos GmbH
in Hamburg, Germany